ANTIVIRAL DRUGS – ASPECTS OF CLINICAL USE AND RECENT ADVANCES

Edited by **Patrick Arbuthnot**

Antiviral Drugs – Aspects of Clinical Use and Recent Advances
Edited by Patrick Arbuthnot

Published by InTech

Janeza Trdine 9, 51000 Rijeka, Croatia

Publishing Process Manager Ana Skalamera

Technical Editor Teodora Smiljanic

Cover Designer InTech Design Team

Additional hard copies can be obtained from orders@intechopen.com

Antiviral Drugs – Aspects of Clinical Use and Recent Advances, Edited by Patrick Arbuthnot
p. cm.
ISBN 978-953-51-0256-4

For EU product safety concerns:
IN TECH d.o.o., Prolaz Marije Krucifikse Kozulić 3, 51000 Rijeka, Croatia,
info@intechopen.com or visit our website at intechopen.com.

Meet the editor

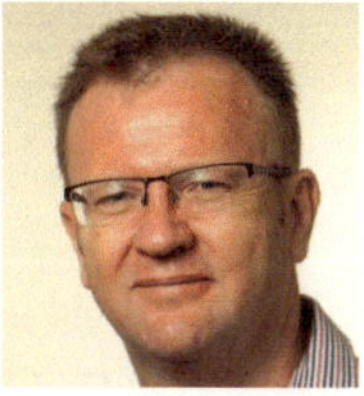

Patrick Arbuthnot is Personal Professor and Director of the Antiviral Gene Therapy Research Unit of the University of the Witwatersrand (Wits) in South Africa. After graduating with a medical degree from Wits, Patrick Arbuthnot completed a PhD in 1992. From 1993 to 1994, he worked as a post-doctoral researcher at Necker Hospital in Paris, and investigated the development of gene therapy for treating liver cancer and hepatitis B virus (HBV) infection. On returning to South Africa, Patrick Arbuthnot established the Antiviral Gene Therapy Research Unit. This unit is now a Centre of Excellence of the African Network for Drug and Diagnostic Innovation (ANDI). The unit has a research interest in HBV infection, liver cancer, HIV-1 infection and developing new methods of treating these diseases.

Contents

Preface XI

Part 1 Clinical Management of Viral Infection 1

Chapter 1 **Antiviral Therapy in HCV-Infected Decompensated Cirrhotics 3**
Fazal-I-Akbar Danish

Chapter 2 **Virus Diagnostics and Antiviral Therapy in Acute Retinal Necrosis (ARN) 17**
Peter Rautenberg, Jost Hillenkamp, Livia Grančičova, Bernhard Nölle, Johann Roider and Helmut Fickenscher

Chapter 3 **Leflunomide an Immunosuppressive Drug for Antiviral Purpose in Treatment for BK Virus-Associated Nephropathy After Kidney Transplantation 35**
Christophe Bazin

Chapter 4 **Modeling Virologic Response in HIV-1 Infected Patients to Assess Medication Adherence 51**
Yangxin Huang

Part 2 Developing New Antivirals 69

Chapter 5 **Use of Animal Models for Anti-HIV Drug Development 71**
Zandrea Ambrose

Chapter 6 **Discovery of Novel Antiviral Agents Directed Against the Influenza A Virus Nucleoprotein 99**
Yoko Aida, Yutaka Sasaki and Kyoji Hagiwara

Chapter 7 **Targeting Norovirus: Strategies for the Discovery of New Antiviral Drugs 121**
Joana Rocha-Pereira and Maria São José Nascimento

Chapter 8 **Single Domain Camelid Antibodies that Neutralize Negative Strand Viruses 151**
Francisco Miguel Lopez Cardoso, Lorena Itatí Ibañez, Bert Schepens and Xavier Saelens

Chapter 9 **Treatment of Herpes Simplex Virus with Lignin-Carbohydrate Complex Tablet, an Alternative Therapeutic Formula 171**
Blanca Silvia González López, Masaji Yamamoto and Hiroshi Sakagami

Preface

Viral infections remain common causes of serious public health problems throughout the world. Viruses have highly varied mechanisms of propagation and the diseases that they cause are consequently very different. Approaches to countering virus infection therefore need to be tailored according to specific viral characteristics. Understanding the fundamentals of virus-related disease pathogenesis is critically important to improving treatment. The articles that appear in *Antiviral Drugs – Aspects of Clinical Use and Recent Advances* cover a broad collection of topics that reflect the fascinating range of viral characteristics and the measures that are being employed to counter the diseases that viruses cause.

Clinical management and new developments in the treatment of virus-related diseases are the two main topics covered in the book. The first section reviews the treatment of hepatitis C virus (HCV) infection in cirrhotic patients, the management of virus-related acute retinal necrosis, the use of leflunomide therapy for BK virus-related nephropathy in renal transplant patients ,and the mathematical modeling of HIV-1 responses to antiviral therapies. Useful general concepts are provided in each chapter and will be helpful to physicians with general and specialized expertise. Chapters dealing with commonly occurring infections, such as those caused by HCV and HIV, are of wide interest. HCV infection occurs in approximately 170 million people in the world and ensuring that available licensed drugs are used in optimal treatment regimens is critical to minimizing risks associated with the virus infection. A complex, often misunderstood, topic is whether decompensation resulting from complicating cirrhosis is a contraindication to HCV treatment. In the chapter entitled *Antiviral Therapy in HCV-infected Decompensated Cirrhotics,* comprehensive and valuable treatment guidelines are provided. Another topic of global significance is the understanding of variable responses that HIV-infected individuals have to treatment. Adherence to the treatment regimens and also virus drug susceptibility are some of the important factors that influence patients' treatment responses. Measurement of patient adherence to therapy may be difficult. Evaluation is typically based on patient questionnaires and data derived from electronic medication monitoring caps or Medication Event Monitoring Systems (MEMS). The chapter entitled *Modeling Virologic Response in HIV-1 Infected Patients to Assess Medication Adherence* proposes a mechanism-based dynamic model to assess how adherence data based on questionnaires and the MEMS can be used to predict virologic responses. The modeling offers a means of assessing the effect of adherence on antiviral responses. Analysis was carried out in different situations and provides clinicians with a tool that will assist with making patient treatment decisions.

Basic applied research topics are dealt with in the second half of the book. Many interesting and promising new developments are covered and these include advances in the treatment of the influenza virus, animal models for the study of HIV-1 drug development, the use of single chain camelid antibodies to counter negative strand RNA viruses, new strategies for inhibition of norovirus infection, as well as the use of plant extracts to treat herpes simplex virus infection. The importance of structural insights for drug development is reinforced in the chapters dealing with advancing new norovirus and influenza virus treatments. Widening the range of drugs available for the treatment of HIV infection is a highly active and critically important field of research. The preclinical steps of drug development require careful planning to yield results that mitigate risks of testing in clinical trial settings. The chapter entitled *Use of Animal Models for Anti-HIV Drug Development* addresses many of these considerations and provides useful information on the appropriate selection of animal models for testing new HIV drugs. In another chapter, the antiviral utility of engineered protein derivatives of single domain binding camelid antibodies (HCAbs) is explored. Interestingly the epitope-binding domain of HCAbs, called single variable domain or VHH, retain their specificity when produced alone. These so-called nanobodies (Nbs) may be conveniently engineered and expressed in large numbers using standard recombinant procedures. The potential for neutralizing negative strand viruses, particularly influenza, respiratory syncytial and rabies viruses, is explored in the chapter entitled *Single domain camelid antibodies that neutralize negative strand viruses*.

The wide-ranging topics covered in *Antiviral Drugs – Aspects of Clinical Use and Recent Advances* provide a useful cross section within the field of antiviral drug development. Topics of general and specialized interest have been covered. The content of the book is not intended to be comprehensive, but aims to provide the reader with insights into selected aspects of established and new viral therapies. Students, clinicians, teachers, and basic scientists who have interests in advances in antiviral therapies will no doubt find the book helpful.

Patrick Arbuthnot
Antiviral Gene Therapy Research Unit, School of Pathology,
Faculty of Health Sciences,
University of the Witwatersrand,
South Africa

Part 1

Clinical Management of Viral Infection

1

Antiviral Therapy in HCV-Infected Decompensated Cirrhotics

Fazal-I-Akbar Danish
Quaid-e-Azam University, Islamabad, Pakistan

1. Introduction

What we are dealing with: Hepatitis C virus (HCV) infection is the commonest blood-borne infection, one of the commonest cause of chronic liver disease (CLD) & hepatocellular carcinoma (HCC) and one of the commonest reason for liver transplantation (LT) the world over.

What is the meaning of decompensation: Fibrosis is the histopathological hallmark of chronic hepatitis causing progressive derangement of normal liver architecture with consequent reduction in hepatic synthetic function. CLD is said to be decompensated when one or the other complication of CLD has developed - ascites, variceal bleeding (secondary to portal hypertension), impaired hepatic synthetic function (hypoalbuminemia), jaundice, and/or hepatic encephalopathy. Five years survival rate in decompensated cirrhotics is estimated to be 50%.[1]

Decompensated cirrhosis is NOT a contraindication to antiviral therapy: Decompensated cirrhosis has traditionally been considered a contraindication to interferon and ribavirin therapy. Whereas, the same may be true for advanced cirrhosis (which is only successfully amenable to LT), there are reports in the literature in which antiviral therapy was given *successfully* in selected cases of *early* hepatic decompensation with an aim to attain sustained viral clearance (SVR), halt disease progression and expect potential (though often partial) recovery of hepatic metabolic function. Antiviral therapy may also be instituted to prevent hepatitis C recurrence post-transplantation. If HCV is not eradicated pre-transplantation, reinfection with HCV occurs in *all* transplant recipients *as a rule,* with secondary cirrhosis developing in approximately 30% of cases within 5 years.[2] Pre-transplantation HCV eradication is however associated with less likelihood of reinfection and this forms the rationale for treating decompensated cirrhotics awaiting LT with antiviral therapy.[3] Initiating pre-emptive post-transplantation antiviral therapy, and treating established post-transplant HCV hepatitis are other options in LT patients. The aim of instituting pre-transplantation antiviral therapy is either to attain a sustained virological response (SVR) at transplantation, or an *on-treatment* HCV RNA clearance at transplantation. Mere reduction of viral load should *not* be the aim because, unlike HBV cirrhotics, this has not been shown to decrease the rate &/or severity of post-transplant HCV recurrence.

Thus decompensation per se is not an absolute contraindication for antiviral therapy. Although the final SVR rates attained in such patients are lower,[21,23] successful antiviral therapy is potentially lifesaving which supports the rationale for implementing HCV treatment in these patients.

In this chapter, the pros and cons of antiviral therapy in decompensated liver cirrhosis are reviewed with special emphasis on how to avoid antiviral dose reductions/ withdrawals secondary to the development of haematologic side effects by using haematopoietic growth factors (HGF's).

2. Discussion

2.1 Therapeutic options in decompensated cirrhosis

In selected cases, HCV-infected decompensated cirrhosis may be treated surgically (i.e. with LT) &/or medically (i.e. with antiviral therapy).

2.2 Surgical option

LT: How feasible is this option? LT is not a feasible option in the great majority of cirrhotics. This is not only because of the limited number of organ donors available at a given time, but also because of the age-related cardiovascular, renal, and pulmonary derangements that practically make going for this option rather *irrational* at times. Additionally, old age (≥65 years) is generally considered an exclusion criterion for LT.

2.3 Medical option

Historical reasons for reluctance to institute medical therapy in decompensated cirrhotics: Historically, despite the known theoretical benefits of antiviral therapy (improvement in liver histology, partial reversal of established cirrhosis, and prevention of life-threatening complications), most decompensated cirrhotics have not been offered antiviral therapy. Primarily, this has been due to the concerns regarding the therapeutic efficacy and safety of antiviral therapy in such cases. Peginterferon-ribavirin combination therapy is known to have *limited efficacy* in decompensated cirrhotics.[4,5] Also, compared to non-cirrhotics, such patients are more prone to develop *hematologic side effects* (neutropenia, thrombocytopenia & anemia) with antiviral therapy.[6] In fact, patients who already have severe neutropenia or thrombocytopenia (neutrophil count <1500/mm^3 or platelets count <75,000/mm^3) are highly prone to develop life-threatening infections after starting antiviral therapy, particularly if they have Child–Pugh class C disease.[7,8] Also, it is generally thought that age-related derangements in cardiovascular and pulmonary functions make the cirrhotic patients less tolerant to ribavirin-induced hemolytic anemia. Finally, there are concerns that decompensation may worsen with antiviral therapy as is the case with decompensated chronic hepatitis B cases.[9]

Do the reasons for reluctance evidence-based: Current literature reviews shows that because of the unstandardized dosage schedules being administered over variable periods of time in the past studies, we may have actually under/ overestimated the potential benefits and risks of antiviral therapy respectively in decompensated cirrhotics. There are now several reports in the literature in which antiviral therapy was relatively well tolerated by decompensated cirrhotics with reasonable rates of attainment of end-of-treatment response (ETR) & sustained virological response (SVR):[4,7,10,11]

1. In one study,[7] 39% of the patients receiving low, accelerating regimen of non-pegylated interferon plus ribavirin experienced clearance of HCV-RNA, & 21% attained an SVR. Results with pegylated interferon are even better. In the first study[12] *proving* the benefits of antiviral therapy in cirrhotics with signs of portal hypertension, 51 cirrhotics received 1mg/kg/wk of pegylated-interferon alpha-2b plus oral ribavirin at a fixed dose of 800mg/d for 52 wks. By intention-to-treat analysis, SVR was achieved in 21.6% patients. As otherwise, patients with genotypes 2 & 3 showed better results (83.3%) than genotype 1 cases (13.3%). Although antiviral therapy was stopped in 5 of the patients because of neutrophil counts falling below 0.75×10^3/dL, none of them developed superadded infections. The disease deteriorated in only 6% of those who attained SVR compared to 38% of the non-responders.
2. In another study,[10] Peg-IFN alpha-2b (1.0 mg/kg/wk) plus standard dose of ribavirin were administered to all patients for 24 wks *regardless of the genotype*. The overall SVR rate attained even with this *suboptimal dose* regimen was 19.7%. Except patients with very advanced liver disease (CTP score >10), none experienced life-threatening complications. Peg-IFN and ribavirin in the standard dosage (Peg-IFN alpha-2b 1.5mg/kg & ribavirin 800-1000mg for genotypes 2 and 3, and 1000-1200mg for genotypes 1 and 4) for the standard duration of time (48 & 24 wks for genotype 1 & non-1, respectively) has also been tried.
3. In another study,[13] 35% of end-stage cirrhotics cleared the HCV infection (16% genotype 1 & 4, and 59% genotype 2 & 3 cases). 60% of all patients tolerated the antiviral therapy without any major untoward effects; treatment was discontinued in 19.1% of the patients with 4 among those ending up having severe superadded infections.
4. In yet another study[14] a 48 week course was planned for patients who demonstrated EVR with a standard regimen of PEG-IFN alfa-2a (135µg, once a week) plus ribavirin (1000-1200 mg/day). Results showed 60% patients completing the course with ETR & SVR achieved in 45% & 35% cases, respectively.
5. In a recent study[15] aimed to evaluate both the prevention of post-transplantation HCV recurrence & the risk of bacterial infections during therapy, 47% patients achieved HCV RNA negativity *during* treatment, 29% were HCV RNA negative *at the time of transplantation* (drop outs n=3, deaths n=4, viral relapse n=2) and 20% achieved an SVR *post-transplantation*. Importantly, none of the patients who achieved SVR pre-transplantation developed a recurrence post-transplantation.

3. Evidence-based pharmacotherapy of HCV infection in decompensated cirrhotics

Child–Pugh (sometimes called Child-Turcotte-Pugh [CTP]) scoring - see table 1 - helps determine the need and utility of instituting antiviral therapy:

1. The ideal candidate for antiviral therapy remains a patient with Child–Pugh class A disease in whom the risk of drug-induced side effects is almost identical to that of the controls. Nonetheless, all cirrhotic patients with a CTP score ≤9 and a decompensated event that abated with routine management may be considered for antiviral therapy.

2. Whether or not to institute antiviral therapy in Child–Pugh class B patients should be individualized on case-to-case basis giving due consideration to factors like genotype (2 & 3 better than 1) & pre-treatment viral loads (< 800,000 IU/mL better than higher loads). In all such cases, antiviral therapy probably should be discontinued after 4 or 12 weeks if there is no virological response.
3. Patients with Child–Pugh class C (CTP score ≥10 or MELD score 18 [table 2]) disease are not considered appropriate candidates to institute antiviral therapy.

Measure	**1 point**	**2 points**	**3 points**
Total bilirubin, µmol/l (mg/dl)	<34 (<2)	34-50 (2-3)	>50 (>3)
Serum albumin, g/l	>35	28-35	<28
INR	<1.7	1.71-2.20	> 2.20
Ascites	None	Mild	Severe
Hepatic encephalopathy	None	Grade I-II	Grade III-IV

Table 1. Child–Pugh Score

Points	**Class**	**One year survival**	**Two year survival**
5-6	A	100%	85%
7-9	B	81%	57%
10-15	C	45%	35%

Table 1.a Interpretation of Child–Pugh Score

MELD = 3.78[Ln serum bilirubin (mg/dL)] + 11.2[Ln INR] + 9.57[Ln serum creatinine (mg/dL)] + 6.43

NB:

1. If the patient has had dialysis at least twice in the past week, then the value for serum creatinine used should be 4.0
2. Any value less than one is given a value of 1 (i.e. if bilirubin is 0.8, a value of 1.0 is used). This helps prevent the occurrence of scores below 0 (the natural logarithm of 1 is 0, and any value below 1 would yield a negative result).

Ln = natural logarithm

Table 2. MELD Score (Model For End-Stage Liver Disease) (12 and older):

MELD Score:	3 month mortality:
≥40	71.3%
30–39	52.6%
20–29	19.6%
10–19	6.0%
≤9	1.9%

Table 2.a Interpretation MELD Score

Peginterferon-ribavirin combination therapy (table 3) is now considered the standard drug regimen in cases of HCV infection. In peginterferon, an inert polyethylene glycol moiety is inserted into the interferon molecule. This causes a decrease in renal clearance and thus an increase in the plasma half life (80 hrs) of the peginterferon molecule. Because of the prolonged half life, whereas the non-pegylated interferons need to be administered thrice weekly, pegylated interferons are administered once weekly. The two formulations of peginterferon currently available are peginterferon alpha-2a and 2b. They differ in the size and configuration of the polyethylene glycol moiety attached to the interferon molecule. Although the two peginterferon formulations have not yet been compared head-to-head in the published controlled trails, they are generally believed to be equivalent therapies and thus can be used interchangeably.

Drug:	**Recommended Dosage:**
Peginterferon alfa-2a (40 kD)† (Inj Pegasys 180 μg)	180 μg SQ once weekly regardless of the weight
Peginterferon alfa-2b (12 kD) (Inj Peg-Intron 50/80/100/120/180 μg)	1.5 μg/kg SQ once weekly
Ribavirin∂	*Genotype 1*: Higher weight-adjusted dosage has shown better response rates (1000mg if ≤75kg∆ orally in two divided doses; 1200mg if >75kg)∞. *Genotype 2&3*: Higher dosage has not been shown in published studies to be consistently associated with better response rates. Therefore, 800mg/day orally in two divided doses is the current dosage of choice regardless of the weight.⌂

Abbreviations: kD, kilodaltons; μg, micrograms; SQ, subcutaneously; kg, kilograms; mg, milligrams.
† Peginterferons are therapeutically superior to non-pegylated interferons.
∂ Peginterferon-ribavirin combination therapy is therapeutically superior to peginterferon monotherapy as well as non-pegylated interferon-ribavirin combination therapy.
∆ More studies are needed to ascertain whether or not the treatment outcomes with 1000mg and 800mg ribavirin in patient's ≤75kg weight are comparable.
∞ It is not yet clear whether or not patients heavier than 88 kg will have better outcomes on 1400mg of ribavirin than 1200mg.
⌂ More studies are needed to ascertain that whether or not heavier patients yield better results with >800mg of ribavirin dose in genotypes 2 & 3 cases.

Table 3. Peginterferon-Ribavirin Combination Dosage Regimen: The Current Standard

After starting antiviral therapy, HCV RNA assay needs to be repeated at specific intervals to determine the treatment responses. Depending upon the results of the repeat HCV RNA assays, different treatment responses have been defined (table 4).

Rapid virologic response (RVR)	Qualitative HCV RNA assay done at 4 weeks comes back to be negative (<50IU/mL)
Early virologic response (EVR)	Quantitative HCV RNA assay done at 12 weeks: • Comes back to be negative - called early virologic clearance (EVC) or aviremic response • Shows a decline in the HCV RNA titre (compared with the pre-treatment assay) of ≥ 2 log - called partial virologic response (PVR) or viremic response
Nonresponders	Quantitative HCV RNA assay done at 12 weeks showing either no decline in the HCV RNA titre (compared with the pre-treatment assay) or a decline of < 2 log
End of treatment response (ETR)	Qualitative HCV RNA assay done on completion of the recommended duration of the treatment course comes back to be negative
Sustained virologic response (SVR)*	Qualitative HCV RNA assay done 24 weeks after completion of the recommended duration of the treatment course comes back to be negative
Relapsers	Qualitative HCV RNA assay done on completion of the recommended duration of the treatment course was negative (ETR achieved), but 24 weeks later it becomes positive again (SVR not achieved). .

*Achievement of SVR is generally considered as the marker of eradication of HCV infection. Almost all such patients show EVC or PVR on 12 weeks assay.

Table 4. Definitions of Treatment Responses

Positive and negative predictors of therapeutic response:

1. *Positive predictors:* As otherwise, attainment of a rapid/ early virological response and genotypes 2 & 3 are the most robust predictors of viral clearance with antiviral therapy.[10,12] Child-Pugh class A and lower pre-transplantation viral loads (< 800,000 IU/mL) are other positive predictors.
2. *Negative predictors:* A reduction in the viral load of ≤2 1 log^{10} between baseline & week 4, Child-Pugh class C or MELD >18 have a strong negative predictive value. In the absence of a ≥2 log^{10} reduction in HCV RNA at week 4, probably the best approach to reduce the risk of complications is to stop antiviral therapy at this point.

The exact treatment protocol instituted in a given patient depends upon the genotype. Genotypes 2&3 are more responsive to interferon therapy than genotype 1 and therefore the recommended duration of antiviral therapy in former is 06 months as compared to one year in the latter. Although more data and experience is needed to establish definite protocols in genotypes 4, 5 & 6 cases, current evidence suggests treating them as genotype 1 cases.[23] Tables 5 & 6 summarize the current standards of treatment depending upon the genotype.

HCV RNA Assay:	**Recommendations according to the PCR results:**
Week 4 qualitative HCV RNA assay:†	
Negative assay (<50IU/mL) i.e. a case of RVR	Shorten the standard treatment course of 24 weeks to 12-16 weeks. Ribavirin is given at higher weight-adjusted dosage in the short courses (1000mg if ≤75 kg orally in two divided doses; 1200mg if >75 kg)‡,∂
Positive assay	Give treatment for the standard duration of 24 weeks∆ (may be 36-48 weeks)
Week 24 qualitative HCV RNA assay:	
Negative assay i.e. a case of ETR	Successful therapy. Needs a repeat qualitative HCV RNA assay at week 48 (24 weeks after ETR) to establish SVR
Positive assay	Treatment failed
Week 48 qualitative HCV RNA assay:	
Negative assay i.e. a case of SVR	HCV infection eradicated
Positive assay i.e. a case of relapse	*Previously treated with non-pegylated interferon:* Treat with peginterferon and ribavirin. If EVR is not achieved at week 12, stop the treatment *Previously treated with pegylated interferon:* Retreatment is not indicated even if a different type of peginterferon is administered. Consensus interferon has shown to improve responses in such cases, but it is too premature to recommend it.

† The newly recommended week 4 qualitative HCV RNA assay helps modify the duration of the therapy based on viral kinetics. On one hand, this approach helps maximize the SVR rates and on the other hand, limits the toxicities and cost associated with the extended treatment courses. Achievement of RVR means that we can consider shortening the treatment course.
‡ With the shortened treatment courses in subjects who show RVR, SVR rates of 80-100% have been reported in genotype 2 cases and 77-85% in genotype 3 cases.
∂ In case of relapse, retreatment with the standard 24 weeks course is recommended.
∆ SVR rates achieved in this subgroup are poor, particularly in genotype 3 cases – 41-58%. In genotype 2 cases, the results are relatively better - 50-89%. Because of the poor SVR rates, prolonged therapy (>24 weeks) may be considered in this subgroup, although more evidence is needed at this time for a definite recommendation.

Table 5. Summary of Current Standards in the Management of Genotypes 2&3 Cases:

HCV RNA Assay:	Recommendations as per the PCR results:
Week 4 qualitative HCV RNA assay:	
Negative assay (<50IU/mL) i.e. a case of RVR	*Predictors of poor response absent:*† Shorten the treatment duration to a total of 24 weeks‡,∂ *Predictors of poor response present:* Give treatment for the standard duration of 48 weeks
Positive assay	Continue treatment and repeat HCV RNA at 12 weeks
Week 12 qualitative HCV RNA assay:	
Negative assay i.e. a case of EVC	Continue treatment for a total of 48 weeks
HCV RNA fall by ≥ 2 logs i.e. a case of PVR	Continue treatment & repeat qualitative HCV RNA at 24 weeks.
HCV RNA fall by < 2 logs i.e. a case of non-responder	Stop treatment
Week 24 qualitative HCV RNA assay (only done in cases which show PVR at week 12 assay):	
Negative assay (this subgroup is called 'slow responders')	Continue treatment for a total of 48-72 weeks. 72 weeks therapy has generally shown superior results as compared to 48 weeks therapy in slow responders.
Positive assay	Stop treatment as probability of attaining SVR is negligible
Week 48 qualitative HCV RNA assay:	
Negative assay i.e. a case of ETR	Successful therapy. Needs a repeat qualitative HCV RNA assay at week 72 (24 weeks after ETR) to establish SVR
Positive assay	Treatment failed
Week 72 qualitative HCV RNA assay:	
Negative assay i.e. a case of SVR	HCV infection got eradicated
Positive assay i.e. a case of relapse	*Previously treated with non-pegylated interferon:* Treat with peginterferon and ribavirin. If EVR is not achieved at week 12, stop the treatment *Previously treated with pegylated interferon:* Retreatment is not indicated even if a different type of peginterferon is administered. Consensus interferon has shown to improve responses in such cases, but it is too premature to recommend it.

† Old age (>50yrs); male gender; African American race; obesity; alcoholism; HIV confection or immunosuppression; more-than-portal fibrosis on liver biopsy (Metavir ≥2 or Ishak ≥ 3); a pretreatment viral load of >800,000IU/mL.

‡ SVR rates of 80-89% can be achieved in this subgroup.

∂ In case of relapse, retreatment with the standard 48 weeks course is recommended.

Table 6. Summary of Current Standards in the Management of Genotype 1 Cases

Monitoring the antiviral therapy not only involves asking repeat HCV RNA assays at specific intervals to determine therapeutic response, but also a battery of other blood tests to rule out the development of any adverse effects (see table 7).

Fortnightly:	CBC at weeks 1, 2, 4, 6, 8 and then monthly
Week 4:	Qualitative HCV RNA assay at week 4 in both genotype 1 and 2&3 cases to assess for RVR
Every month:	Pregnancy assay in a sexually-active female of child bearing age
Week 12:	Quantitative HCV RNA test at week 12 in genotype 1 cases only to assess for EVR
Every 3 months:	LFTs, INR, albumin, creatinine, urinalysis, glucose and TSH
Week 24:	• Qualitative HCV RNA assay at week 24 in only those genotype 1 cases who attained EVR at week 12 • Qualitative HCV RNA assay at week 24 in genotype 2&3 cases to determine ETR
Week 48	• Qualitative HCV RNA assay at week 48 in genotype 2&3 cases to determine SVR • Qualitative HCV RNA assay at week 48 in genotype 1 cases to determine ETR
Week 72	• Qualitative HCV RNA assay at week 72 in genotype 1 cases to determine SVR

Table 7. Monitoring of Anti-viral Therapy

4. Pharmacotherapy of side effects

As a general rule, decompensated cirrhotics are more prone to develop drug-induced side-effects compared to patients with compensated disease. Important side effects in decompensated cirrhotics include:[16]

1. Drug-induced hematological side effects: neutropenia (50–60%), thrombocytopenia (30–50%), hemolytic anemia (30–50%).
2. Superadded infections: spontaneous bacterial peritonitis (SBP), spontaneous bacteraemia/ septicaemia/ septic shock (due to Gram-negative bacilli) etc (4–13%).
3. Worsening of hepatic decompensation with therapy (11–20%).

4.1 Drug-induced hematological side effects

4.1.1 Ribavirin-induced hemolytic anemia

The minimum effective dose of ribavirin appears to be 10.6 mg/kg/day. In case hemolytic anemia develops, it is recommended to first reduce the dose of ribavirin to the minimum effective level. If no or little improvement in hemoglobin (Hb) level occurs, initiating concomitant erythropoietin (EPO) therapy may be considered.[17,18]

Possible indications:	1. Fall in Hb level by >4 g/dL. 2. Hb levels of <8g/dL. 3. Development of symptoms and signs attributable to anemia (palpitations, dyspnea, easy fatigability, pallor).[21,22]
Dosage regimens:	1. 20,000-40,000IU/week given in three divided doses subcutaneously (max. 60,000IU/week) with an aim to achieve & maintain Hb level of ≥10g/dL (return to the pretreatment level is NOT the aim).[23] 2. Another study suggested starting EPO therapy at a lower dose of 4,000IU subcutaneously thrice weekly (12,000IU/week) and then increasing the dose depending upon the response.[24]

Table 8. Erythropoietin (EPO) therapy

Monitoring EPO therapy: The first evidence of response to the thrice weekly EPO administration is an increase in the reticulocyte count within 10 days.[25] Since erythroid progenitors take several days to mature, a clinically significant increase in hematocrit is usually not observed in less than 2 weeks and may require up to 6 weeks in some patients.[26] If the rate of rise of hemoglobin is greater than 1 g/dL over 2 weeks, it generally warrants decreasing EPO dose. This is because a greater than 1 g/dL rise in *any* 2 weeks during the course of the therapy has been associated with an increased risk of thromboembolic phenomenon, predisposing to myocardial infarction, stoke and even death.[27] Also, according to manufacturer's recommendations, a Hb level of greater than 12g/dL should not be aimed, the reason being potentially increased risk of thromboembolic phenomenon.[28] Once adequate Hb level (≥10g/dL) is achieved, ribavirin dose can be increased to the optimum level.[20] Once started, adjunct EPO therapy may be required until the end of the treatment. In one study,[24] the median duration of EPO treatment was 24 weeks (range 6–39).

4.1.2 Interferon-induced neutropenia/ thrombocytopenia

The minimum effective dose of pegylated interferon appears to be 1 μg/kg/wk. It is recommended to reduce IFN dose to the minimum effective level if neutrophil count falls to $<0.5x10^9/L$, and discontinue it if it falls to $<0.3x10^9/L$.[17] Regarding platelet count, IFN dose should be reduced to the minimum effective level if platelet count falls to $<30x10^9/L$, and discontinued if it falls to $<20x10^9/L$.[17] If no or little improvement in neutrophil/ platelet counts occur, initiating concomitant granulocyte-colony-stimulating-factor (G-CSF) or granulocyte-monocyte-colony-stimulating-factor (GM-CSF) therapy may be considered[19,20] with an aim to avoid using the suboptimal drug doses.

Possible indications:	1.	Neutrophil count <0.5x10⁹/L.
	2.	Platelet count <30x10⁹/L
Dosage regimens:	3.	30MU subcutaneously once weekly and then adjusting the dose as per the response/ requirement.

Table 9. Granulocyte-colony-stimulating-factor (G-CSF) therapy

Monitoring G-CSF therapy: Complete blood counts should be requested twice or thrice weekly and response to therapy judged. Once adequate neutrophil count is achieved, IFN dose can be *increased* to the optimum level.[21] Once started, adjunct G-CSF therapy may be required till the end of the treatment. In one study,[24] the median duration of G-CSF therapy was 20 weeks (range 9–45).

4.2 Pharmacotherapy of superadded infections

Norfloxacin prophylaxis has been shown to reduce the incidence of superadded infections.[15,16] In cases of established nosocomial SBP (often caused by bacteria resistant to 3rd-generation cephalosporins and/or amoxicillin-clavulanic acid), broad-spectrum antibiotics like carbapenems or glycopeptides should be prescribed.

Although it is not yet clear how much survival benefit antiviral therapy confers, a standardized mortality rate analysis in one study reported a lower liver-related mortality among cirrhotics with SVR (0.6: CI: 0.0-3.1) compared to untreated patients.[29] In post-liver transplant cases, avoidance of allograft failure due to recurrence of HCV infection has also been reported in the literature although it needs further studies and validation.[30]

5. Conclusion

One thing that has become increasingly clear from the existing trials data is that cirrhotic patients who are treated with antiviral therapy and who achieve SVR are less likely to develop liver-related complications as compared to the non-responders. Despite the many encouraging studies on this subject, data on the long-term disease progression, avoidance of transplantation, and most importantly, improvement of life expectancy is however still sparse. Although liver functions have clearly been shown to improve with antiviral therapy (as indicated by significant reductions in CTP and MELD scores), the same are more likely to deteriorate within a few years in patients with advanced cirrhosis thus explaining the need to accumulate data on the possible survival benefit conferred by antiviral therapy in cirrhotic patients.

6. References

[1] Fattovich G, Giustina G, Degos F, Diodati G, Tremolada F, Nevens F, et al. Effectiveness of interferon alfa on incidence of hepatocellular carcinoma and decompensation in

cirrhosis type C. European Concerted Action on Viral Hepatitis (EUROHEP). J Hepatol 1997; 27: 201-205

[2] Terrault NA, Berenguer M. Treating hepatitis C infection in liver transplant recipients. Liver Transpl. 2006;12:1192–1204.

[3] Everson GT, Trouillot T, Trotter J, Skilbred J, Halprin A, McKinley C, et al. Treatment of decompensated cirrhotics with a low-accelerating dose regimen (LADR) of interferon-alfa-2b plus ribavirin: safety and efficacy [Abstract]. HEPATOLOGY 2000;32:308A.

[4] Everson GT, Trotter J, Forman L. Treatment of advanced hepatitis C with a low-accelerating dosage regimen of antiviral therapy. Hepatology 2005;42:255-62.

[5] Everson GT. Treatment of chronic hepatitis C in patients with decompensated cirrhosis. Rev Gastroenterol Disord 2004;4(Suppl 1):S31-8.

[6] Everson GT. Treatment of patients with hepatitis C on the waiting list. Liver Transpl 2003;9:S90–S94.

[7] Crippin JS, McCashland T, Terrault N, Sheiner P, Charlton MR. A pilot study of the tolerability and efficacy of antiviral therapy in hepatitis C virus-infected patients awaiting liver transplantation. Liver Transpl 2002; 8:350–355.

[8] Heathcote EJ, Shiffman ML, Cooksley WG, Dusheiko GM, Lee SS, Balart L, et al. Peginterferon alfa-2a in patients with chronic hepatitis C and cirrhosis. N Engl J Med 2000;343:1673–1680.

[9] Hoofnagle JH, Di Bisceglie AM, Waggoner JG, Park Y. Interferon alfa for patients with clinically apparent cirrhosis due to chronic hepatitis B. Gastroenterology 1993;104:1116–1121.

[10] Iacobellis A, Siciliano M, Perri F, Annicchiarico BE, Leandro G, Caruso N, et al. Peginterferon alfa-2b and ribavirin in patients with hepatitis C virus and decompensated cirrhosis: a controlled study. J Hepatol 2007; 46: 206-212

[11] Thomas RM, Brems JJ, Guzman-Hartman C, Yong S, Cavaliere P, Van Thiel DH. Infection with chronic hepatitis C virus and liver transplantation: a role for interferon therapy before transplantation. Liver Transpl 2003; 9: 905-915

[12] Di Marco V, Almasio PL, Ferraro D, Calvaruso V, Alaimo G, Peralta S, et al. Peg-interferon alone or combined with ribavirin in HCV cirrhosis with portal hypertension: a randomized controlled trial. J Hepatol 2007; 47: 484-491

[13] Angelo Iacobellis, Antonio Ippolito, Angelo Andriulli. Antiviral therapy in hepatitis C virus cirrhotic patients in compensated and decompensated condition. World J Gastroenterol 2008; 14(42): 6467-6472.

[14] Tekin F, Gunsar F, Karasu Z, Akarca U, Ersoz G. Safety, tolerability, and efficacy of pegylated-interferon alfa-2a plus ribavirin in HCV-related decompensated cirrhotics. Aliment Pharmacol Ther. 2008 Jun 1;27(11):1081-5.

[15] Carrión JA, Martínez-Bauer E, Crespo G, Ramírez S, Pérez-del-Pulgar S, García-Valdecasas JC, et al. Antiviral therapy increases the risk of bacterial infections in HCV-infected cirrhotic patients awaiting liver transplantation: A retrospective study. J Hepatol. 2009;50:719–728.

[16] Bruno Roche, Didier Samuel. Antiviral therapy in HCV-infected cirrhotics awaiting liver transplantation: A costly strategy for mixed virological results. J Hepatol. 2009;50 (4): 652-654.

[17] Kasper C. Recombinant human erythropoietin in the treatment of anemic patients with hematological malignancies. Ann Hematol 2001;80:319–329.

[18] Itri LM. The use of epoetin alfa in chemotherapy patients: a consistent profile of efficacy and safety. Semin Oncol 2002;29(suppl 8):81–87.

[19] Hubel K, Dale DC, Liles WC. Therapeutic use of cytokines to modulate phagocyte function for the treatment of infectious diseases: current status of granulocyte colony-stimulating factor, granulocyte-macrophage colony stimulating factor, macrophage colony-stimulating factor, and interferon gamma. J Infect Dis 2002;185:1490–1501.

[20] Berghmans T, Paesmans M, Lafitte JJ, Mascaux C, Meert AP, Jacquy C, et al. Therapeutic use of granulocyte and granulocyte-macrophage colony-stimulating factors in febrile neutropenic cancer patients. A systematic review of the literature with meta-analysis. Support Care Cancer 2002;10:181–188.

[21] Danish FA, Koul SS, Subhani FR, Rabbani AE, Yasmin S. Role of haematopoietic growth factors as adjuncts in the treatment of chronic hepatitis C patients. Saudi J Gastroenterol 2008;14:151-7.

[22] Afdhal NH, Dieterich DT, Pockros PJ, Schiff ER, Shiffman ML, Sulkowski MS, et al. Proactive Study Group. Epoetin alfa maintains ribavirin dose in HCV-infected patients: a prospective, double-blind, randomized controlled study. Gastroenterology 2004; 126:1302–1311.

[23] M Sherman, S Shafran, K Burak. Management of chronic hepatitis C: Consensus guidelines. Can J Gastroenterol 2007 ;21(Suppl C):25C-34C.

[24] Lebray P, Nalpas B, Vallet-Pichard A. The impact of haematopoietic growth factors on the management and efficacy of antiviral treatment in patients with hepatitis C virus. Antivir Ther 2005;10:769-76.

[25] Eschbach JW, Egrie JC, Downing MR, et al. Correction of the Anemia of End-Stage Renal Disease with Recombinant Human Erythropoietin. NEJM. 1987;316:73-78.

[26] Eschbach JW, Abdulhadi MH, Browne JK. Recombinant Human Erythropoietin in Anemic Patients with End-Stage Renal Disease. Ann Intern Med. 1989;111:992-1000.

[27] Singh AK, Szczech L, Tang KL. Correction of Anemia with Epoetin Alfa in Chronic Kidney Disease, N Engl j Med. 2006; 355:2085-98.

[28] Besarab A, Bolton WK, Browne JK. The effects of normal as compared with low haematocrit values in patients with cardiac disease who are receiving haemodialysis and epoetin. NEJM. 1998;339:584-90.

[29] Yoshida H, Arakawa Y, Sata M, Nishiguchi S, Yano M, Fujiyama S, Yamada G, et al. Interferon therapy prolonged life expectancy among chronic hepatitis C patients. Gastroenterology 2002; 123: 483-491

[30] Forns X, Garcia-Retortillo M, Serrano T, Feliu A, Suarez F, de la Mata M, et al. Antiviral therapy of patients with decompensated cirrhosis to prevent recurrence of hepatitis C after liver transplantation. J Hepatol 2003; 39: 389-396

2

Virus Diagnostics and Antiviral Therapy in Acute Retinal Necrosis (ARN)

Peter Rautenberg[1], Jost Hillenkamp[2], Livia Grančičova[1], Bernhard Nölle[2], Johann Roider[2] and Helmut Fickenscher[1]*

[1]Institute for Infection Medicine,
[2]Department for Ophthalmology, Christian Albrecht University of Kiel and University Medical Center Schleswig-Holstein, Kiel, Germany

1. Introduction

Acute retinal necrosis (ARN) is a fulminant necrotizing form of retinitis of viral origin. Without treatment, ARN leads to the irreversible blindness by destruction of the retina and the optic nerve. The clinical observation was first described under the term *Kirisawa uveitis* (Urayama et al., 1971) while the term *acute retinal necrosis* was introduced by Young & Bird (1978). The international diagnostic standard criteria were defined by Holland et al. (1994). ARN is a rare disease occurring world-wide in approximately one per 1.5-2.0 million persons per year (Muthiah et al., 2007; Vandercam et al., 2008). The rareness of this disease precludes randomized prospective clinical studies. Most observations are derived from small case series and homogenous international guidelines for therapy are still lacking. A few studies, however, allow statements on the causative agents and therapeutic principles.

Initially, herpesvirus particles were detected by electron microscopy in the retina of enucleated eyes with ARN. The causative role of herpesviruses was further established by showing local virus-specific antibody production, by demonstrating viral nucleic acids with the polymerase chain reaction (PCR), and by therapeutic success with antiviral drugs (Culbertson & Atherton, 1993). The disease is mainly caused by the α-herpesviruses varicella-zoster virus (VZV) or herpes-simplex virus (HSV) in 70% and 30% of the cases, respectively (*e.g.*, Culbertson et al., 1986; Rummelt et al., 1992). While the β-herpesvirus cytomegalovirus (CMV) plays a marginal role in the pathogenesis of ARN, the role of the γ-herpesvirus Epstein-Barr virus (EBV) remains controversial. Meta-analysis shows that men are affected slightly more frequently than women (Rautenberg et al., 2009).

The early ARN diagnosis is primarily based on the virus-specific polymerase-chain reaction in punctuate fluid from the anterior chamber or the vitreous and can be supported by the detection of specific antibody titers from punctate fluid and serum using the Goldmann-Witmer coefficient. Detection of virus DNA provides the basis for the early antiviral therapy which limits disease progression and risk for complications. Retinal infections by VZV or HSV are treated with aciclovir, valaciclovir, or famciclovir. Ganciclovir and valganciclovir are primarily used for the therapy of retinal CMV infections. In the case of resistance development against antiviral drugs, foscarnet or cidofovir are available as second-line antiviral drugs. The early specific antiviral therapy is the crucial prerequisite for the optimal clinical outcome. The pros and cons of the different application routes (oral, intraveneous, intravitreal) are discussed in order to provide sufficient drug levels in the eye. The antiviral therapy of ARN must be combined with ophthalmological and surgical procedures. Early vitrectomy has been shown to lead to a significant reduction of secondary retinal detachment. The early and combined strategy is essential for the clinical outcome of the rare ARN (Hillenkamp et al., 2009a, b, 2010; Pleyer et al., 2009).

2. Pathogenesis, epidemiology, and clinical course of ARN

2.1 Viral pathogenesis

The establishment of latency after primary infection is a common feature of herpesviruses. During latency, the entire, mostly inactive virus genome is maintained in the nuclei of host cells. The α-herpesviruses VZV, HSV-1, and HSV-2 are characterized by their tropism for sensory neurones and epithelia. Via mucosal or cutaneous entry sites, the neurotropic herpesviruses gain access to the peripheral endings of sensory neurones. After virus uptake and axonal transport of the nucleocapsids, the virus establishes latency within approximately 14 days in the nucleus of autonomous or sensory ganglia. The viral genome persists there in circular, extrachromosomal form (Steiner et al., 2007).

In case of HSV, production of latency-associated viral transcripts seems to block virus replication and neuronal cell death. HSV-1 was shown to induce a local, CD8+ T cell-mediated, non-lytical inflammation in human trigeminal ganglia (Mott et al., 2009; Theil et al., 2003). These CD8+ T cells seem to block HSV reactivation via release of granzyme B which selectively degrades one of the regulatory proteins of HSV-1 and inhibits reactivation already in the very early phase (Khanna et al., 2004; Knickelbein et al., 2008). Thus, a well balanced equilibrium between host defense and viral immune evasion mechanisms is formed during herpesviral latency. Since virus particles are not produced during latency, virus elimination by antiviral drugs is not feasible.

The factors are not well defined which induce the reactivation of herpesvirus replication and the axonal transport of the viral nucleocapsids from the ganglion to the periphery. For HSV, ultraviolet light, neurosurgical procedures, periocular trauma and high-dosed steroid medication are known to cause reactiviation. During peripheral virus replication, clinical symptoms are observed in the region innervated by the respective sensory nerve, mostly in the form of oroacial herpes or as herpes zoster (shingles) and by far more rarely as ocular herpes (Liesegang, 2001; Lorette et al., 2006; Malvy et al., 2007).

The extremely low incidence of the ocular herpes manifestations can be explained through epidemiology as well as neuroanatomy. HSV-1 and HSV-2 have strongly different capabilities of establishing latency in trigeminal or sacral sensory ganglia and of inducing reactivation. Whereas 41% of the cases with latent trigeminal HSV-1 reactivate the virus, this occurs only in 4% of the trigeminal HSV-2 infections. In latent sacral HSV-2 infections, 89% of the patients develop recurrent genital herpes, in contrast to 25% of the cases with sacral HSV-1 latency (Lafferty et al., 1987). The rate for the symptomatic recurrence of orofacial HSV-1 is 0.12 per month in contrast to 0.001 for orofacial HSV-2 (Lafferty et al., 1987). The different rates of reactivation from different anatomical regions correspond to the mRNA prevalence as detected by by PCR in trigeminal ganglia, 79% for VZV, 53% for HSV-1, and 7% for HSV-2, respectively (Pevenstein et al., 1999). Moreover, the HSV-specific latency-associated transcripts and HSV-reactive CD8+ T cells were clearly less frequent in the neurones projecting to the ophthalmic nerve as in the other branches of the trigeminal nerve (Hüfner et al., 2009). These findings indicate that HSV reactivations occur more rarely in the eye than in the other orofacial regions.

As the latency site of CMV, hematopoetic myelomonocytic progenitor cells are considered, from which systemic dissemination occurs via monocytes (Crough et al., 2009; Sinclair, 2008; Sinclair & Sissons, 2006). EBV replicates primarily in the pharyngeal and tonsillar epithelium and in B cells. EBV latency is localized to quiescent B lymphocytes (Miyashita et al., 1995). Both viruses can be reactivated spontaneously or, drastically more frequently, during immunosuppression. Correspondingly, the simultaneous demonstration of DNA of different herpesviruses is possible in retinitis or ARN (Hasselbach et al., 2008; Hillenkamp et al., 2009a; Lau et al., 2007; Sugita et al., 2008).

The mechanisms are not yet sufficiently clarified which lead to the viral infection of the retina and finally to ARN. In a murine model, retinitis of the contralateral eye was observed within three days after intravitreal inoculation with a highly neurovirulent HSV-1 strain (Labetoulle et al., 2000). The time course of virus spread and immunohistological findings support the theory of non-synaptic virus transfer between neurones and glia cells in the chiasma opticum leading to the infection of the contralateral eye (Labetoulle et al., 2000). This is clinically relevant, since specific antiviral therapy reduces the risk for bilateral ARN (Palay et al., 1991).

For rare diseases such as herpesviral encephalitis or ARN, causative immunological defects have been discussed. In one study, plasmacytoid dendritic cells from nine ARN patients were significantly fewer than in healthy controls, as well as interferon-α production and CD8+ cell responses were clearly diminished. This could contribute to the impaired control of latent herpesvirus infections and subsequent development of ARN (Kittan et al., 2007).

2.2 Epidemiology

ARN is an extremely rare disease. Patients with endogenous uveitis had ARN in 1.3% (41 of 3060; 95% confidence interval [CI]: 0.97-1.83%; Goto et al., 2007). During a prospective study in Great Britain over a period of 12 months, an ARN incidence of 0.5-0.6 per million was determined (Muthiah et al., 2007). Retrospective results were obtained for the Netherlands with a similar incidence of 1.1-1.6 per million (Vandercam et al., 2008). Approximately 55% of ARN patients are men (Fig. 1; Rautenberg et al., 2009: ratio men/women: 1.18; 95% CI: 1.06-1.29). In contrast, only 37.7% of the patients with orofacial herpes are men (95% CI: 33-43%; Lorette et al., 2006), while HSV seroprevalence is identical in both genders (Malkin et al., 2002).

More than 97% (95% CI: 96-99%) of all ARN cases are caused by the α-herpesviruses VZV, HSV-1, and HSV-2. VZV is the most common causative agent of ARN in approximately 70% (Fig. 2; Rautenberg et al., 2009; 95% CI: 66-76%) of ARN cases, followed by HSV-2 and HSV-1. The age of ARN manifestation depends on the causative agent. Patients with VZV-induced ARN were 48.8±19.6 years old (mean ±1 standard deviation; Fig. 3). The mean age of HSV-1- or HSV-2-induced ARN patients was 31.1±17.5 or was 47.8+-19.2 or 31.1+-17.5 years, respectively

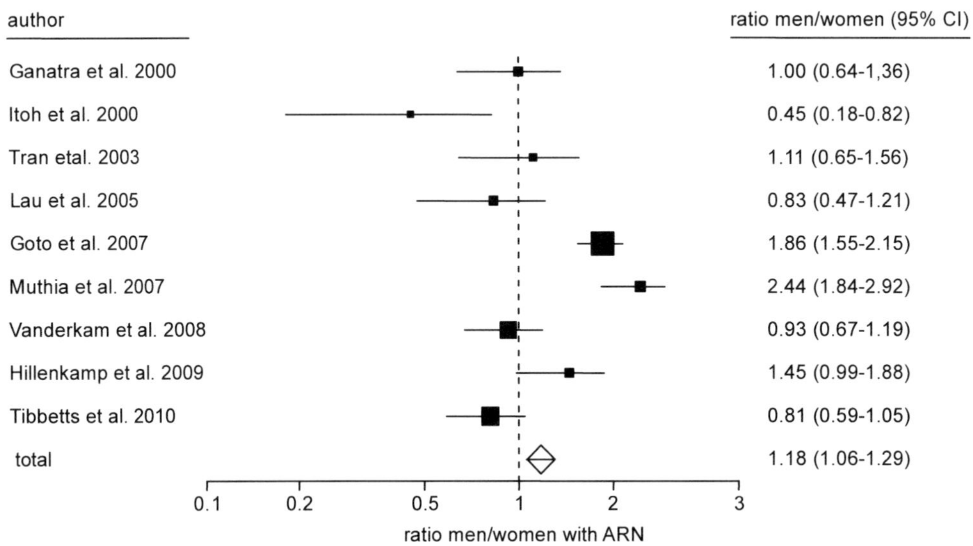

Fig. 1. Gender distribution in ARN patients. The total value (diamond) indicates slightly more men than women (54% men vs. 46% women).

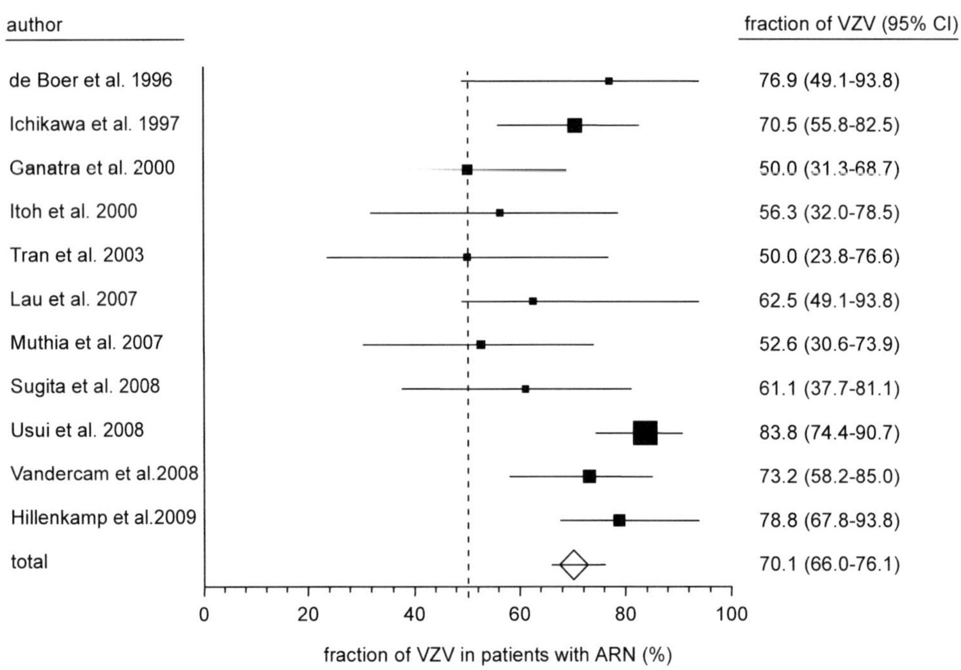

Fig. 2. Fraction of patients with VZV-induced ARN. The total value (diamond) indicates a favourite role of VZV (about 70%) in this rare disease.

(Ganatra et al., 2000; Itoh et al., 2000; Kychenthal et al., 2001; Rahhal et al., 1996; Schlingemann et al., 1996; Tran et al., 2003b; van Gelder et al., 2001). According to these results, a cut-off value of 36 years allows to discriminate HSV-2 from the other herpesvius-induced ARN (Fig. 3; sensitivity: 64%; specificity: 83%; positive predictive value at 30% prevalence: 56%; negative predictive value at 30% prevalence: 84%). The diagnostic discrimination between ARN caused by HSV-1, HSV-2, or VZV is not highly relevant, since the therapy is identical in these cases, primarily by aciclovir.

In contrast, the virological and clinical discrimination of CMV retinitis from ARN caused by the three α-herpesviruses is very important, since the drug of choice is ganciclovir in CMV infections. CMV as the causative agent of a viral retinitis in absence of immunsuppressive therapy in immunocompetent patients is extremely rare. To our knowledge, only four such cases were documented in the literature (Silverstein et al., 1997; Tajunisah et al., 2009; Urayama et al., 1971; Voros et al., 2006).

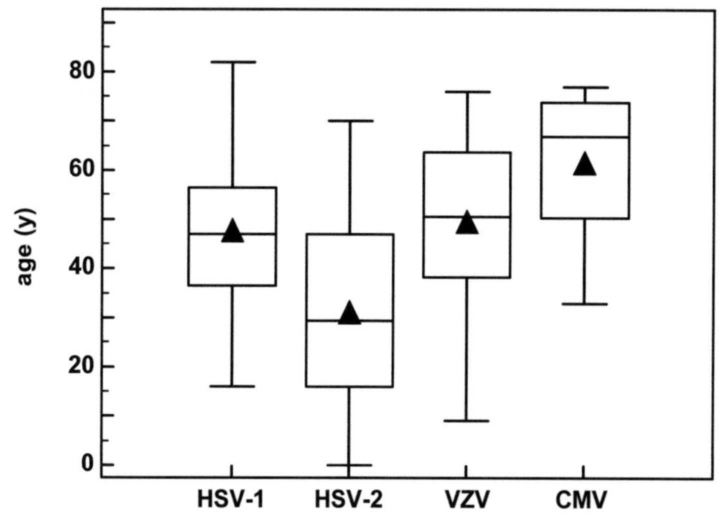

Fig. 3. Age-distribution of patients who contracted ARN by different herpesviruses. Analysis showed a significant younger age in patients who were infected by HSV-2 as compared to the other herpesviruses. The triangle within the box indicates the mean.

The controversial role of EBV for ARN was investigated in a case control study (Ongkosuwito et al., 1998). By qualitative PCR, EBV was detected in one out of 24 ocular ARN samples. However, three of 46 vitreous samples from a control group also contained EBV DNA (odds ratio: 0.62; 95% CI: 0.06-6.34). Therefore, an association between the demonstration of EBV DNA and ARN could not be determined. Only a few studies analysed EBV DNA prevalence in ARN (Abe et al., 1996; Hillenkamp et al., 2009a; Itoh et al., 2000; Lau et al., 2007; Ongkosuwito et al., 1998; Sugita et al., 2008; Tran et al., 2003a; Yamamoto et al., 2008). In nine of 134 ARN patients, EBV DNA was detected from ocular samples. In seven of these nine ARN patients (78%; 95% CI: 40-96%) VZV DNA was detected in addition to EBV by PCR (Hillenkamp et al., 2009a; Lau et al., 2007; Sugita et al., 2008). In theory, quantitative PCR methods could contribute to a clarification. However, there are no standard values for clinically relevant DNA concentrations in ocular materials and neither the diagnostic samples nor the PCR methods are sufficiently standardized. In summary, EBV seems to play no or -if at all- only a minor role in ARN development.

2.3 Clinical course

Almost 90% of all ARN cases remain unilateral (Hillenkamp et al., 2009a; Muthiah et al., 2007; Usui et al., 2008; Vandercam et al., 2008). In approximately 10% of the patients, also the contralateral eye is affected within one to six weeks, in an extreme case after up to 34 years (Falcone & Brockhurst, 1993; Saari et al., 1982; Schlingemann et al., 1996). A case-control study revealed that aciclovir therapy considerably reduces the risk for the contralateral eye (Palay et al., 1991). As soon as the ARN diagnosis is made, antiviral therapy should be started in order to avoid disease progression. Longer termed aciclovir prophylaxis should be considered (Cordero-Coma et al., 2007).

An increased ARN risk was discovered for the HLA alleles DQw7, DR4, and Bw62 (odds ratio: 5.2 and 7.3 respectively; Holland et al., 1989). Moreover, there is a 20-fold increased risk ($p=0.05$) for a fulminant ARN course in the presense of the HLA DR9 allele (Matsuo & Matsuo, 1991). Several case reports describe ARN following HSV encephalitis (Bristow et al., 2006; de la Blanchardiere et al., 2000; Gain et al., 2002; Ganatra et al., 2000; Gaynor et al., 2001; Hadden & Berry, 2002; Kim & Yoon, 2002; Maertzdorf et al., 2001; Pavésio et al., 1997; Yamamoto et al., 2007). In a retrospective study, thirteen of 52 patients showed infectious or non-infectious neurological diseases in the medical history (Vandercam et al., 2008). Four of eleven patients had HSV encephalitis 20.6 months (mean) prior to ARN. Two of 28 patients had VZV encephalitis 28 months (mean) before. The HSV patients showed a unilateral ARN, whereas both immunosuppressed VZV patients developed bilateral ARN. Besides various case reports, these results clearly demonstrate herpes encephalitis as a risk factor for ARN which needs attention in neurology and ophthalmology.

3. Virus diagnostics

3.1 Preanalytical conditions

Diagnostic samples can be generated in early stages by puncture of the anterior chamber, by paracentesis, by fine needle aspiration of vitreous fluid, or in advanced conditions by therapeutic pars plana vitrectomy (Winterhalter et al., 2007). The rapid PCR demonstration of virus DNA is highly important for the therapy, because specific antiviral drugs are used. Since herpesviruses and their DNA genomes are rather stable, the transport of fluid from the anterior chamber or from the vitreous does not need special precautions. Only in the case of prolonged transport times, the samples should be shipped in cooled conditions. The major diagnostic test is the PCR for herpesviral DNA for the direct demonstration of the causative agent. Virus-specific serologic tests can serve as indirect methods in order to show local antibody production at delayed time points. The major advantage of PCR testing is the low sample volume required and the independence of time-delayed immune reaction. Due to the rareness of ARN and to the critical contribution of antiviral therapy, the authors recommend the genotypic sensitivity test after demonstration of herpesvirus DNA. In case of failure of the antiviral therapy, this allows the rapid decision for either switching to cidofovir or foscarnet or for increasing aciclovir dosage in case of preserved drug sensitivity.

3.2 Nucleic acid diagnostics

The clinical ARN diagnosis needs the critical validation by virus-specific PCR. During the initial stage, only PCR allows rapid and valid results. Time-delayed PCR diagnostics lead to diminished test sensitivity (de Boer et al., 1996; Knox et al., 1998). Due to the high test sensitivity of the PCR, 20-50 µl sample volume is sufficient in most cases. The PCR discrimination beween HSV-1 and HSV-2 is an established method. Real-time PCR methods allow the quantitation of viral loads in copy number per ml. Although there are no standards available for a clinically relevant virus load value, the quantitation is relevant to discriminate between the major causative agent and an additional, perhaps weak reactivation of another herpesvirus, *e. g.*, under immunosuppression (Hasselbach et al., 2008).

3.3 Antibody assays

The quantitative determination of antibody titers from the anterior chamber or the vitreous in comparison to the serum levels is an indirect and supporting procedure for virus-specific diagnostics at delayed time points. For the determination of the Goldmann-Witmer coefficient (antibody index, AI; Goldmann & Witmer, 1954), the intraocular and serum antibody titers and total IgG values are included in the following formula:

AI = (antibody titer punctate/antibody titer serum) / (total IgG punctate/total IgG serum)

Most authors consider an AI > 2-3 an obvious indicator of intraocular antibody production (de Boer et al., 1994; Dussaix et al., 1987; Fekkar et al., 2008; Pepose et al., 1992). Serological procedures have the disadvantages that significant antibody levels can be expected only after one to two weeks and that a false-negative AI can result from massive disturbance of the blood-eye barrier. In the case of latently peristing herpesviruses, an ocular reactivation does not necessarily lead to a significant AI increase. Moreover, there are serological cross-reactivites between HSV and VZV (Pepose et al., 1992). Finally, the intraocular antibody generation can be variable in immunosuppressed or HIV-infected patients (de Boer et al., 1996; Doornenbal et al., 1996; Kijlstra et al., 1989, 1990).

4. Therapy

4.1 Drugs directed against α-herpesviruses

Aciclovir by the parenteral route is the drug of choice in severe, acute HSV or VZV infections. The acyclic guanosine derivate aciclovir is specifically activated by the viral enzyme thymidine kinase of HSV or VZV to its monophosphate. Ubiquitous cellular kinases are responsible for the conversion to aciclovir triphosphate which is a specific inhibitor for the viral DNA polymerase (de Clercq, 2004). The dosage is based on tissue culture-derived determinations of the 50%-inhibitory concentration (IC50) of aciclovir against HSV-1, HSV-2, or VZV. Due to a lack of standardisation of the assay conditions and the test viruses, these values are variable, up to several orders of magnitude. The IC50 values were 0.02 to 13.5 µg/ml for HSV-1, 0.01 to 9.9 µg/ml for HSV-2 and 0.12 to 10.8 µg/ml for VZV (O'Brien & Campoli-Richards, 1989). Due to the three hours half life of aciclovir, it should be administered intraveneously at 10 mg/kg for ten to 14 days three times daily. Consecutively, the oral application of five times daily 800 mg for further six weeks is recommended (Blumenkranz et al., 1986; Duker & Blumenkranz, 1991; Morse & Mizoguchi, 1995; Palay et al., 1991). This recommendation is based on a case-control study in which most of the bilateral ARN cases ocurred within a period of six weeks and in which 90% of the bilateral ARN cases could have been avoided by aciclovir therapy (Palay et al., 1991). After the start of the antiviral therapy, new lesions should not occur from the second day on. From the fourth or fifth day on, the retinal infiltrates should show a tendence for regression. After one month, a complete remission should be achieved (Blumenkranz et al., 1986). If this is not accomplished, either there was an insufficient drug dosage, or antiviral resistance has developed which is more frequently seen in immunosuppressed patients. The side effects of aciclovir are rather weak and rare and may include mild serum creatinine increase, nausea, and vomiting. Presently, the authors recommend aciclovir as first-line therapy of choice in the early phase of the disease. This is based on the long-termed experience with this drug. Moreover, this excludes influences from the intra- and interindividual variability of the oral bioavailability of valaciclovir (Hillenkamp et al., 2009a, b, 2010; Phan et al., 2003). The management of ARN by antiviral drugs has been summarized in a recent review article (Tam eta al., 2010).

Valaciclovir is the valyl ester of aciclovir, which is quickly taken up into enterocytes after oral administration via enteric aminoacid transport systems and which is then hydrolyzed to the active prodrug aciclovir (Granero & Amidon, 2006; Katragadda et al., 2005). The oral bioavailability of valaciclovir of 54% is three times higher than that of aciclovir (Soul-Lawton et al., 1995). When 1000 mg valaciclovir were administered three times daily, aciclovir serum levels of 4.41 µg/ml and aciclovir levels in the vitreous of 1.03 µg/ml were reached. These concentrations are in the IC50 range for most HSV or VZV isolates. The lower peak concentrations during oral in comparison to parenteral aciclovir therapy minimize the risk for renal side effects (Huynh et al., 2008).

Famciclovir is an orally available di-acetyl derivate of penciclovir. By deacetylation, famciclovir is metabolized in the liver to the active prodrug penciclovir which is secreted without modification by the kidneys (Chakrabarty et al., 2004). The oral bioavailability of famciclovir is 77% and, thus, approximately 1.5-fold higher than that of valaciclovir (Soul-Lawton et al., 1995) or 3.4-fold higher than that of aciclovir (15–30%; Fletcher & Bean, 1985). By oral administration of 500 mg every eight hours, intravitreal penciclovir concentrations of 1.2 µg/ml can be reached (Chong et al., 2009), which is appropriate for the therapy of non-resistant HSV-1, HSV-2, or VZV strains. In some single case reports, famciclovir was active against aciclovir-resistant VZV strains (Figueroa et al., 1997). However, the main reasons for aciclovir resistance are mutations of the viral thymidine kinase gene, which would typically also result in penciclovir resistance.

Based on case reports with orally available prodrugs of aciclovir (Emerson et al., 2006; Savant et al., 2004), a pilot study was performed with ten eyes of eight patients (Aizman et al., 2007). Under the oral therapy with 1 g valganciclovir or 500 mg famaciclovir three times daily, the ARN regression occurred within six days and the maximal improvement within 17 days without any case of contralateral ARN during further 36 weeks of observation. As long as randomized prospective studies on the efficiency of the oral aciclovir alternatives are not yet available, the initial standard therapy should be performed with intraveneous aciclovir, only.

Resistance mutations. Especially in immunosuppressed patients, resistance development against aciclovir is observed frequently. However, underdosage must be excluded first. Under optimal conditions, the genotypic viral resistance can be determined by DNA PCR and sequencing of the viral gene for thymidine kinase and by the sequence comparison with known resistant viruses within a few days. The cultural resistance testing depends on the successful virus isolation. This procedure is slower, hardly standardized and only possible in a few reference laboratories. More than 90% of the resistance cases result from mutations of the thymidine kinase gene. In case of resistance, cidofovir and foscarnet are usually the only available alternatives, since their activity mechanism is independent of the viral thymidine kinase. Both drugs can also be used for ganciclovir-resistant CMV strains.

Cidofovir is an acyclic nucleosid phosphonate with a broad activity spectrum against DNA viruses (de Clercq & Holý, 2005). Host cell kinases convert cidofovir to the active diphosphonyl ester which acts as a competitive inhibitor of the viral DNA polymerases and induces viral DNA chain termination. Aciclovir-resistant virus strain may be susceptible to cidofovir. The drug is administered intraveneously since its oral bioavailability is only 5%. The peculiarity of cidofovir is its very high intracellular half-life time of more than 24 hours (de Clercq & Holý, 2005). Cidofovir should be used only as a drug of second choice. It is infused in a dose of 5 mg/kg over one hour once weekly in two weeks. For maintenance, the infusion is then repeated every second week in the same dosage. The major disadvantage of cidofovir is its nephrotoxicity which is due to the accumulation of this drug by an anion transporter system of the proximal tubuli of the renal cortex (Ho et al., 2000). Since cidofovir is renally secreted, it must be combined with probenecid for kidney protection.

Foscarnet. In the case of a proven resistance against aciclovir, ganciclovir, or their prodrugs, foscarnet is the drug of choice. Foscarnet is a pyrophosphate analogon which occupies the pyrophosphate binding site on the herpesviral DNA polymerase and inhibits the release of pyrophosphate from the terminal nucleotide triphosphate of the growing viral DNA chain (Biron, 2006). Due to the very low oral bioavailability of 20%, the drug is administered by large-volume intraveneous infusions. Foscarnet is used in a dosage of 60 mg/kg every eight hours. Foscarnet is renally eliminated without any metabolic modification. In patients with diminished renal function, the dosis must be adjusted to the creatinine clearance value. The major side effect of foscarnet is its nephrotoxicity.

Intravitreal application. Vitreous concentrations of aciclovir following intravenous administration has not yet been tested on a broad basis. Therefore, in patients, who do not respond to intravenous therapy, the intravitreal application of the respective antiviral drug should be considered in order to rapidly achieve high concentrations of the drug and, thus, an improved prognosis (Hillenkamp et al., 2009a, 2010; Scott et al., 2002; Velez et al., 2001; Zambarakji et al., 2002). This strategy allows high intraocular drug levels under reduced systemic exposure. Studies on repeated injections are not yet available.

4.2 Drugs directed against cytomegalovirus

In contrast to the α-herpesviruses, CMV lacks a viral thymidine kinase. Presently, four drugs are licensed for CMV therapy: ganciclovir, valganciclovir, cidofovir, and foscarnet. All of them target the viral DNA polymerase and inhibit the viral DNA synthesis.

Ganciclovir and its orally available valyl ester-derivate valganciclovir are the drugs of first choice for the therapy of CMV-induced diseases (de Clercq, 2004). The substances are monophosphorylated in CMV-infected cells by the CMV-specific protein kinase UL97, and subsequently triphosphorylated by cellular kinases. The incorporation of the acyclic ganciclovir triphosphate into the growing viral DNA chain results in the blockade of polymerase translocation (Reid et al., 1988). Since the oral bioavailability of ganiclovir is only approximately 5%, the drug should be administered intravenously during the ganciclovir disease. In most cases, 10 mg/kg i.v. daily should be sufficient for the CMV therapy in ARN cases. The oral bioavailability of valganciclovir is approximately 60%. A daily dose of 900 mg will yield serum concentrations comparable to 5 mg/kg intraveneous ganciclovir or a 1,7-fold serum concentration in comparison to 1000 mg oral ganciclovir (Cvetković & Wellington, 2005). The major side effect of systemic ganciclovir therapy is neutropenia in approximately 8% of the patients. Therefore, ganciclovir therapy needs the regular control of blood counts, as well as the surveillance of renal function (Paya et al., 2004).

UL97 resistance mutations. Mutations of the UL97 protein kinase of CMV are the major cause of resistance against ganciclovir and its derivates. The resistence is determined genotypically by sequencing if the viral genes for the UL97 kinase and for the DNA polymerase. The most frequent ganciclovir resistence mutations in UL97 (codons 460, 520, 590-607) inhibit ganciclovir phosphorylation which is the prerequsite for antiviral activity (Chou et al., 2008). The activity of cidofovir and foscarnet is independent of the protein kinase UL97 and appropriate for the therapy of many DNA viruses.

4.3 Differential diagnosis

During the early disease stages, additional infectious agents, rheumatological disorders, autoimmune uveitis, or intraocular lymphomas have to be considered (Table 1). Whereas

Disease	Diagnosis	First-line therapy
ARN by varicella zoster virus	PCR	aciclovir
ARN by herpes simplex virus	PCR	aciclovir
ARN by cytomegalovirus	PCR	ganciclovir
ARN by Epstein-Barr virus	PCR	not available
Progressive outer retina necrosis	PCR, serology	dependent on the agent
Cytomegalovirus retinitis	PCR	ganciclovir
Lyme borreliosis	serology, PCR	cephalosporin
Syphilis	serology	penicillin
Toxoplasmosis retinitis	serology, PCR	pyrimethamine/sulfonamide
Tuberculosis	culture, PCR	antimycobacterial therapy
Endogeneous endophthalmitis	culture, PCR	dependent on the agent
Bacterial eye infection	culture, PCR	dependent on the agent
Fungal eye infection	culture, PCR, Antigen	Candida: Fluconazol Aspergillus: Voriconazol
Behçet's disease	clinic, pathergia test	immunosuppression
Sarcoidosis	histology	immunosuppression
Idiopathic chorioretinitis	exclusion diagnosis	immunosuppression
Idiopathic retinovasculitis	exclusion diagnosis	immunosuppression
Intraocular lymphoma	cytology, tumor genetics	radiochemotherapy

Table 1. Differential diagnosis of acute retinal necrosis.

the start of ARN therapy is critical for the outcome the initiation of the therapy for most alternative causes is by far less urgent. Due to the similar clinical appearance, toxoplasmosis chorioretinitis is an important differential diagnosis (Balansard et al., 2005; Hasselbach et al., 2008; Moshfeghi et al., 2004). An ocular manifestation of syphilis can show many different symptoms and can mimick various diseases. In contrast to ARN, CMV retinitis shows weak inflammation signs in the anterior chamber and the vitreous. Patients with CMV retinitis are usually infected with human immunodeficiency virus (HIV) with less than 50 CD4+ T cells/µl. CMV retinitis is resistant to aciclovir therapy. Therefore, the early PCR test for virus DNA is necessary.

Finally, progressive outer retina necrosis (PORN) forms another differential diagnosis, which was mainly described in HIV patients (Forster et al., 1990). Typically, the outer retinal layers are primarily affected multifocally, while the inner retinal layers are less concerned. In contrast to ARN, there is no vasculitis component. The course of PORN disease is extremely rapid, spreading to the the deep retinal layers and leading to retinal detachment. Patients with PORN usually show coinfection with HIV and VZV.

5. Conclusion

ARN occurs in up to one per million persons per year. The virus-caused disease remains unilateral in approximately 90% of the cases. Without treatment, ARN shows poor prognosis. The immediate calculated antiviral therapy by aciclovir or its prodrugs is justified, since approximately 70% of the cases are caused by VZV and 30% by HSV. The causative role of EBV remains controversial; often, EBV reactivation occurs concomitantly with VZV reactivation. While EBV reactivation cannot be treated efficiently, aciclovir is appropriate for VZV and HSV reactivations. The very rare case of CMV in ARN is an indication for ganciclovir or its prodrug. The virus-specific DNA PCR test from fluid of the anterior chamber or the vitreous provides the critical indication for the specific therapy. Disease progression and complications rates can be limited by additional immediate conservative and surgical therapy.

6. Acknowledgements

The scientific work underlying this manuscript was supported in part by the Deutsche Forschungsgemeinschaft (Bonn), the Excellence Cluster Inflammation at Interfaces (Kiel), and the Varicella-Zoster Virus Research Foundation (New York).

7. References

Abe, T.; Tsuchida, K.; Tamai, M. (1996). A comparative study of the polymerase chain reaction and local antibody production in acute retinal necrosis syndrome and cytomegalovirus retinitis. *Graefes Archive for Clinical and Experimental Ophthalmology*, Vol. 234, No. 7, pp. 419-424

Aizman, A.; Johnson, M. W.; Elner, S. G. (2007). Treatment of acute retinal necrosis syndrome with oral antiviral medications. *Ophthalmology*, Vol. 114, No. 2, pp. 307-312

Balansard, B.; Bodaghi, B.; Cassoux, N.; Fardeau, C.; Romand, S.; Rozenberg, F.; Rao, N. A.; Lehoang, P. (2005). Necrotising retinopathies simulating acute retinal necrosis syndrome. *British Journal of Ophthalmology*, Vol. 89, No. 1, pp. 96-101

Biron, K. K. (2006). Antiviral drugs for cytomegalovirus diseases. *Antiviral Research,* Vol. 71, No. 2-3, pp. 154-163

Blumenkranz, M. S.; Culbertson, W. W.; Clarkson, J. G.; Dix, R. (1986). Treatment of the acute retinal necrosis syndrome with intravenous acyclovir. *Ophthalmology,* Vol. 93, No. 3, 296-300

Bristow, E. A.; Cottrell, D., G.; Pandit, R. J. (2006). Bilateral acute retinal necrosis syndrome following herpes simplex type 1 encephalitis. *Eye (London),* Vol. 20, No. 11, pp. 1327-1330

Chakrabarty, A.; Tyring, S. K.; Beutner, K.; Rauser, M. (2004). Recent clinical experience with famciclovir, a "third generation" nucleoside prodrug. *Antiviral Chemistry and Chemotherapy,* Vol. 15, No. 5, pp. 251-253

Chong, D. Y.; Johnson, M. W.; Huynh, T. H.; Hall, E. F.; Comer, G. M.; Fish, D. N. (2009). Vitreous penetration of orally administered famciclovir. *American Journal of Ophthalmology,* Vol. 148, No. 1, pp. 38-42

Chou, S. (2008). Cytomegalovirus UL97 mutations in the era of ganciclovir and maribavir. *Reviews in Medical Virology,* Vol. 18, No. 4, pp. 233-246

Cordero-Coma, M.; Anzaar, F.; Yilmaz, T.; Foster, C. S. (2007). Herpetic retinitis. *Herpes,* Vol. 14, No. 1, pp. 4-10.

Crough T, Khanna R (2009) Immunobiology of human cytomegalovirus: from bench to bedside. *Clinical Microbiology Reviews,* Vol. 22, No. 1, pp. 76-98

Culbertson, W. W.; Atherton, S. S. (1993). Acute retinal necrosis and similar retinitis syndromes. *International Ophthalmology Clinics,* Vol. 33, No. 1, pp. 129-143

Culbertson, W. W.; Blumenkranz, M. S.; Pepose, J. S.; Stewart, J. A.; Curtin, V. T. (1986). Varicella zoster virus is a cause of the acute retinal necrosis syndrome. *Ophthalmology,* Vol. 93, No. 5, 559-569

Cvetković, R. S.; Wellington, K. (2005). Valganciclovir: a review of its use in the management of CMV infection and disease in immunocompromised patients. *Drugs,* Vol. 65, No. 6, pp. 859-878

de Boer, J. H.; Luyendijk, L.; Rothova, A.; Baarsma, G. S.; de Jong, P. T.; Bollemeijer, J. G.; Rademakers, A. J.; van der Lelij, A.; Zaal, M.J.; Kijlstra, A. (1994). Detection of intraocular antibody production to herpesviruses in acute retinal necrosis syndrome. *American Journal of Ophthalmology,* Vol. 117, No. 2, 201-210

de Boer, J. H.; Verhagen, C.; Bruinenberg, M.; Rothova, A.; de Jong, P. T.; Baarsma, G. S.; van der Lelij, A.; Ooyman, F. M.; Bollemeijer, J. G.; Derhaag, P. J.; Kijlstra, A. (1996). Serologic and polymerase chain reaction analysis of intraocular fluids in the diagnosis of infectious uveitis. *American Journal of Ophthalmology,* Vol. 121, No. 6, pp. 650-658

de Clercq, E. (2004). Antiviral drugs in current clinical use. *Journal of Clinical Virology,* Vol. 30, No. 2, pp. 115-133

de Clercq, E.; Holý, A. (2005). Acyclic nucleoside phosphonates: a key class of antiviral drugs. *Nature Reviews Drug Discovery,* Vol. 4, No. 11, pp. 928-940

de la Blanchardiere, A.; Rozenberg, F.; Caumes, E.; Picard, O.; Lionnet, F.; Livartowski, J.; Coste, J.; Sicard, D.; Lebon, P.; Salmon-Cèron, D. (2000). Neurological complications of varicella-zoster virus infection in adults with human immunodeficiency virus infection. *Scandinavian Journal of Infectious Diseases,* Vol. 32, No. 3, pp. 263-269

Doornenbal, P.; Seerp Baarsma, G.; Quint, W. G.; Kijlstra, A.; Rothbarth, P. H.; Niesters, H. G. (1996). Diagnostic assays in cytomegalovirus retinitis: detection of herpesvirus by simultaneous application of the polymerase chain reaction and local antibody analysis on ocular fluid. *British Journal of Ophthalmology,* Vol. 80, No. 3, pp. 235-240

Duker, J. S.; Blumenkranz, M. S. (1991). Diagnosis and management of the acute retinal necrosis (ARN) syndrome. *Survey of Ophthalmology,* Vol. 35, No. 5, pp. 327-343

Dussaix, E.; Cerqueti, P. M.; Pontet, F.; Bloch-Michel, E. (1987). New approaches to the detection of locally produced antiviral antibodies in the aqueous of patients with endogenous uveitis. *Ophthalmologica,* Vol. 194, No. 2-3, pp. 145-149

Emerson, G. G.; Smith, J. R.; Wilson, D. J.; Rosenbaum, J. T.; Flaxel, C. J. (2006). Primary treatment of acute retinal necrosis with oral antiviral therapy. *Ophthalmology,* Vol. 113, No. 12, pp. 2259-2261

Falcone, P. M.; Brockhurst, R. J. (1993). Delayed onset of bilateral acute retinal necrosis syndrome: a 34-year interval. *Annals of Ophthalmology,* Vol. 25, No. 10, pp. 373-374

Fekkar, A.; Bodaghi, B.; Touafek, F.; Le Hoang, P.; Mazier, D.; Paris, L. (2008). Comparison of immunoblotting, calculation of the Goldmann-Witmer coefficient, and real-time PCR using aqueous humor samples for diagnosis of ocular toxoplasmosis. *Journal of Clinical Microbiology,* Vol. 46, No. 6, pp. 1965-1967

Figueroa, M. S.; Garabito, I.; Gutierrez, C.; Fortun, J. (1997). Famciclovir for the treatment of acute retinal necrosis (ARN) syndrome. *American Journal of Ophthalmology,* Vol. 123, No. 2, pp. 255-257

Fletcher, C.; Bean, B. (1985). Evaluation of oral acyclovir therapy. *Drug Intelligence and Clinical Pharmacology,* Vol. 19, No. 7-8, pp. 518-524

Forster, D. J.; Dugel, P. U.; Frangieh, G. T.; Liggett, P. E.; Rao, N. A. (1990). Rapidly progresssive outer retinal necrosis in the acquired immunodeficiency syndrome. *American Journal of Ophthalmology,* Vol. 110, No. 4, pp. 341-348

Gain, P.; Chiquet, C.; Thuret, G.; Drouet, E.; Antoine, J. C. (2002). Herpes simplex virus type 1 encephalitis associated with acute retinal necrosis syndrome in an immunocompetent patient. *Acta Ophthalmologica Scandinavica,* Vol. 80, No. 5, pp. 546-549

Ganatra, J. B.; Chandler, D.; Santos, C.; Kuppermann, B.; Margolis, T. P. (2000). Viral causes of the acute retinal necrosis syndrome. *American Journal of Ophthalmology,* Vol. 129, No. 2, pp. 166-172

Gaynor, B. D.; Wade, N. K.; Cunningham, E. T. Jr. (2001). Herpes simplex virus type 1 associated acute retinal necrosis following encephalitis. *Retina,* Vol. 21, No. 6, pp. 688-690

Goldmann, H.; Witmer, R. (1954). Antibodies in the aqueous humor. *Ophthalmologica,* Vol. 127, No. 4-5, pp. 323-330

Goto, H.; Mochizuki, M.; Yamaki, K.; Kotake, S.; Usui, M.; Ohno, S. (2007). Epidemiological survey of intraocular inflammation in Japan. *Japanese Journal of Ophthalmology,* Vol. 51, No. 1, pp. 41-44

Granero, G. E.; Amidon, G. L. (2006). Stability of valacyclovir: implications for its oral bioavailability. *International Journal of Pharmaceutics,* Vol. 317, No. 1, pp. 14-18

Hadden, P. W.; Barry, C. J. (2002). Herpetic encephalitis and acute retinal necrosis. *New England Journal of Medicine,* Vol. 347, No. 24, p. 1932

Hasselbach, H. C.; Fickenscher, H.; Nölle, B; Roider, J. (2008) Atypical ocular toxoplasmosis with concomitant ocular reactivation of varicella-zoster virus and cytomegalovirus in an immunocompromised host. *Klinische Monatsblätter für Augenheilkunde,* Vol. 225, No. 3, pp. 236-239

Hillenkamp, J., Nölle, B., Bruns, C., Rautenberg, P., Fickenscher, H., Roider, J. (2009a). Acute retinal necrosis: clinical features, early vitrectomy, and outcomes. *Ophthalmology,* Vol. 116, No. 10, pp. 1971-1975

Hillenkamp, J., Nölle, B., Bruns, C., Rautenberg, P., Fickenscher, H., Roider, J. (2010). Acute retinal necrosis: clinical features, early vitrectomy, and outcomes. Author reply. *Ophthalmology,* Vol. 117, No. 8, pp. 1660-1661

Hillenkamp, J., Nölle, B., Rautenberg, P., Fickenscher, H., Roider, J. (2009b) Acute retinal necrosis: Clinical features and therapy options. *Ophthalmologe,* Vol. 106, No. 12, pp. 1058-1064

Ho, E. S.; Lin, D. C.; Mendel, D. B.; Cihlar, T. (2000). Cytotoxicity of antiviral nucleotides adefovir and cidofovir is induced by the expression of human renal organic anion transporter 1. *Journal of the American Society for Nephrology,* No. 11, Vol. 3, pp. 383-393

Holland, G. N.; Cornell, P. J.; Park, M. S.; Barbetti, A.; Yuge, J.; Kreiger, A. E.; Kaplan, H. J.; Pepose, J. S.; Heckenlively, J. R.; Culbertson, W. W.; Terasaki. P. I. (1989). An association between acute retinal necrosis syndrome and HLA-DQw7 and phenotype Bw62, DR4. *American Journal of Ophthalmology,* Vol. 108, No. 4, pp. 370-374

Holland GN, Executive committee of the American uveitis society (1994). Standard diagnostic criteria for the acute retinal necrosis syndrome. *American Journal of Ophthalmology,* Vol. 117, No. 5, pp. 663-667

Hüfner, K.; Horn, A.; Derfuss, T.; Glon, C.; Sinicina, I.; Arbusow, V.; Strupp, M.; Brandt, T.; Theil, D. (2009). Fewer latent herpes simplex virus type 1 and cytotoxic T cells occur in the ophthalmic division than in the maxillary and mandibular divisions of the human trigeminal ganglion and nerve. *Journal of Virology,* Vol. 83, No. 8, pp. 3696-3703.

Huynh, T. H.; Johnson, M. W.; Comer, G. M.; Fish, D. N. (2008). Vitreous penetration of orally administered valacyclovir. *American Journal of Ophthalmology,* Vol. 145, No. 4, pp. 682-686

Ichikawa, T.; Sakai, J.; Yamauchi, Y.; Minoda, H.; Usui, M. (1997). A study of 44 patients with Kirisawa type uveitis. *Nippon Ganka Gakkai Zasshi,* Vol. 101, No. 3, pp. 243-247

Itoh, N.; Matsumura, N.; Ogi, A.; Nishide, T.; Imai, Y.; Kanai, H.; Ohno, S. (2000). High prevalence of herpes simplex virus type 2 in acute retinal necrosis syndrome associated with herpes simplex virus in Japan. *American Journal of Ophthalmology,* Vol. 129, No. 3, pp. 404-405

Katragadda, S.; Talluri, R. S.; Pal, D.; Mitra, A. K. (2005). Identification and characterization of a Na+-dependent neutral amino acid transporter, ASCT1, in rabbit corneal epithelial cell culture and rabbit cornea. *Current Eye Research,* Vol. 30, No. 11, pp. 989-1002

Khanna, K. M.; Lepisto, A. J.; Decman, V.; Hendricks, R. L. (2004). Immune control of herpes simplex virus during latency. *Current Opinion in Immunology,* Vol. 16, No. 4, pp. 463-469

Kijlstra, A.; Luyendijk, L.; Baarsma, G. S.; Rothova, A.; Schweitzer, C. M.; Timmerman, Z.; de Vries, J.; Breebaart, A. C. (1989). Aqueous humor analysis as a diagnostic tool in toxoplasma uveitis. *International Ophthalmology,* Vol. 13, No. 6, pp. 383-386

Kijlstra, A.; van den Horn, G. J.; Luyendijk, L.; Baarsma, G. S.; Schweitzer, C. M.; Zaal, M. J.; Timmerman, Z.; Beintema, M.; Rothova, A. (1990). Laboratory tests in uveitis. New developments in the analysis of local antibody production. *Documenta Ophthalmologica,* Vol. 75, No. 3-4, pp. 225-231

Kim, C.; Yoon, Y. H. (2002). Unilateral acute retinal necrosis occurring 2 years after herpes simplex type 1 encephalitis. *Ophthalmic Surgery, Lasers and Imaging,* Vol. 33, No. 3, pp. 250-252

Kittan, N. A.; Bergua, A.; Haupt, S.; Donhauser, N.; Schuster, P.; Korn, K.; Harrer, T.; Schmidt, B. (2007). Impaired plasmacytoid dendritic cell innate immune responses in patients with herpesvirus-associated acute retinal necrosis. *Journal of Immunology,* Vol. 179, No. 6, pp. 4219-30.

Knickelbein, J. E.; Khanna, K. M.; Yee, M. B.; Baty, C. J.; Kinchington, P. R.; Hendricks, R. L. (2008) Noncytotoxic lytic granule-mediated CD8+ T cell inhibition of HSV-1 reactivation from neuronal latency. *Science,* Vol. 322, No. 5899, pp. 268-271

Knox, C. M.; Chandler, D.; Short, G. A.; Margolis, T. P. (1998). Polymerase chain reaction-based assays of vitreous samples for the diagnosis of viral retinitis. Use in diagnostic dilemmas. *Ophthalmology,* Vol. 105, No. 1, pp. 37-44

Kychenthal, A.; Coombes, A.; Greenwood, J.; Pavesio, C.; Aylward, G. W. (2001). Bilateral acute retinal necrosis and herpes simplex type 2 encephalitis in a neonate. *British Journal of Ophthalmology,* Vol. 85, No. 5, pp. 629-630

Labetoulle, M.; Kucera, P.; Ugolini, G.; Lafay, F.; Frau, E.; Offret, H.; Flamand, A. (2000). Neuronal pathways for the propagation of herpes simplex virus type 1 from one retina to the other in a murine model. *Journal of General Virology,* Vol. 81, No. 5, pp. 1201-1210

Lafferty, W. E.; Coombs, R. W.; Benedetti, J.; Critchlow, C.; Corey, L. (1987). Recurrences after oral and genital herpes simplex virus infection. Influence of site of infection and viral type. *New England Journal of Medicine,* Vol. 316, No. 23, 1444-1449

Lau, C. H.; Missotten, T.; Salzmann, J.; Lightman, S. L. (2007). Acute retinal necrosis features, management, and outcomes. *Ophthalmology,* Vol. 114, No. 4, pp. 756-762

Liesegang, T. J. (2001). Herpes simplex virus epidemiology and ocular importance. *Cornea,* Vol. 20, No. 1, pp. 1-13

Lorette, G.; Crochard, A.; Mimaud, V.; Wolkenstein, P.; Stalder, J. F.; El Hasnaoui, A. (2006). A survey on the prevalence of orofacial herpes in France: the INSTANT study. *Journal of the American Academy of Dermatology,* Vol. 55, No. 2, pp. 225-232

Maertzdorf, J.; van der Lelij, A.; Baarsma, G. S.; Osterhaus, A. D.; Verjans, G. M. (2001). Herpes simplex virus type 1 (HSV-1)-induced retinitis following herpes simplex encephalitis: indications for brain-to-eye transmission of HSV-1. *Annals of Neurology,* Vol. 49, No. 1, pp. 104-106

Malkin, J. E.; Morand, P.; Malvy, D.; Ly, T.D.; Chanzy, B.; de Labareyre, C.; El Hasnaoui,A.; Hercberg, S. (2002). Seroprevalence of HSV-1 and HSV-2 infection in the general French population. *Sexually Transmitted Infections,* Vol. 78, No. 3, 201-203

Malvy, D.; Ezzedine, K.; Lançon, F.; Halioua, B.; Rezvani, A.; Bertrais, S.; Chanzy, B.; Malkin, J. E.; Morand, P.; de Labareyre, C.; Hercberg, S.; El Hasnaoui, A. (2007). Epidemiology of orofacial herpes simplex virus infections in the general population in France: results of the HERPIMAX study. *Journal of the European Academy of Dermatology and Venereology,* Vol. 21, No. 10, pp. 1398-1403

Matsuo, T.; Matsuo, N. (1991). HLA-DR9 associated with the severity of acute retinal necrosis syndrome. *Ophthalmologica,* Vol. 203, No. 3, pp. 133-137

Miyashita, E. M.; Yang, B.; Lam, K. M.; Crawford, D. H.; Thorley-Lawson, D. A. (1995). A novel form of Epstein-Barr virus latency in normal B cells in vivo. *Cell,* Vol. 80, No. 4, pp. 593-601

Morse, L. S.; Mizoguchi, M. (1995). Diagnosis and management of viral retinitis in the acute retinal necrosis syndrome. *Seminars in Ophthalmology,* Vol. 10, No. 1, pp. 28-41

Moshfeghi, D. M.; Dodds, E. M.; Couto, C. A.; Santos, C. I.; Nicholson, D. H.; Lowder, C. Y.; Davis, J. L. (2004). Diagnostic approaches to severe, atypical toxoplasmosis mimicking acute retinal necrosis. *Ophthalmology,* Vol. 111, No. 4, pp. 716-725

Mott, K. R.; Bresee, C. J.; Allen, S, J; Ben Mohamed, L.; Wechsler, S. L.; Ghiasi, H. (2009). Level of herpes simplex virus type 1 latency correlates with severity of corneal scarring and exhaustion of CD8+ T cells in trigeminal ganglia of latently infected mice. *Journal of Virology,* Vol. 83, No. 5, pp. 2246-2254

Muthiah, M. N.; Michaelides, M.; Child, C. S.; Mitchell, S. M. (2007). Acute retinal necrosis: a national population-based study to assess the incidence, methods of diagnosis, treatment strategies and outcomes in the UK. *British Journal of Ophthalmology,* Vol. 91, No. 11, pp. 1452-1455

O'Brien, J. J. ; Campoli-Richards, D. M. (1989). Acyclovir. An updated review of its antiviral activity, pharmacokinetic properties and therapeutic efficacy. *Drugs,* Vol. 37, No. 3, pp. 233-309

Ongkosuwito, J. V.; van der Lelij, A.; Bruinenberg, M.; Wienesen-van Doorn, M.; Feron, E. J.; Hoyng, C. B.; de Keizer, R. J.; Klok, A. M.; Kijlstra, A. (1998). Increased presence of Epstein-Barr virus DNA in ocular fluid samples from HIV negative immunocompromised patients with uveitis. British Journal of Ophthalmology, Vol. 82, No. 3, pp. 245-251

Palay, D. A.; Sternberg, P. Jr.; Davis, J.; Lewis, H.; Holland, G. N.; Mieler, W. F.; Jabs, D. A.; Drews, C. (1991). Decrease in the risk of bilateral acute retinal necrosis by acyclovir therapy. *American Journal of Ophthalmology,* Vol. 112, No. 3, pp. 250-255

Pavésio, C. E.; Conrad, D. K.; McCluskey, P. J.; Mitchell, S. M.; Towler, H. M.; Lightman, S. (1997). Delayed acute retinal necrosis after herpetic encephalitis. *British Journal of Ophthalmology,* Vol. 81, No. 5, pp. 415-416

Paya, C.; Humar, A.; Dominguez, E.; Washburn, K.; Blumberg, E.; Alexander, B.; Freeman, R.; Heaton, N.; Pescovitz, M. D.; valganciclovir solid organ transplant study group (2004). Efficacy and safety of valganciclovir vs. oral ganciclovir for prevention of cytomegalovirus disease in solid organ transplant recipients. *American Journal of Transplantation,* Vol. 4, No. 4, pp. 611-620

Pepose, J. S.; Flowers, B.; Stewart, J. A.; Grose, C.; Levy, D. S.; Culbertson, W. W.; Kreiger, A. E. (1992). Herpesvirus antibody levels in the etiologic diagnosis of the acute retinal necrosis syndrome. *American Journal of Ophthalmology,* Vol. 113, No. 3, pp. 248-256

Pevenstein, S. R.; Williams, R. K.; McChesney, D.; Mont, E. K.; Smialek, J. E.; Straus, S. E. (1999). Quantitation of latent varicella-zoster virus and herpes simplex virus genomes in human trigeminal ganglia. *Journal of Virology,* Vol. 73, No. 12, pp. 10514-10518

Phan, D. D.; Chin-Hong, P.; Lin, E. T.; Anderle, P.; Sadee, W.; Guglielmo, B. J. (2003). Intra- and interindividual variabilities of valacyclovir oral bioavailability and effect of co-administration of an hPEPT1 inhibitor. *Antimicrobial Agents and Chemotherapy,* Vol. 47, No. 7, pp. 2351-2353

Pleyer, U.; Metzner, S.; Hofmann, J. (2009). Diagnostics and differential diagnosis of acute retinal necrosis. *Ophthalmologe,* Vol. 106, No. 12, pp. 1074-1082

Rahhal, F. M.; Siegel, L. M.; Russak, V.; Wiley, C. A.; Tedder, D. G.; Weinberg, A.; Rickman, L.; Freeman, W. R. (1996). Clinicopathologic correlations in acute retinal necrosis caused by herpes simplex virus type 2. *Archives of Ophthalmology,* Vol. 114, No. 11, pp. 1416-1419

Rautenberg, P.; Grančičova, L.; Hillenkamp, J.; Nölle, B.; Roider, J.; Fickenscher, H. (2009). Acute retinal necrosis from the virologist's perspective. *Ophthalmologe,* Vol. 106, No. 12, pp. 1065-1073

Reid, R.; Mar, E.C.; Huang, E. S.; Topal, M. D. (1988). Insertion and extension of acyclic, dideoxy, and ara nucleotides by herpesviridae, human alpha and human beta polymerases. A unique inhibition mechanism for 9-(1,3-dihydroxy-2-propoxymethyl)-guanine triphosphate. *Journal of Biological Chemistry,* No. 263, No. 8, pp. 3898-3904

Rummelt, V.; Wenkel, H.; Rummelt, C.; Jahn, G.; Meyer, H. J.; Naumann, G. O. (1992). Detection of varicella zoster virus DNA and viral antigen in the late stage of bilateral acute retinal necrosis syndrome. *Archives of Ophthalmology,* Vol. 110, No. 8, 1132-1136

Saari, K. M.; Böke, W.; Manthey, K. F.; Algvere, P.; Hellquist, H.; Kättström, O.; Räsänen, O.; Paavola, M. (1982). Bilateral acute retinal necrosis. *American Journal of Ophthalmology,* Vol. 93, No. 4, pp. 403-411

Savant, V.; Saeed, T.; Denniston, A.; Murray, P. I. (2004). Oral valganciclovir treatment of varicella zoster virus acute retinal necrosis. *Eye (London),* Vol. 18, No. 5, pp. 544-545

Schlingemann, R. O.; Bruinenberg, M.; Wertheim-van Dillen, P.; Feron, E. (1996). Twenty years' delay of fellow eye involvement in herpes simplex virus type 2-associated bilateral acute retinal necrosis syndrome. *American Journal of Ophthalmology,* Vol. 122, No. 6, pp. 891-892

Scott, I. U.; Luu, K. M.; Davis, J. L. (2002). Intravitreal antivirals in the management of patients with aquired immunodeficiency syndrome with progressive outer retinal necrosis. *Archives of Ophthalmology,* Vol. 120, No. 9, pp. 1219-1222

Silverstein, B. E.; Conrad, D.; Margolis, T. P.; Wong, I. G. (1997). Cytomegalovirus-associated acute retinal necrosis syndrome. *American Journal of Ophthalmology,* Vol. 123, No. 2, pp. 257-258

Sinclair, J. (2008). Human cytomegalovirus: Latency and reactivation in the myeloid lineage. *Journal of Clinical Virology,* Vol. 41, No. 3, pp. 180-185

Sinclair, J.; Sissons, P. (2006). Latency and reactivation of human cytomegalovirus. *Journal of General Virology,* Vol. 87, No. 7, pp. 1763-1779

Soul-Lawton, J.; Seaber, E.; On, N.; Wootton, R.; Rolan, P.; Posner, J. (1995). Absolute bioavailability and metabolic disposition of valaciclovir, the L-valyl ester of acyclovir, following oral administration to humans. *Antimicrobial Agents and Chemotherapy,* Vol. 39, No. 12, pp. 2759-2764

Steiner, I.; Kennedy, P. G.; Pachner, A. R. (2007). The neurotropic herpes viruses: herpes simplex and varicella-zoster. *Lancet Neurology,* Vol. 6, No. 11, pp. 1015-1028

Sugita, S.; Shimizu, N.; Watanabe, K.; Mizukami, M.; Morio,T.; Sugamoto, Y.; Mochizuki, M. (2008). Use of multiplex PCR and real-time PCR to detect human herpesvirus genome in ocular fluids of patients with uveitis. *British Journal of Ophthalmology,* Vol. 92, No. 7, pp. 928-932

Tajunisah, I.; Reddy, S. C.; Tan, L. H. (2009). Acute retinal necrosis by cytomegalovirus in an immunocompetent adult: case report and review of the literature. *International Ophthalmology,* Vol. 29, No. 2, pp. 85-90

Tam, P. M.; Hooper, C. Y.; Lightman, S. (2010). Antiviral selection in the management of acute retinal necrosis. Clinical Ophthalmology, Vol.4, pp. 11-20

Theil, D.; Derfuss, T.; Paripovic, I.; Herberger, S.; Meinl, E.; Schueler, O.; Strupp, M.; Arbusow, V.; Brandt, T. (2003). Latent herpesvirus infection in human trigeminal ganglia causes chronic immune response. *American Journal of Pathology,* Vol. 163, No. 6, pp. 2179-2184

Tibbetts, M. D.; Shah, C. P.; Young, L. H.; Duker, J. S.; Maguire, J. I.; Morley, M. G. (2010). Treatment of acute retinal necrosis. *Ophthalmology,* Vol. 117, No. 4, pp. 818-824

Tran, T. H.; Rozenberg, F.; Cassoux, N.; Rao, N. A.; LeHoang, P.; Bodaghi, B. (2003a). Polymerase chain reaction analysis of aqueous humour samples in necrotising retinitis. *British Journal of Ophthalmology,* Vol. 87, No. 1, pp. 79-83.

Tran, T. H.; Stanescu, D.; Caspers-Velu, L.; Rozenberg, F.; Liesnard, C.; Gaudric, A.; Lehoang, P.; Bodaghi, B. (2003b). Clinical characteristics of acute HSV-2 retinal necrosis. *American Journal of Ophthalmology,* Vol. 137, No. 5, pp. 872-879

Urayama, A.; Yamada, N.; Sasaki, T. (1971). Unilateral acute uveitis with periarteritis and detachment. *Japanese Journal of Clinical Ophthalmology,* Vol. 25, pp. 607-619

Usui, Y.; Takeuchi, M.; Goto, H.; Mori, H.; Kezuka, T.; Sakai, J.; Usui, M. (2008). Acute retinal necrosis in Japan. *Ophthalmology,* Vol. 115, No. 9, pp. 1632-1633

Vandercam, T.; Hintzen, R. Q.; de Boer, J. H.; van der Lelij, A. (2008). Herpetic encephalitis is a risk factor for acute retinal necrosis. *Neurology,* Vol. 71, No. 16, pp. 1268-1274

van Gelder, R. N.; Willig, J. L.; Holland, G. N.; Kaplan, H. J. (2001). Herpes simplex virus type 2 as a cause of acute retinal necrosis syndrome in young patients. *Ophthalmology,* Vol. 108, No. 5, pp. 869-876

Velez, G.; Roy, C. E.; Whitcup, S. M.; Chan, C. C.; Robinson, M. R. (2001). High-dose intravitreal ganciclovir and foscarnet for cytomegalovirus retinitis. *American Journal of Ophthalmology,* Vol. 131, No. 3, pp. 396-397

Voros, G. M.; Pandit, R.; Snow, M.; Griffiths, P. G. (2006). Unilateral recurrent acute retinal necrosis syndrome caused by cytomegalovirus in an immune-competent adult. *European Journal of Ophthalmology,* Vol. 16, No. 3, pp. 484-486

Winterhalter, S.; Adams, O.; Althaus, Ch.; Stammen, J.; Schöler, E. M.; Joussen, A. M. (2007). Acute retinal necrosis. *Klinische Monatsblätter für Augenheilkunde,* Vol. 224, No. 7, pp. 567-574

Yamamoto, S.; Nakao, T.; Kajiyama, K. (2007). Acute retinal necrosis following herpes simplex encephalitis. *Archives of Neurology,* Vol. 64, No. 2, pp. 283

Yamamoto, S.; Sugita, S.; Sugamoto, Y.; Shimizu, N.; Morio, T.; Mochizuki, M. (2008). Quantitative PCR for the detection of genomic DNA of Epstein-Barr virus in ocular fluids of patients with uveitis. *Japanese Journal of Ophthalmology,* Vol. 52, No. 6, pp. 463-467

Young, N. J.; Bird, A. C. (1978). Bilateral acute retinal necrosis. *British Journal of Ophthalmology,* Vol. 62, No. 9, pp. 581-590

Zambarakji, H. J.; Obi, A. A.; Mitchell, S. M. (2002). Successful treatment of varicella-zoster virus retinitis with aggressive intravitreal and systemic antiviral therapy. *Ocular Immunology and Inflammation,* Vol. 10, No. 1, pp. 41-46

3

Leflunomide an Immunosuppressive Drug for Antiviral Purpose in Treatment for BK Virus-Associated Nephropathy After Kidney Transplantation

Christophe Bazin
Hôpital Européen Georges-Pompidou, Assistance Publique – Hôpitaux de Paris
France

1. Introduction

1.1 BK Virus

BK virus is a polyomavirus belonging to the *papovaviridae* branch. In addition to BK, the human polyomavirus family includes John Cunningham virus (JCV), Washington University virus (WUV), Karolinska Institute virus (KIV) and Merkel cell viruses (Boothpur et al. 2010). BK virus is a virus without a shell and it has a double-stranded circular non-enveloped DNA. It was first discovered and isolated in 1971 just like JC virus, responsible for Progressive Multifocal Leukoencephalopathy (PML). Contamination usually occurs during early childhood through the airway without clinical symptoms. BK virus seroprevalence in general population is around 60%. The main latency areas are the kidney and the urothelium. Asymptomatic BK virus infection is often acquired in childhood and the virus persists in a dormant state in urothelium and kidneys of healthy and immunocompetent individuals, where it can be reactivated under immunosuppression (Nickeleit et al. 2000a; Brocker et al. 2011).

1.2 Prevalence and incidence

Urinary viral prevalence for BK virus is between 0.3% and 6% in general population, and increases in functions of immunosuppression degree; between 10% and 45% in patients after renal transplant, 30% in patients after bone marrow graft and 25% in patients with Human immunodeficiency virus. In patients with renal graft, the annual incidence of the nephropathy is between 3% and 5% (Randhawa et al. 2000; Pavlakis et al. 2006).

1.3 Risk factors

BK virus-associated nephropathy seems to be promoted by the concurrent presence of several risk factors. The immunosuppressive regimen strength, with high level blood concentrations, is the first factor involved. Most patients affected by BK virus-associated nephropathy previously had an intensification of immunosuppressive regimen due to a rejection event or a treatment including tacrolimus and/or mycophenolate mofetil combined with monoclonal or polyclonal antibodies (De Luca et al. 2000; Nickeleit et al. 2000b; Randhawa et al. 2000; Hirsch et al. 2001). Conversely, no cases have been reported in patients treated with cyclosporine and corticosteroids (Binet et al. 1999; Mengel et al. 2003).

The other risk factors identified comprise donor characteristics, such as female gender, deceased donation, ischemia-reperfusion injury, high BK virus specific antibody titres, HLA mismatch and African-American ethnicity. The recipient characteristics in cause are older age, male gender, white race, diabetes, obesity, retransplantation, lack of HLA C-7, low or absent BK virus specific T-cell activity. Lastly, in addition to high immunosuppressive drug levels and tacrolimus based combinations, other post-transplant factors can be mentioned as acute rejection and antirejection treatment, cumulative steroid exposure and lymphocyte depleting antibodies (Gupta & Gupta, 2011).

Although immunosuppression increases the probability of latent BK virus reactivation, clinical manifestation of disease is rare. When symptoms occur, on the clinical point of view, a progressive decline of the renal functions can be observed up to 45 % of patients, usually 9 to 12 months after the renal transplant (Nickeleit et al. 2000a; Randhawa et al. 2000). The most serious form of the infection turns out to be the interstitial nephritis; although the BK virus was discovered in the 70's, this serious complication has first been seen in 1995. This fact can probably be explained by the commercialization of two drugs in 1995 and 1996, tacrolimus and mycophenolate mofetil.

Interestingly, BK virus-associated nephropathy happens hardly only in patients with renal graft. Some explanations could be found, such as the role of vesico-urethral reflux, quite usual in renal transplantation, with the systemic pathway of collecting tubes in peritubular capillary and the tubular localization of the infection. Some authors evoked easiness in the viral antigens presentation in a context of allograft, cold ischemia, tubular necrosis and graft rejection. For that matter BK virus-associated nephropathy is generally related to rejection, both events being linked in time; most cases of nephropathy are falsely tagged and treated just like a rejection. This confusion suggests that rejection is a risk factor on its own. Viral antigens could probably lead to rejection and conversely a rejection event could reactivate viral replication. In mice, Atencio et al proved an inductive effect of tubular damage upon BK virus linked interstitial nephritis (Atencio et al. 1993).

1.4 Clinical aspects

BK virus infection may lead to encephalitis, retinitis, pneumonitis, damage of the kidneys, bleeding of the bladder, and blockage of urine passageways. Minor infections are most of the time asymptomatic and can lead to urethral stenosis. This infection occurs 1 to 45 months (average 12.5 months) after the graft. It is linked to the conjunction of multiple factors, including an intense immunosuppressive regimen, viral reactivation, existence of an immune-allogenic conditions, and a suffering tubular due to ischemia or rejection (Nickeleit et al. 2003).

1.5 Genotypes

BK virus comes in the form of 4 different genotypes, type I being the most common seen. The coding regions for non structural proteins T and t antigens (pathogenic viral power), viral capsid proteins (cellular tropism) and a regulatory non coding zone have a vital importance. Some authors have brought to light emerging mutations which could explain the renal physiopathologic effects of these viruses (Chen et al. 2001). Virus selection in patients with renal graft results in rearrangements in the T antigen region, mutations in the non coding regulatory zone, and above all variations in VP1 protein (Smith et al. 1998; Baksh et al. 2001; Randhawa et al. 2002). Heterogeneity and genetic instability in a same patient seem to favor renal damage and the risk of escaping immunologic surveillance (Chen et al. 2001; Randhawa et al. 2002).

1.6 Histology

BK virus is usually associated with changes in the kidney and sometimes haemorrhagic cystitis and urethral stenosis. The virus affects tubular epithelial cells that show characteristic intranuclear inclusion bodies. Diagnosis relies upon urinary cytology, detection of viral DNA in fluids and renal biopsy. The nephropathy diagnosis can only be made histologically in a graft biopsy. Intranuclear viral inclusions are exclusively seen in epithelial cells and tubular cells reveal focal necrosis. Four different variants of intranuclear inclusion bodies can be seen throughout the entire nephron. Type 1 is the most frequently observed; it is an amorphous basophilic ground-glass variant. Type 2 is an eosinophilic granular type, halo surrounded. Type 3 is a finely granular form lacking a halo. And finally type 4 is a vesicular variant presenting markedly enlarged nuclei and irregular chromatin. Infected cells which are rounded-up and extruded from the epithelial cell layer into tubular lumens are frequently observed. Viral replication often causes tubular epithelial cell necrosis with denudation of basement membranes. Although cytopathic signs can be seen along the entire nephron, they are mostly abundant in distal tubular parts and collecting ducts (Nickeleit et al. 2000a).

1.7 Interstitial inflammation

Interstitial inflammation in BK virus-associated nephropathy still remains controversial and needs to be fully explained. The major outcome is to distinguish between virally induced interstitial nephritis and cellular rejection. As lowering immunosuppression is the first option which can be chosen in the treatment, this choice requires two conditions, first the absence of rejection and second the BK virus should not trigger rejection. BK virus is frequently accompanied by an heterogeneous inflammatory reaction (Drachenberg et al. 1999). This inflammation can be minimal or absent in up to 17% of biopsies (Nickeleit et al. 2000a). When inflammation is encountered, the inflammatory cell infiltrate is composed of lymphocytes, macrophages and occasional plasma cells. Polymorphonuclear leukocytes can be seen in response to markedly damaged tubules with urinary leakage (Drachenberg et al. 1999). About 50% of biopsies performed during persistent BK virus-associated nephropathy show evidence of cellular rejection as conventionally defined with abundant tubulitis and transplant endarteritis in about 25%. Typically, mononuclear cell infiltrates and tubulitis are pronounced in areas without viral inclusions making virally induced interstitial nephritis highly unlikely (Nickeleit et al. 2000a).

The upregulation of MCH-class II (HLA-DR) and ICAM-1 on tubular epithelial cells is a typical finding in graft biopsies with cellular rejection and can serve as an adjunct diagnostic tool (Seron et al. 1989; Nickeleit et al. 1998). HLA-DR expression can stimulate an allogenic lymphocytic reaction and also enhance T cell mediated lysis (Rosenberg et al. 1992). Consequently, BK virus could probably trigger rejection episodes by inducing HLA-DR upregulation as previously proposed for CMV (von Willebrand et al. 1986). However, no association could be found between BK virus infection and tubular HLA-DR expression based on immunofluorescence double labeling staining techniques. It is only in biopsies showing characteristic morphological evidence of rejection with marked tubulitis that typical upregulation of HLA-DR and ICAM-1 could be observed (Nickeleit et al. 2000a). Therefore, BK virus does not stimulate HLA-DR expression. Consequently no significant difference can be found between the prevalence of rejection in tissue samples taken during persistent BK virus-associated nephropathy and time matched controls without BK virus nephropathy. Thus, BK virus does not seem to provoke a constant and pronounced interstitial inflammatory reaction and should probably not be considered as associated with an increased prevalence of rejection episodes (Nickeleit et al. 2000a).

1.8 PCR

BK-virus DNA in the plasma and the urine, which can be detected by PCR (Polymerase Chain Reaction), is closely associated with nephropathy. Quantitative PCR can be used to follow the disease evolution and the treatment efficiency (Randhawa et al. 2004).

As for BK virus infection, this technique has proven a 100% sensivity, a 88% specificity and above all a negative predictive test of 100%. Hirsch et al. have even shown a correlation between viral load and nephropathy and proposed a cut-off above which the risk of nephropathy is significant: all patients with more than 7700 copies/mL in plasma had typical BK virus-associated nephropathy lesions on the biopsy (Hirsch et al. 2002).

The nephropathy evolution is very poor with a cytopathogenic effect persistent in up to 70% of patients, a graft loss in 45% of cases; and major sequel fibrosis in 75% of cases, even if viremia can be controlled (Nickeleit et al. 2000a; Randhawa et al. 2000; Mylonakis et al. 2001; Mengel et al. 2003).

2. Classical treatments for BKV nephropathy

Therapeutic alternatives are quite few in number. Despite the absence of randomized clinical trials, the current approach generally includes reduction of immunosuppression (Brennan et al. 2005; Hardinger et al. 2010). The rational is to allow host immune function to combat the virus, with the risk to increase acute and subclinical rejection. Lowering immunosuppression with smaller dosage and/or less drugs is partially efficient and seems to be the first thing to do. Except from lowering immunosuppression, to date no treatment seem to be efficient enough to be recommended to all patients, and new research have to be performed because of the poor evidence in small series of patients (Johnston et al. 2010).

2.1 Lowering immunosuppression

Reduction of immunosuppression is to date the only consensus regarding the treatment of BK virus-associated nephropathy. Lowering tacrolimus dosage of 41% and mycophenolate mofetil dosage of 44% allowed to eradicate 24 patients' viremia in 6 months (Saad et al. 2008).

In a previous study, mycophenolate mofetil was stopped the day leflunomide treatment was initiated; tacrolimus and everolimus were respectively reduced of 50% and 12.5%. Therapeutic drug monitoring target for tacrolimus was lowered to 4 - 6 ng/mL on immunoenzymatic techniques on whole blood. Corticosteroids were kept with average dosage of 5 to 10 mg per day (Bazin et al. 2009). Other authors recommend even lower targets with 3 ng/mL for tacrolimus and 100 ng/mL for cyclosporine (Gupta & Gupta, 2011).

Besides, lowering immunosuppressive regimens together with a specific treatment for BK virus-associated nephropathy recently turns out to be effective to prolong graft survival, and moreover a safe treatment with acute rejection rates not increased significantly after lowering immunosuppression (Dheir et al. 2011).

Two different therapeutic strategies have been evaluated: the immunosuppression withdrawal (3-drug to 2-drug immunosuppression) within the first month versus reduction of immunosuppression. The regimen modifications and results are presented in table 1 and figure 1. The Withdrawal cohort had significantly better graft survival at 1 year compared with the Reduction cohort (1-year graft survival 87.8% versus 56.2%, P = 0.03) (Weiss et al. 2008).

	Withdrawal cohort (n = 17)	Reduction cohort (n = 18)	p
CNI, sirolimus, prednisone at diagnosis	12	11	0.56
CNI, MMF, prednisone at diagnosis	5	7	0.56
Median serum creatinine at diagnosis (mg/dl)	2.5	2.2	0.30
Agent withdrawal within 1 mo of diagnosis			
CNI withdrawal	14	-	-
AP withdrawal	3	-	-
Dose reduction within 1 mo of diagnosis			
CNI reduction, AP reduction < 50%	-	8	-
CNI reduction, AP reduction ≥ 50%	-	7	-
Tac to CsA switch, AP reduction < 50%	-	3	-
Ancillary therapy			
Cidofovir	2	5	0.40
Intravenous Ig	8	8	0.88
Leflunomide	4	5	1.0
Acute rejection after diagnosis	1	1	1.0

Table 1. Immunosuppression modifications comparing immunosuppression withdrawal *versus* immunosuppression reduction after diagnosis of BK virus-associated nephropathy. CNI, calcineurin inhibitor; MMF, mycophenolate; AP, antiproliferative; Tac, tacrolimus; CsA, cyclosporine A (Weiss et al. 2008).

2.2 Cidofovir

Cidofovir (Vistide®) is an injectable antiviral drug. It belongs to nucleoside analogues. It is used in infections due to human Cytomegalovirus (CMV) in adults suffering of AIDS (Acquired immune deficiency syndrome) without renal insufficiency, and it should only be used when other treatments are considered as inappropriate. Cidofovir counters CMV replication thanks to a selective inhibition of viral DNA polymerase in *herpesviridae* viruses

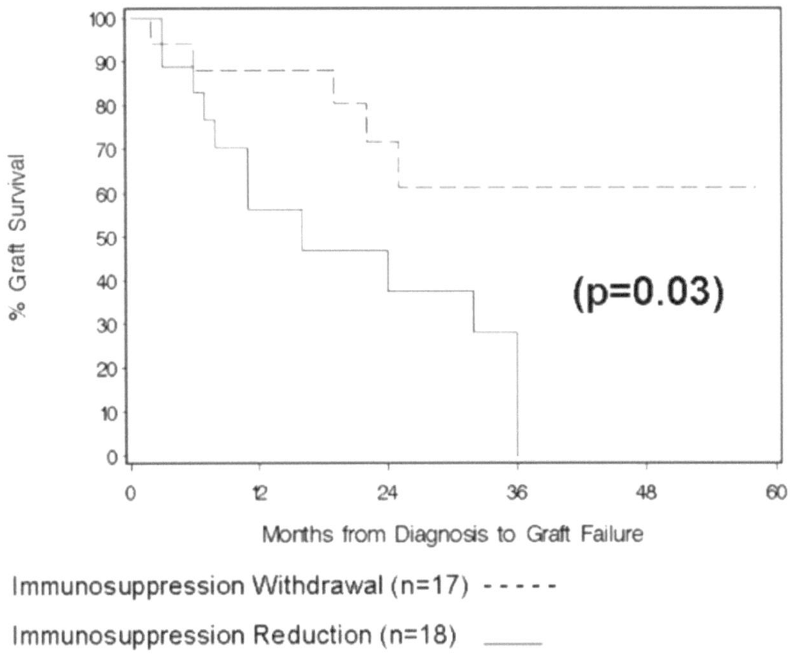

Fig. 1. Immunosuppression withdrawal preserves graft function compared with reduction (Weiss et al. 2008).

(Gilead 2010). Cidofovir has also demonstrated *in vitro* activity against murine and simian polyomavirus strains and appears to have activity against JC virus *in vivo* (De Luca et al. 2000). Pharmacokinetic studies have demonstrated that cidofovir is highly concentrated in urine and renal tissue which are the primary sites of BK virus infection (Kadambi et al. 2003). This fact highlights the possibility that low doses might be sufficient for treating an infectious process, such as BK virus-associated nephropathy, that appears to be largely localized to the kidney and genitourinary tract.

The treatment consists in a low-dose treatment, 0.25 mg/kg/day intravenous during 2 weeks, associated to a prior hydration of 1 litre of saline solution. Cidofovir seems to be efficient in BK virus as well, but it tends to concentrate itself inside the kidney and can be responsible of a nephrotoxicity mostly for tubular cells leading to renal insufficiency.

Few cases have been described in literature and no conclusion can be given on the real efficacy of cidofovir. Indeed, despite viremia control, viruria remains detectable and the treatment is not able to avoid the evolution towards fibrosis and renal insufficiency (Kadambi et al. 2003; Kuypers et al. 2005).

In some cases, cidofovir may also become deleterious (Pallet et al. 2010; Talmon et al. 2010).

3. Leflunomide

3.1 Drug generalities

Leflunomide (Arava®) is a disease-modifying antirheumatic drug (DMARD) used in adult patients with methotrexate intolerance, failure or loss of efficiency; it is also used in a second line to treat severe and active forms of psoriatic arthritis (Maddison et al. 2005; Sanofi-Aventis 2009).

3.2 Pharmacodynamy

Its immunosuppressive action lies in the dihydroorotate dehydrogenase (DHOH) inhibition, an enzyme necessary for de novo synthesis of pyrimidic bases in lymphocytes. It also has an anti-proliferative action (Williamson et al. 1995; Fox et al. 1999).

Besides, leflunomide has proven abilities to reduce the viral proliferation for Human Cytomegalovirus (CMV), Herpes Simplex Viruses (HSV) *in vitro* (Knight et al. 2001) and respiratory syncytial virus (RSV) *in vitro* and *in vivo* (Dunn et al. 2011).

3.3 Pharmacokinetics

After per os administration, leflunomide is promptly and almost fully metabolized into its active form, terflunomide or A77 1726. This metabolism happens during first pass and consists in a carbon cycle opening in the intestinal wall and the liver. 95% of leflunomide is turned into A77 1726 this way, the remains into minor metabolites. Terflunomide is the drug responsible for the activity and side effects of leflunomide.

Leflunomide bioavailability is about 82% in healthy volunteers (Sanofi-Aventis 2009). Elimination plasma half-life of A77 1726 is quite considerable, with some 15 days in average. Patients are so compelled to take a 100 mg charging dose for 3 days before a 10 to 20 mg maintenance dose per day.

After a unique charging dose, A77 1726 Tmax is comprised between 6 and 12 hours, with a high inter-individual variability in patients with rheumatoid arthritis (Rozman 2002).

The volume of distribution (Vd) is quite low, with about 12.7 L (6 to 30.8 L), which is logical with its high affinity and linkage to albumin (99.4% in healthy volunteers) (Rozman 2002). Elimination of A77 1726 is slow, it is characterized by an apparent clearance of 0.051 L/h (Rozman 2002). This elimination is mostly renal (43%) and biliary (48%), as a consequence renal insufficiency alone does not significantly impair A77 1726 plasma concentrations (Beaman et al. 2002). Furthermore haemodialysis does not modify concentrations or clearance of A77 1726, which allows the patients to be on a dialysis without any dose adjustment. In vitro studies showed that cytochroms P450, in particular cytochroms 1A2, 2C19, 3A4 and 3A5 were involved in leflunomide metabolism (Kalgutkar et al. 2003). A pharmacogenetic study also showed the link between a polymorphism of cytochrom 1A2 and a risk of toxicity for patients with rheumatoid arthritis (Bohanec Grabar et al. 2008).

3.4 Predictive efficiency

In rheumatoid arthritis, plasma concentrations above 13 μg/mL seem to be efficient. These concentrations are usually reached with 20 mg per day dosage (van Roon et al. 2005). Some authors tried to establish a relation between plasma concentrations and efficiency in patients with BK virus nephropathy, showing a tendency but with no absolute proof. Finally to date, no link between plasma concentrations and side effects has been shown (Bazin et al. 2009). Yet *in vitro* studies seem to show a predictive correlation between concentrations and the viral inhibitory effect: 10 µg/mL reduced the extracellular BKV load by 90% (IC_{90}) but with significant host cytostatic effects (see figure 2) (Bernhoff et al. 2010).

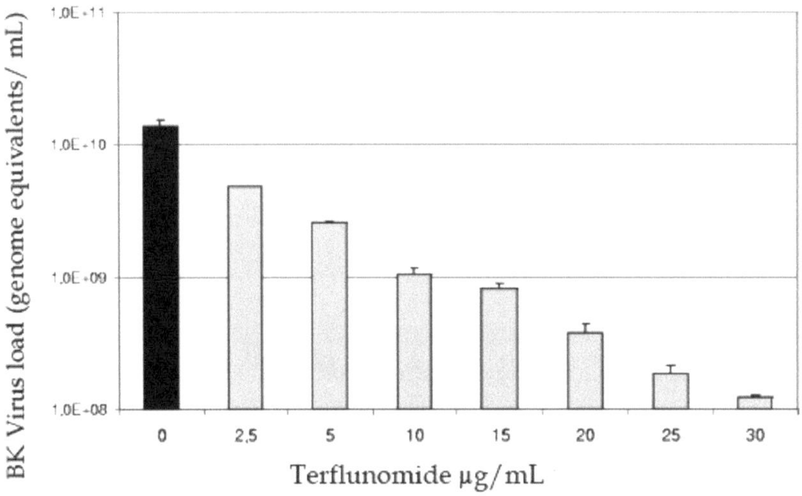

Fig. 2. Effect of Terflunomide on BK Virus load *in vitro* (Bernhoff et al. 2010)

3.5 Mechanism of action

Researches about the mechanism of leflunomide have recently been brightened. Leflunomide has two mechanisms of action: inhibition of dihydroorotate dehydrogenase, a key enzyme in the pyrimidine synthesis pathway, and tyrosine kinase inhibition. Dihydroorotate dehydrogenase inhibition is the primary mechanism involved in rheumatoid arthritis treatment. Interactions between the BK virus and the cellular protein kinase AKt / mammalian target of rapamycin (mTOR) pathway have been discovered (Liacini et al. 2010). These interactions are described in figure 3.

Akt (protein kinase B) is a serine/threonine kinase activated by growth factors, cytokines and mitogens (Fayard et al. 2010). The mTOR pathway which controls protein synthesis is located downstream of Akt. Akt indirectly activates mTOR. Two mTOR complexes have yet been described, mTOR complex 1 (mTORC1) which controls translation initiation, and mTOR complex 2 (mTORC2) which controls cytoskeletal changes and is also a 3'-phosphoinositide-dependent kinase-2 (PDK2), phosphorylating Akt, which may alter its substrate specificity (Bhaskar et al. 2007). Liacini et al showed that BK virus infecting renal tubular epithelial cells was able to activate the Akt/mTOR pathway; that leflunomide active metabolite, A77 1726 could inhibit PDK1 and Akt phosphorylation in a dose-dependent manner and in this way to reduce BK large T antigen expression and DNA replication. The combination of serine/threonine kinase inhibition of mTOR and tyrosine kinase inhibition significantly reduce the ability of the virus to survive and to produce new virions. More interesting though seems to be the combination of leflunomide and sirolimus targeting the Akt/mTOR pathway on different sites. Because both leflunomide and sirolimus possess immunosuppressive activity, this combination may allow treatment of BK virus-associated nephropathy without reduction of immunosuppression (Liacini et al. 2010).

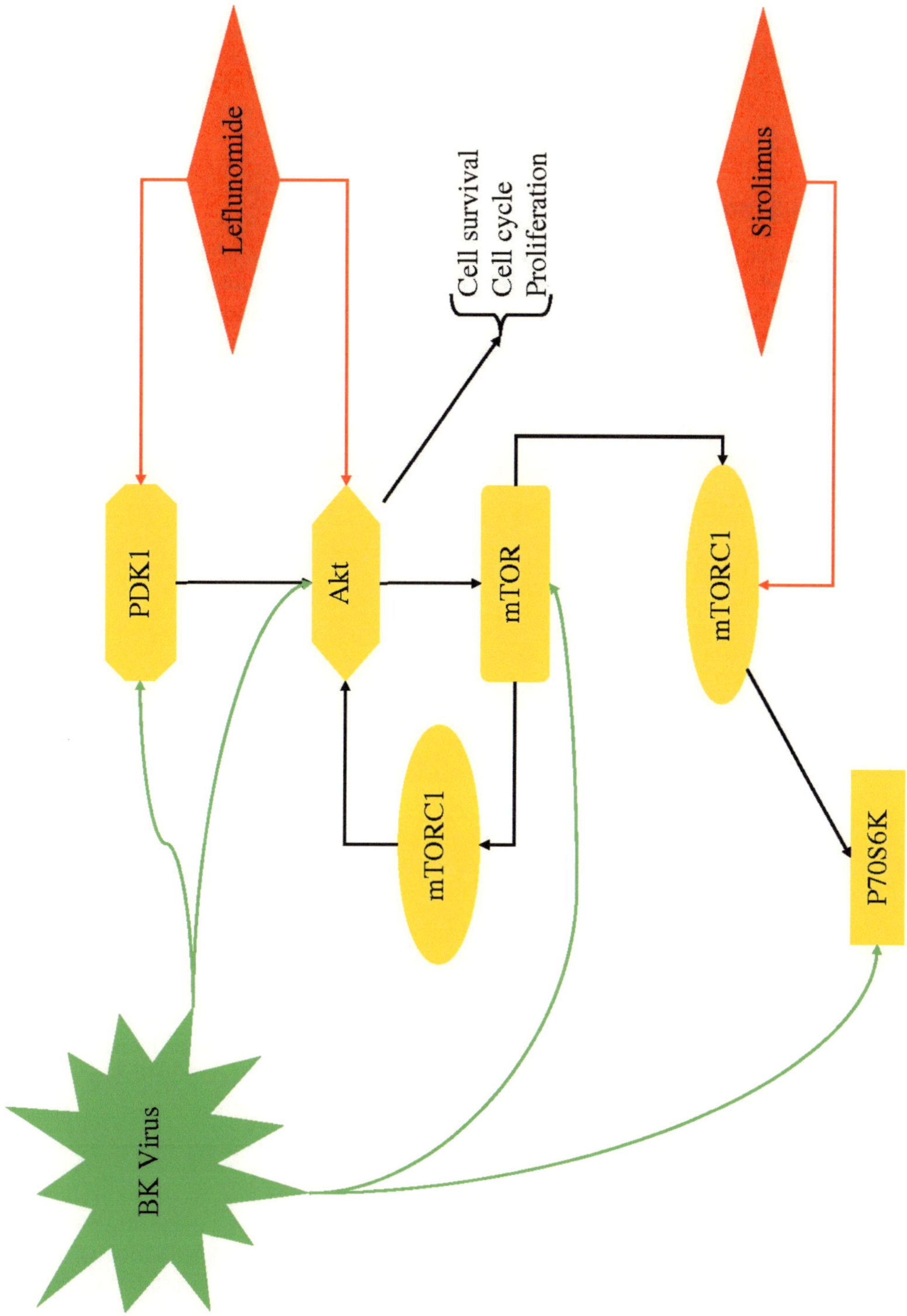

Fig. 3. Interactions between BK virus and inhibitors, sirolimus and leflunomide (Liacini et al. 2010)

Results in terms of biological evolution in patients speak for itself. In a mean monitoring time of 16 months (12-24 months), viral load with leflunomide can be reduced about up to 50%, and even be brought to undetectable, in blood like in urine. But more important is the lowering of renal failure and graft rejection thanks to this treatment. Creatinine clearance (Cockroft-Gault) can be stabilized and even improved (Bazin et al. 2009).

3.6 Therapeutic drug monitoring

Initial dosage for leflunomide is 20 mg once a day, and can be raised to 30 or 40 mg for patients with viral loads remaining important. Plasma concentrations in therapeutic drug monitoring fluctuate between 15 and 135 µg/mL. These concentrations set out low intra-individual but high inter-individual variability, and moreover without apparent correlation with prescribed dosage. It is interesting to notice that these concentrations were outside usual targets used in most studies - 50 to 100 µg/mL - which are supposed to offer the best efficiency and to limit the hepatotoxicity risk which can be lethal. Besides, the patient with the highest concentration - 135 µg/mL - had its viremia turned undetectable after only a two months treatment and showed no side effect of any kind. This result suggests that higher concentrations lead to higher efficacy and vice versa (Bazin et al. 2009).

3.7 Tolerance

Concerning tolerance, very few patients suffer from serious side effects. Loss of taste or lethargy can be observed but without any correlation with plasma concentrations. These side effects can prompt the treatment to be stopped, but in most cases viremia tends to increase strongly (Bazin et al. 2009).

4. Discussion

The main risk factor for BK virus-associated nephropathy is undeniably the immunosuppressive regimen intensity, in particular an intensification due to an acute rejection event (Binet et al. 1999; Nickeleit et al. 2000a; Barri et al. 2001; Nickeleit et al. 2003). Drugs in cause for these events seem to be the combination of tacrolimus, mycophenolate mofetil and monoclonal or polyclonal antibodies (Binet et al. 1999; Nickeleit et al. 1999; Nickeleit et al. 2000a; Nickeleit et al. 2003; Benavides et al. 2007). The organ and the graft type also play a role. For instance, Benavides et al. showed that the incidence of BK virus-associated nephropathy is higher in patients with kidney and pancreas rather than kidney alone; and that an alive donor would had a protective effect, probably explained by a lighter immunosuppressive regimen (Benavides et al. 2007).

Other risk factors have been evoked, like age and sex: nephropathy incidence seem to be greater for aged men (Ramos et al. 2002).

Furthermore many patients improve their symptoms at a distance of the surgery with the lowering of immunosuppression. We already have at our disposal a few experimental studies testing leflunomide on chronic or acute graft rejection (Williams et al. 1994; Xiao et al. 1995; Shen et al. 1998). More recently the inhibitory effects of leflunomide upon HSV, CMV and BK virus have been proved *in vitro* like *in vivo* (Waldman et al. 1999; Waldman et al. 1999; Knight et al. 2001; Farasati et al. 2005). Indeed a study suggests leflunomide is at least as efficient as ganciclovir in CMV infections and does not seem to be affected by resistant viruses (John et al. 2004). Leflunomide has even be successfully used in a patient with bone marrow graft and infected by a resistant virus to ganciclovir, foscarnet and cidofovir (Avery et al. 2004).

The studies where leflunomide is used as an immunosuppressive drug in renal and hepatic graft are more and more, because leflunomide allows to reduce anti-calcineurin drugs which have the major inconvenient of nephrotoxicity, and potentially protects aside from CMV, HSV and BK virus infections (Hardinger et al. 2002; Williams et al. 2002). Moreover leflunomide seems to be an interesting alternative in BK virus-associated nephropathy in renal transplant by eradicating detectable viremia in some patients. Leflunomide also allows avoiding rejection in most cases in spite of classical immunosuppressive drugs dosage reduction. Besides one of leflunomide's main asset is its absence of renal toxicity, contrary to cidofovir (Williams et al. 2005; Josephson et al. 2006; Teschner et al. 2006; Faguer et al. 2007).

Thanks to the encountered success in renal transplant, leflunomide is now used to treat hemorrhagic cystitis linked to BK virus in bone marrow transplant (Dropulic et al. 2008). However, due to the absence of randomized clinical trials with a sufficient number of patients, some authors consider its use in a first-line drug not recommended (Chon et al. 2011).

Leflunomide pharmacokinetics is characterized by a great inter-individual variability with terflunomide concentrations from 15 to 130 µg/mL obtained with the same dosage (Bazin et al. 2009). In BK virus infection, terflunomide concentrations between 15-30 µg/mL and 35-100 µg/mL are sufficient to suppress respectively 50% and 90% of the replication for CMV and BK virus *in vitro*. That is why a therapeutic margin between 50 and 100 µg/mL has been proposed in this indication (Josephson et al. 2006). However, current strategic therapy so as to limit BK virus incidence tends to manage an early reduction of immunosuppressive regimen to avoid the apparition of a nephropathy. A prospective study with a significant number of patients would be probably necessary to definitely conclude about this relation between plasma concentrations and efficacy or in terms of rapidity of viral load eradication.

5. Conclusion

Leflunomide appears to be an alternative treatment in nephropathy due to BK virus in addition to lower immunosuppression regimen. In case of leflunomide use, a major standard seems to be high plasma terflunomide concentrations so as to obtain rapid virus eradication. Concentrations comprised between 15 and 60 µg/mL appear to be pertinent; these concentrations are usually reached with 20-40 mg per day. In patients with insufficient concentrations, further studies should be carried out to determine whether exists a benefit to use higher dosage up to 60 or 80 mg a day. Even if tolerance is quite satisfying, it will probably be the most important parameter in such high-dose treatments.

Despite the small number of studies and the weak number of patients in each of them, a correlation seems to exist between plasma terflunomide concentrations and the treatment efficacy. This relation has not yet been proved with tolerance.

Due to its great inter-individual variability and alongside classical virological and clinical follow-up therapeutic drug monitoring appears to be an important step to take into care patients with BK virus related nephropathy.

6. Acknowledgment

The author would like to acknowledge the staff of Henri-Mondor and Bicetre University Hospital Pharmacology laboratories and especially Anne Hulin, PharmD, PhD, Valerie Furlan, PharmD, PhD and Caroline Barau, PharmD.

7. References

Atencio, I. A., Shadan, F. F., Zhou, X. J., Vaziri, N. D. and Villarreal, L. P. (1993). "Adult mouse kidneys become permissive to acute polyomavirus infection and reactivate persistent infections in response to cellular damage and regeneration." *J Virol* 67(3): 1424-32.

Avery, R. K., Bolwell, B. J., Yen-Lieberman, B., Lurain, N., Waldman, W. J., Longworth, D. L., Taege, A. J., Mossad, S. B., Kohn, D., Long, J. R., Curtis, J., Kalaycio, M., Pohlman, B. and Williams, J. W. (2004). "Use of leflunomide in an allogeneic bone marrow transplant recipient with refractory cytomegalovirus infection." *Bone Marrow Transplant* 34(12): 1071-5.

Baksh, F. K., Finkelstein, S. D., Swalsky, P. A., Stoner, G. L., Ryschkewitsch, C. F. and Randhawa, P. (2001). "Molecular genotyping of BK and JC viruses in human polyomavirus-associated interstitial nephritis after renal transplantation." *Am J Kidney Dis* 38(2): 354-65.

Barri, Y. M., Ahmad, I., Ketel, B. L., Barone, G. W., Walker, P. D., Bonsib, S. M. and Abul-Ezz, S. R. (2001). "Polyoma viral infection in renal transplantation: the role of immunosuppressive therapy." *Clin Transplant* 15(4): 240-6.

Bazin, C., Barau, C., Grimbert, P., François, H., Blanchet, B., Astier, A., Furlan, V. and Hulin, A. (2009). "Etude pilote du suivi thérapeutique du Léflunomide en transplantation rénale." *J Pharm Clin* 28(1): 21-6.

Beaman, J. M., Hackett, L. P., Luxton, G. and Illett, K. F. (2002). "Effect of hemodialysis on leflunomide plasma concentrations." *Ann Pharmacother* 36(1): 75-7.

Benavides, C. A., Pollard, V. B., Mauiyyedi, S., Podder, H., Knight, R. and Kahan, B. D. (2007). "BK virus-associated nephropathy in sirolimus-treated renal transplant patients: incidence, course, and clinical outcomes." *Transplantation* 84(1): 83-8.

Bernhoff, E., Tylden, G. D., Kjerpeseth, L. J., Gutteberg, T. J., Hirsch, H. H. and Rinaldo, C. H. (2010). "Leflunomide inhibition of BK virus replication in renal tubular epithelial cells." *J Virol* 84(4): 2150-6.

Bhaskar, P. T. and Hay, N. (2007). "The two TORCs and Akt." *Dev Cell* 12(4): 487-502.

Binet, I., Nickeleit, V., Hirsch, H. H., Prince, O., Dalquen, P., Gudat, F., Mihatsch, M. J. and Thiel, G. (1999). "Polyomavirus disease under new immunosuppressive drugs: a cause of renal graft dysfunction and graft loss." *Transplantation* 67(6): 918-22.

Bohanec Grabar, P., Rozman, B., Tomsic, M., Suput, D., Logar, D. and Dolzan, V. (2008). "Genetic polymorphism of CYP1A2 and the toxicity of leflunomide treatment in rheumatoid arthritis patients." *Eur J Clin Pharmacol* 64(9): 871-6.

Boothpur, R. and Brennan, D. C. (2010). "Human polyoma viruses and disease with emphasis on clinical BK and JC." *J Clin Virol* 47(4): 306-12.

Brennan, D. C., Agha, I., Bohl, D. L., Schnitzler, M. A., Hardinger, K. L., Lockwood, M., Torrence, S., Schuessler, R., Roby, T., Gaudreault-Keener, M. and Storch, G. A. (2005). "Incidence of BK with tacrolimus versus cyclosporine and impact of preemptive immunosuppression reduction." *Am J Transplant* 5(3): 582-94.

Brocker, V., Schwarz, A. and Becker, J. U. (2011). "[BK virus nephropathy after kidney transplantation.]." *Pathologe*.

Chen, C. H., Wen, M. C., Wang, M., Lian, J. D., Wu, M. J., Cheng, C. H., Shu, K. H. and Chang, D. (2001). "A regulatory region rearranged BK virus is associated with tubulointerstitial nephritis in a rejected renal allograft." *J Med Virol* 64(1): 82-8.

Chon, W. J. and Josephson, M. A. (2011). "Leflunomide in renal transplantation." *Expert Rev Clin Immunol* 7(3): 273-81.

De Luca, A., Giancola, M. L., Ammassari, A., Grisetti, S., Cingolani, A., Paglia, M. G., Govoni, A., Murri, R., Testa, L., Monforte, A. D. and Antinori, A. (2000). "Cidofovir added to HAART improves virological and clinical outcome in AIDS-associated progressive multifocal leukoencephalopathy." *Aids* 14(14): F117-21.

Dheir, H., Sahin, S., Uyar, M., Gurkan, A., Turunc, V., Kacar, S., Bayirli Turan, D. and Basdemir, G. (2011). "Intensive polyoma virus nephropathy treatment as a preferable approach for graft surveillance." *Transplant Proc* 43(3): 867-70.

Drachenberg, C. B., Beskow, C. O., Cangro, C. B., Bourquin, P. M., Simsir, A., Fink, J., Weir, M. R., Klassen, D. K., Bartlett, S. T. and Papadimitriou, J. C. (1999). "Human polyoma virus in renal allograft biopsies: morphological findings and correlation with urine cytology." *Hum Pathol* 30(8): 970-7.

Dropulic, L. K. and Jones, R. J. (2008). "Polyomavirus BK infection in blood and marrow transplant recipients." *Bone Marrow Transplant* 41(1): 11-8.

Dunn, M. C., Knight, D. A. and Waldman, W. J. (2011). "Inhibition of respiratory syncytial virus in vitro and in vivo by the immunosuppressive agent leflunomide." *Antivir Ther* 16(3): 309-17.

Faguer, S., Hirsch, H. H., Kamar, N., Guilbeau-Frugier, C., Ribes, D., Guitard, J., Esposito, L., Cointault, O., Modesto, A., Lavit, M., Mengelle, C. and Rostaing, L. (2007). "Leflunomide treatment for polyomavirus BK-associated nephropathy after kidney transplantation." *Transpl Int* 20(11): 962-9.

Farasati, N. A., Shapiro, R., Vats, A. and Randhawa, P. (2005). "Effect of leflunomide and cidofovir on replication of BK virus in an in vitro culture system." *Transplantation* 79(1): 116-8.

Fayard, E., Xue, G., Parcellier, A., Bozulic, L. and Hemmings, B. A. (2010). "Protein kinase B (PKB/Akt), a key mediator of the PI3K signaling pathway." *Curr Top Microbiol Immunol* 346: 31-56.

Fox, R. I., Herrmann, M. L., Frangou, C. G., Wahl, G. M., Morris, R. E., Strand, V. and Kirschbaum, B. J. (1999). "Mechanism of action for leflunomide in rheumatoid arthritis." *Clin Immunol* 93(3): 198-208.

Gilead (2010). "Vistide®." *Résumé des Caractéristiques du Produit*.

Gupta, A. and Gupta, P. (2011). "BK virus associated nephropathy in renal transplantation: where do we stand." *Minerva Urol Nefrol* 63(2): 155-67.

Hardinger, K. L., Koch, M. J., Bohl, D. J., Storch, G. A. and Brennan, D. C. (2010). "BK-virus and the impact of pre-emptive immunosuppression reduction: 5-year results." *Am J Transplant* 10(2): 407-15.

Hardinger, K. L., Wang, C. D., Schnitzler, M. A., Miller, B. W., Jendrisak, M. D., Shenoy, S., Lowell, J. A. and Brennan, D. C. (2002). "Prospective, pilot, open-label, short-term study of conversion to leflunomide reverses chronic renal allograft dysfunction." *Am J Transplant* 2(9): 867-71.

Hirsch, H. H., Knowles, W., Dickenmann, M., Passweg, J., Klimkait, T., Mihatsch, M. J. and Steiger, J. (2002). "Prospective study of polyomavirus type BK replication and nephropathy in renal-transplant recipients." *N Engl J Med* 347(7): 488-96.

Hirsch, H. H., Mohaupt, M. and Klimkait, T. (2001). "Prospective monitoring of BK virus load after discontinuing sirolimus treatment in a renal transplant patient with BK virus nephropathy." *J Infect Dis* 184(11): 1494-5; author reply 1495-6.

John, G. T., Manivannan, J., Chandy, S., Peter, S. and Jacob, C. K. (2004). "Leflunomide therapy for cytomegalovirus disease in renal allograft recepients." *Transplantation* 77(9): 1460-1.

Johnston, O., Jaswal, D., Gill, J. S., Doucette, S., Fergusson, D. A. and Knoll, G. A. (2010). "Treatment of polyomavirus infection in kidney transplant recipients: a systematic review." *Transplantation* 89(9): 1057-70.

Josephson, M. A., Gillen, D., Javaid, B., Kadambi, P., Meehan, S., Foster, P., Harland, R., Thistlethwaite, R. J., Garfinkel, M., Atwood, W., Jordan, J., Sadhu, M., Millis, M. J. and Williams, J. (2006). "Treatment of renal allograft polyoma BK virus infection with leflunomide." *Transplantation* 81(5): 704-10.

Kadambi, P. V., Josephson, M. A., Williams, J., Corey, L., Jerome, K. R., Meehan, S. M. and Limaye, A. P. (2003). "Treatment of refractory BK virus-associated nephropathy with cidofovir." *Am J Transplant* 3(2): 186-91.

Kalgutkar, A. S., Nguyen, H. T., Vaz, A. D., Doan, A., Dalvie, D. K., McLeod, D. G. and Murray, J. C. (2003). "In vitro metabolism studies on the isoxazole ring scission in the anti-inflammatory agent lefluonomide to its active alpha-cyanoenol metabolite A771726: mechanistic similarities with the cytochrome P450-catalyzed dehydration of aldoximes." *Drug Metab Dispos* 31(10): 1240-50.

Knight, D. A., Hejmanowski, A. Q., Dierksheide, J. E., Williams, J. W., Chong, A. S. and Waldman, W. J. (2001). "Inhibition of herpes simplex virus type 1 by the experimental immunosuppressive agent leflunomide." *Transplantation* 71(1): 170-4.

Kuypers, D. R., Vandooren, A. K., Lerut, E., Evenepoel, P., Claes, K., Snoeck, R., Naesens, L. and Vanrenterghem, Y. (2005). "Adjuvant low-dose cidofovir therapy for BK polyomavirus interstitial nephritis in renal transplant recipients." *Am J Transplant* 5(8): 1997-2004.

Liacini, A., Seamone, M. E., Muruve, D. A. and Tibbles, L. A. (2010). "Anti-BK virus mechanisms of sirolimus and leflunomide alone and in combination: toward a new therapy for BK virus infection." *Transplantation* 90(12): 1450-7.

Maddison, P., Kiely, P., Kirkham, B., Lawson, T., Moots, R., Proudfoot, D., Reece, R., Scott, D., Sword, R., Taggart, A., Thwaites, C. and Williams, E. (2005). "Leflunomide in rheumatoid arthritis: recommendations through a process of consensus." *Rheumatology (Oxford)* 44(3): 280-6.

Mengel, M., Marwedel, M., Radermacher, J., Eden, G., Schwarz, A., Haller, H. and Kreipe, H. (2003). "Incidence of polyomavirus-nephropathy in renal allografts: influence of modern immunosuppressive drugs." *Nephrol Dial Transplant* 18(6): 1190-6.

Mylonakis, E., Goes, N., Rubin, R. H., Cosimi, A. B., Colvin, R. B. and Fishman, J. A. (2001). "BK virus in solid organ transplant recipients: an emerging syndrome." *Transplantation* 72(10): 1587-92.

Nickeleit, V., Hirsch, H. H., Binet, I. F., Gudat, F., Prince, O., Dalquen, P., Thiel, G. and Mihatsch, M. J. (1999). "Polyomavirus infection of renal allograft recipients: from latent infection to manifest disease." *J Am Soc Nephrol* 10(5): 1080-9.

Nickeleit, V., Hirsch, H. H., Zeiler, M., Gudat, F., Prince, O., Thiel, G. and Mihatsch, M. J. (2000). "BK-virus nephropathy in renal transplants-tubular necrosis, MHC-class II expression and rejection in a puzzling game." *Nephrol Dial Transplant* 15(3): 324-32.

Nickeleit, V., Klimkait, T., Binet, I. F., Dalquen, P., Del Zenero, V., Thiel, G., Mihatsch, M. J. and Hirsch, H. H. (2000). "Testing for polyomavirus type BK DNA in plasma to identify renal-allograft recipients with viral nephropathy." *N Engl J Med* 342(18): 1309-15.

Nickeleit, V., Singh, H. K. and Mihatsch, M. J. (2003). "Polyomavirus nephropathy: morphology, pathophysiology, and clinical management." *Curr Opin Nephrol Hypertens* 12(6): 599-605.

Nickeleit, V., Zeiler, M., Gudat, F., Thiel, G. and Mihatsch, M. J. (1998). "Histological characteristics of interstitial renal allograft rejection." *Kidney Blood Press Res* 21(2-4): 230-2.

Pallet, N., Burgard, M., Quamouss, O., Rabant, M., Bererhi, L., Martinez, F., Thervet, E., Anglicheau, D., Noel, L. H., Rouzioux, C. and Legendre, C. (2010). "Cidofovir may be deleterious in BK virus-associated nephropathy." *Transplantation* 89(12): 1542-4.

Pavlakis, M., Haririan, A. and Klassen, D. K. (2006). "BK virus infection after non-renal transplantation." *Adv Exp Med Biol* 577: 185-9.

Ramos, E., Drachenberg, C. B., Papadimitriou, J. C., Hamze, O., Fink, J. C., Klassen, D. K., Drachenberg, R. C., Wiland, A., Wali, R., Cangro, C. B., Schweitzer, E., Bartlett, S. T. and Weir, M. R. (2002). "Clinical course of polyoma virus nephropathy in 67 renal transplant patients." *J Am Soc Nephrol* 13(8): 2145-51.

Randhawa, P., Ho, A., Shapiro, R., Vats, A., Swalsky, P., Finkelstein, S., Uhrmacher, J. and Weck, K. (2004). "Correlates of quantitative measurement of BK polyomavirus (BKV) DNA with clinical course of BKV infection in renal transplant patients." *J Clin Microbiol* 42(3): 1176-80.

Randhawa, P. S. and Demetris, A. J. (2000). "Nephropathy due to polyomavirus type BK." *N Engl J Med* 342(18): 1361-3.

Randhawa, P. S., Khaleel-Ur-Rehman, K., Swalsky, P. A., Vats, A., Scantlebury, V., Shapiro, R. and Finkelstein, S. (2002). "DNA sequencing of viral capsid protein VP-1 region in patients with BK virus interstitial nephritis." *Transplantation* 73(7): 1090-4.

Rosenberg, A. S. and Singer, A. (1992). "Cellular basis of skin allograft rejection: an in vivo model of immune-mediated tissue destruction." *Annu Rev Immunol* 10: 333-58.

Rozman, B. (2002). "Clinical pharmacokinetics of leflunomide." *Clin Pharmacokinet* 41(6): 421-30.

Saad, E. R., Bresnahan, B. A., Cohen, E. P., Lu, N., Orentas, R. J., Vasudev, B. and Hariharan, S. (2008). "Successful treatment of BK viremia using reduction in immunosuppression without antiviral therapy." *Transplantation* 85(6): 850-4.

Sanofi-Aventis (2009). "Arava®." *Résumé des Caractéristiques du Produit.*

Seron, D., Alexopoulos, E., Raftery, M. J., Hartley, R. B. and Cameron, J. S. (1989). "Diagnosis of rejection in renal allograft biopsies using the presence of activated and proliferating cells." *Transplantation* 47(5): 811-6.

Shen, J., Chong, A. S., Xiao, F., Liu, W., Huang, W., Blinder, L., Foster, P., Sankary, H., Jensik, S., McChesney, L., Mital, D. and Williams, J. W. (1998). "Histological characterization and pharmacological control of chronic rejection in xenogeneic and allogeneic heart transplantation." *Transplantation* 66(6): 692-8.

Smith, R. D., Galla, J. H., Skahan, K., Anderson, P., Linnemann, C. C., Jr., Ault, G. S., Ryschkewitsch, C. F. and Stoner, G. L. (1998). "Tubulointerstitial nephritis due to a mutant polyomavirus BK virus strain, BKV(Cin), causing end-stage renal disease." *J Clin Microbiol* 36(6): 1660-5.

Talmon, G., Cornell, L. D. and Lager, D. J. (2010). "Mitochondrial changes in cidofovir therapy for BK virus nephropathy." *Transplant Proc* 42(5): 1713-5.

Teschner, S., Geyer, M., Wilpert, J., Schwertfeger, E., Schenk, T., Walz, G. and Donauer, J. (2006). "Remission of polyomavirus-induced graft nephropathy treated with low-dose leflunomide." *Nephrol Dial Transplant* 21(7): 2039-40.

van Roon, E. N., Jansen, T. L., van de Laar, M. A., Janssen, M., Yska, J. P., Keuper, R., Houtman, P. M. and Brouwers, J. R. (2005). "Therapeutic drug monitoring of A77 1726, the active metabolite of leflunomide: serum concentrations predict response to treatment in patients with rheumatoid arthritis." *Ann Rheum Dis* 64(4): 569-74.

von Willebrand, E., Pettersson, E., Ahonen, J. and Hayry, P. (1986). "CMV infection, class II antigen expression, and human kidney allograft rejection." *Transplantation* 42(4): 364-7.

Waldman, W. J., Knight, D. A., Blinder, L., Shen, J., Lurain, N. S., Miller, D. M., Sedmak, D. D., Williams, J. W. and Chong, A. S. (1999). "Inhibition of cytomegalovirus in vitro and in vivo by the experimental immunosuppressive agent leflunomide." *Intervirology* 42(5-6): 412-8.

Waldman, W. J., Knight, D. A., Lurain, N. S., Miller, D. M., Sedmak, D. D., Williams, J. W. and Chong, A. S. (1999). "Novel mechanism of inhibition of cytomegalovirus by the experimental immunosuppressive agent leflunomide." *Transplantation* 68(6): 814-25.

Weiss, A. S., Gralla, J., Chan, L., Klem, P. and Wiseman, A. C. (2008). "Aggressive immunosuppression minimization reduces graft loss following diagnosis of BK virus-associated nephropathy: a comparison of two reduction strategies." *Clin J Am Soc Nephrol* 3(6): 1812-9.

Williams, J. W., Javaid, B., Kadambi, P. V., Gillen, D., Harland, R., Thistlewaite, J. R., Garfinkel, M., Foster, P., Atwood, W., Millis, J. M., Meehan, S. M. and Josephson, M. A. (2005). "Leflunomide for polyomavirus type BK nephropathy." *N Engl J Med* 352(11): 1157-8.

Williams, J. W., Mital, D., Chong, A., Kottayil, A., Millis, M., Longstreth, J., Huang, W., Brady, L. and Jensik, S. (2002). "Experiences with leflunomide in solid organ transplantation." *Transplantation* 73(3): 358-66.

Williams, J. W., Xiao, F., Foster, P., Clardy, C., McChesney, L., Sankary, H. and Chong, A. S. (1994). "Leflunomide in experimental transplantation. Control of rejection and alloantibody production, reversal of acute rejection, and interaction with cyclosporine." *Transplantation* 57(8): 1223-31.

Williamson, R. A., Yea, C. M., Robson, P. A., Curnock, A. P., Gadher, S., Hambleton, A. B., Woodward, K., Bruneau, J. M., Hambleton, P., Moss, D., Thomson, T. A., Spinella-Jaegle, S., Morand, P., Courtin, O., Sautes, C., Westwood, R., Hercend, T., Kuo, E. A. and Ruuth, E. (1995). "Dihydroorotate dehydrogenase is a high affinity binding protein for A77 1726 and mediator of a range of biological effects of the immunomodulatory compound." *J Biol Chem* 270(38): 22467-72.

Xiao, F., Chong, A., Shen, J., Yang, J., Short, J., Foster, P., Sankary, H., Jensik, S., Mital, D., McChesney, L. and et al. (1995). "Pharmacologically induced regression of chronic transplant rejection." *Transplantation* 60(10): 1065-72.

4

Modeling Virologic Response in HIV-1 Infected Patients to Assess Medication Adherence

Yangxin Huang
Department of Epidemiology and Biostatistics, College of Public Health, University of South Florida, Tampa, FL, USA

1. Introduction

Although the advent of highly active antiretroviral therapy (HAART), including potent protease inhibitors (PIs), has profoundly reduced human immunodeficiency virus (HIV) mortality and morbidity (Palella et al., 1998; CDC, 2009), these combination regimens are not a cure for HIV infection and therapy may be life long. While many patients benefit from HAART treatment, others do not benefit or only experience a temporary benefit. There are several reasons why treatment fails, with poor patient adherence to HAART a leading contributing factor (Ickovics & Meisler, 1997; Paterson, 2000). Thus, assessment of medication adherence within AIDS clinical trials is a critical component of the successful evaluation of therapy outcomes. Maintaining adherence may be particularly difficult when the drug regimen is complex or side-effects are common, as is often the case for current HIV therapy especially in highly treatment experienced patients (Ickovics & Meisler, 1997).

The measurement of adherence remains problematic; a standard definition of optimal adherence and completely reliable measures of adherence are lacking. Nevertheless, there has been substantial progress in both of these areas in the past few years. First, it appears that higher levels of adherence are needed for HIV disease than other diseases to achieve the desired therapeutic benefit. Using questionnaires (patient self-reporting and/or face-to-face interview) and electronic compliance monitoring caps (Medication Event Monitoring System [MEMS]), viral suppression is common with at least 54%-100% mean adherence level to antiviral regimens (Bangsberg, 2006). Second, a better appreciation of the value and limitations of different adherence measurements has been addressed (Berg & Arnsten, 2006; Bova et al., 2005). In AIDS clinical trials, adherence to a medication regimen is currently measured by two major methods: by use of questionnaires and by use of MEMS. The MEMS is considered an objective adherence measure. It consists of a microprocessor in the cap of a medication bottle which records the date and time of bottle opening. The results are downloaded to a computer for analysis. Results demonstrate that medication-taking patterns are highly variable among patients (Kastrissios et al., 1998) and that they often give a more precise measure of adherence than self-report (Arnsten et al., 2001a). However, MEMS data are also subject to error and are not widely available in the clinical setting. Adherence assessment by self-report is usually evaluated by a patient's ability to recall their medication dosing during a specific time interval. Often self-reported measures tend to overestimate HIV medication adherence compared to other methods (Arnsten et al., 2001b,

Bangsberg et al. 2000; Levine et al., 2006; Liu et al., 2001). Finally, it is important to note that the measurement of viral load levels is of special utility as an indirect measure of adherence in HIV therapeutics. It has been argued that this is not a good adherence measure because other factors may influence viral load (pharmacokinetics, drug resistance etc.). However, there is a tight correlation between viral load and adherence (Haubrich et al., 1999; Paterson et al., 2000), but results vary by adherence method and summary adherence statistic (Vrijens & Goetghebeur, 1997; Vrijens et al., 2005) . Several recent papers explore the methodological and operational issues when evaluating electronic drug monitoring adherence on viral load (Arnsten et al., 2001b; Fennie et al., 2006; Fletcher et al., 2005; Llabre et al., 2006; Liu et al. , 2006; Liu et al. , 2007; Pearson et al. , 2007; Vrijens et al., 2005). Most importantly, a favorable change in viral load is the desired therapeutic outcome of adherence to HAART.

In this paper, we propose using a viral dynamic model with consideration of long-term medication adherence and drug susceptibility to explore the relationship between adherence to two protease inhibitors, as part of an HAART regimen, and long-term virologic response. In particular, we will use different adherence measures from an AIDS clinical trial study--ACTG398 (Hammer et al., 2002) and compare their performance for predicting virologic response. The dynamic modeling approach (Huang et al., 2006; 2010) allows us to appropriately capture the sophisticated nonlinear relationships and interactions among important factors and virologic response. The complete HIV-1 RNA (viral load) trajectories serve as the virologic response index, which is more informative and sensitive to clinical and drug factors. Thus, this method is more powerful to detect the effect of a clinical or drug factor on the response. Using a Bayesian method (Huang et al., 2006), we fit a long-term viral dynamic model to data from the AIDS clinical trial study to explore the association between adherence and viral load in HIV-infected patients with adjustment of the potential confounding factor, drug susceptibility. In this study, we employed the proposed mechanism-based dynamic model to assess how to efficiently use the adherence data based on questionnaires and the MEMS to predict virologic response. In particular, we intend to address the questions (i) how to summarize the MEMS adherence data for efficient prediction of the virologic response, and (ii) which adherence assessment method, questionnaire or MEMS, is more efficient in predicting the virologic response after accounting for the potential confounding factor, drug resistance. We expect that viral dynamic modeling not only provides a powerful tool to evaluate the effect of adherence on long-term virologic responses, but also can be used to predict antiviral responses for various scenarios that may help with understanding the role of different adherence measure statistics in antiviral activities and assist clinicians in treatment decisions.

2. Materials

In this section, we describe the subject population to be studied and observed data to be used in this research. These measurements include RNA viral load, phenotypic drug sensitivity and medication adherence. We also discuss how to evaluate assessment interval lengths and time frames (delay effect of timing) for the MEMS adherence data.

2.1 Subject population

The subject sample in our analysis was drawn from the AIDS Clinical Trials Group (ACTG) 398 study (Hammer et al., 2002), a randomized, double-blind, placebo-controlled phase II study of amprenavir (APV) as part of several dual protease inhibitor (PI) regimens in subjects with HIV infection in whom initial PI therapy had failed. One of objectives of the ACTG 398 study was to evaluate the genotypic and phenotypic resistance profiles that emerge on treatment and their relationship to the plasma HIV-1 RNA and CD4 cell count responses, and to determine the relationship between drug exposure measured from combined PK and adherence data to the degree and duration of viral response. Subjects in all arms received APV (1200 mg twice a day [q12h]), efavirenz (EFV, 600 mg once a day [qd]), abacavir (300 mg q12h) and adefovir dipivoxil (60 mg qd). A total of 481 subjects were randomized to four treatment arms and received a second PI or placebo: Arm A (n=116) saquinavir (1600 mg q12h); Arm B (n=69) indinavir (1200 mg q12h); Arm C (n=139) nelfinavir (NFV, 1250 mg q12h); and Arm D (n=157) received a placebo matched for one of these three PIs. Assignment of subjects to treatment arms depended on past PI exposure in the arm. Subjects were scheduled for follow-up visits at study (day 0); at weeks 2, 4, 8, 16 and every 8 weeks thereafter until week 72; and at the time of confirmed virologic failure. More detailed descriptions of this study and study results are given by Hammer et al. (2002) and Pfister et al. (2003). Because phenotype sensitivity testing was performed only on a subset of randomly selected subjects, the number of subjects available for our analysis was greatly reduced. We chose to consider only the subjects within Arm C for our analysis because this arm afforded the greatest number of subjects (n=31) with phenotypic drug susceptibility data on the two PIs (APV and NFV) and had available adherence data, as required for our model. Among these 31 subjects, 13 had phenotypic drug susceptibility data at the time of protocol-defined virologic failure.

2.2 Observed measurements

RNA viral load: RNA viral load was measured in copies/mL at study weeks 0, 2, 4, 8 and every 8 weeks thereafter until week 72 by the ultrasensitive reverse transcriptase-polymerase chain reaction HIV-1 RNA assay. Only measurements taken while on protocol-defined treatment were used in the analysis. All viral load values were log (base 10) transformed. Although, the lower limit of assay quantification was 200 copies/mL, when lower values (<200 copies/mL) were detected, these values were used in the analysis. The exact day of viral load measurement (not predefined study week) was used to compute study day in our analysis.

Medication adherence: Medication adherence was measured by two methods-- by the use of questionnaires and by the use of electronic monitoring caps. Subjects completed an adherence questionnaire (AACTG study 398 questionnaire QL0702) at study weeks 4, 8, 12, 16, and every 8 weeks thereafter. The questionnaire was completed by the study participant and/or by a face-to-face interview with study personnel. The subject was asked to specify the number of prescribed doses of each drug that he or she had failed to take on each of the preceding 4 days. Questionnaire adherence rates for APV and NFV were determined at each visit as the number of prescribed doses taken divided by the number prescribed doses during the preceding 4 day interval. For electronically monitored adherence, an MEMS cap (Medication Event Monitoring Systems, Aprex Corp., Menlo CA) was used to monitor APV and EFV compliance only. Subjects were asked to bring their medication bottles and caps to the clinic at each study visit (weeks 2, 4, 8, 12, 16, and every 8 weeks thereafter), where cap data were downloaded to computer files and stored for later analysis. Since APV was prescribed twice daily, a prescribed AM and PM dosing period was defined for each subject. If a subject opened the bottle at least once during a dosing period, then the subject was recorded as having a positive event (x=1), otherwise (x=0). The MEMS adherence rate for APV was determined as the sum of positive dosing events divided by the sum of prescribed dosing events during the specified time interval. A positive dosing event assumes a presumptive dose. If the MEMS cap was recorded as not in use, the MEMS dosing event was set to missing. In our analysis, we assumed that NFV had the same MEMS adherence rate as APV.

		Adherence assessment definition		
Case	MEMS adherence interval notation	Interval length	Time frame length (weeks to RNA measurement)	Example for day 56, adherence computed over
1	M	visit time	0	Days 28 - 55
2	M0.1	1 week	0	Days 49 - 55
3	M0.2	2 weeks	0	Days 42 - 55
4	M0.3	3 weeks	0	Days 35 - 55
5	M1.1	1 week	1 week	Days 43 - 49
6	M1.2	2 weeks	1 week	Days 36 - 49
7	M1.3	3 weeks	1 week	Days 29 - 49
8	M2.1	1 week	2 weeks	Days 36 - 42
9	M2.2	2 weeks	2 weeks	Days 29 - 42
10	M2.3	3 weeks	2 weeks	Days 22 - 42
11	M3.1	1 week	3 weeks	Days 29 - 35
12	M3.2	2 weeks	3 weeks	Days 22 - 35
13	M3.3	3 weeks	3 weeks	Days 15 - 35

Table 1. Summary of the MEMS assessment interval notation and definitions

To determine the best summary metric of the MEMS adherence rate, we evaluated different assessment interval lengths (averaging adherence dosing events over 1, 2, or 3 week intervals) and different assessment time frames (fixing the assessment interval times to end either immediately or 1, 2 or 3 weeks prior to the next measured viral load). Table 1 summarizes the MEMS assessment interval notation and definitions for the 13 models. As an example, M2.2 in Table 1 denotes an MEMS adherence interval length of 2 weeks fixed to end 2 weeks prior to the next viral load measurement; for instance, the MEMS adherence rate for a subject at study week 8 (day 56) was calculated as the number of nominal dosing events divided by the number of prescribed dosing events over study days 29 - 42. The case M serves as a reference and averages all the available MEMS data between viral load measurements.

Phenotypic drug susceptibility: Retrospectively, 200 subjects were randomly selected from the entire ACTG 398 study population for phenotypic sensitivity testing. Of these 139 subjects were tested at baseline based on receiving study treatment for at least 8 weeks and having an available sample. Among these subjects, 59 subjects experienced protocol-defined virologic failure and phenotypic sensitivity testing was performed at the time of failure (Hammer et al., 2002). Phenotypic drug susceptibility was determined by a recombinant virus assay (PhenoSense, ViroLogic, Inc) and values were expressed as the 50% inhibitory concentration (IC_{50}) (Molla et al., 1996). All 31 subjects used in our analysis had baseline APV and NFV IC_{50} values, of which 13 subjects had follow-up APV and NFV IC_{50} values at the time of virologic failure.

3. Mathematical models and statistical methods

We fit the dynamic model to the viral load data from 31 subjects with the following considerations. (i) In the model we incorporate the two clinical factors, drug adherence (questionnaire or MEMS) and drug susceptibility (phenotype IC_{50} values), into a function of treatment efficacy. (ii) We only consider the PI drug effects in the drug efficacy model because the effect of RTI drugs is considered less important compared to the PI drugs and would require a different efficacy model. (iii) We assume that NFV has the same compliance rate as determined for APV by the MEMS method. Details of the mathematical models and statistical methods are described in Huang et al. (2006) and Wu et al. (2005). For completeness, a brief summary of the models and methods is given as follows.

3.1 Drug resistance model

As Molla et al. (1996) suggested, the phenotype marker, median inhibitory concentration (IC_{50}), can be used to quantify agent-specific drug susceptibility. We use the following model to approximate the within-host changes over time in IC_{50} (Huang et al., 2003; Huang et al., 2006; Wu et al., 2005).

$$IC_{50}(t) = \begin{cases} I_0 + \dfrac{I_r - I_0}{t_r} t & \text{for } 0 < t < t_r, \\ I_r & \text{for } t \geq t_r, \end{cases} \tag{1}$$

Where I_0 and I_r are respective values of $IC_{50}(t)$ at baseline and time point t_r at which resistant mutations dominate. In our study, t_r is the time of virologic failure. For subjects without a failure time IC_{50}, baseline IC_{50} was held constant over time.

3.2 Medication adherence model

Poor adherence to a treatment regimen is one of the major causes of treatment failure. (Ickovics abd Meisler, 1997). The following model is used to represent adherence for a time interval $T_k < t \leq T_{k+1}$,

$$A(t) = \begin{cases} 1 & \text{if all doses are taken in } (T_k, T_{k+1}], \\ R_k & \text{if } 100R_k\% \text{ doses are taken in } (T_k, T_{k+1}], \end{cases} \tag{2}$$

where $0 \leq R_k < 1$, with R_k indicating the adherence rate computed for each assessment interval $(T_k, T_{k+1}]$ based on the questionnaire or MEMS data; T_k denotes the adherence assessment time at the kth clinical visit.

3.3 Drug efficacy model

In most viral dynamic studies, investigators assumed that either drug efficacy was constant over treatment time (Perelson and Nelson, 1999; Wu and Ding, 1999; Ding and Wu, 2001) or antiviral regimens had perfect effect in blocking viral replication (Ho et al., 1995; Perelson et al., 1996, 1997). However, the drug efficacy may change as concentrations of antiretroviral drugs and other factors (*e.g.* drug resistance) vary during treatment (Dixit et al., 2004). We employ the following modified E_{max} model (Sheiner, 1985) to represent the time-varying drug efficacy (see Wu et al. (2005) for more discussion about the drug effect E_{max} model) for two antiretroviral agents within a class (for example, the two PI drugs APV and NFV),

$$\gamma(t) = \frac{A_1(t) / IC_{50}^1(t) + A_2(t) / IC_{50}^2(t)}{\phi + A_1(t) / IC_{50}^1(t) + A_2(t) / IC_{50}^2(t)}, \tag{3}$$

where $IC_{50}^k(t)$ $(k = 1,2)$ are median inhibitory concentration change over time for the two agents; $A_k(t)$ $(k = 1,2)$ are adherence profiles of the two drugs measured by questionnaire or the MEMS method. Parameter ϕ can be regarded as a conversion factor between *in vitro* and *in vivo* IC_{50} s and will be estimated from the data. Note that $\gamma(t)$ ranges from 0 to 1.

3.4 Antiviral response model

We consider a simplified HIV dynamic model with antiviral treatment as follows. (Huang et al., 2006; Wu et al., 2005).

$$\begin{aligned} \frac{d}{dt}T &= \lambda - d_T T - [1-\gamma(t)]kTV, \\ \frac{d}{dt}T^* &= [1-\gamma(t)]kTV - \delta T^*, \\ \frac{d}{dt}V &= N\delta T^* - cV, \end{aligned} \tag{4}$$

where the three differential equations represent three compartments: target uninfected cells (T), infected cells (T^*) and free virions (V). Parameter λ represents the rate at which new T cells are generated from sources within the body, such as the thymus, d_T is the death rate of T cells, k is the infection rate without treatment, δ is the death rate of infected cells, N is the number of new virions produced from each of infected cell during its life-time, and c is the clearance rate of free virions. The time-varying parameter $\gamma(t)$ is the antiviral drug efficacy at treatment time t.

3.5 Bayesian modeling approach

Although a number of studies investigated various statistical methods, including Bayesian approaches, of fitting viral dynamic models to predicting virologic responses using short-term viral load data (Wu and Ding, 1999; Ho et al., 1995; Perelson et al., 1996, 1997; Wu et al., 1999; Notermans et al., 1998; Markowitz et al., 2003; Han et al., 2002), little work has been undertaken to investigate long-term virologic responses. In this paper, we used a hierarchical Bayesian modeling approach (Huang et al., 2006) to estimate the dynamic parameters.

We denote the number of subjects by n and the number of measurements on the ith subject by m_i. For notational convenience, let $\mu = (\ln\phi, \ln c, \ln\delta, \ln\lambda, \ln d_T, \ln N, \ln k)^T$,

$\Theta = \{\theta_i, i = 1, \cdots, n\}$, $\theta_i = (\ln\phi_i, \ln c_i, \ln\delta_i, \ln\lambda_i, \ln d_{Ti}, \ln N_i, \ln k_i)^T$, $\Theta_{\{i\}} = \{\theta_l, l \neq i\}$ and $\mathbf{Y} = \{y_{ij}, i = 1, \cdots, n; j = 1, \cdots, m_i\}$. Let $f_{ij}(\theta_i, t_j) = \log_{10}(V_i(\theta_i, t_j))$, where $V_i(\theta_i, t_j)$ denotes the numerical solution of the differential equations (4) for the ith subject at time t_j. Let $y_{ij}(t)$ and $e_i(t_j)$ denote the repeated measurements of common logarithmic viral load and a measurement error with mean zero, respectively. The Bayesian nonlinear mixed-effects model can be written as the following three stages (Davidian and Giltinan, 1995; Huang et al., 2006).

Stage 1. Within-subject variation:

$$\mathbf{y}_i = \mathbf{f}_i(\theta_i) + \mathbf{e}_i, \quad \mathbf{e}_i \mid \sigma^2, \theta_i \sim N(0, \sigma^2 \mathbf{I}_{m_i}) \tag{5}$$

where $\mathbf{y}_i = (y_{i1}(t_1), \cdots, y_{im_i}(t_{m_i}))^T$, $\mathbf{f}_i(\theta_i) = (f_{i1}(\theta_i, t_1), \cdots, f_{im_i}(\theta_i, t_{m_i}))^T$, $\mathbf{e}_i = (e_i(t_1), \cdots, e_i(t_{m_i}))^T$.

Stage 2. Between-subject variation:

$$\theta_i = \mu + \mathbf{b}_i, \quad \mathbf{b}_i \mid \Sigma \sim N(0, \Sigma) \tag{6}$$

Stage 3. Hyperprior distributions:

$$\sigma^{-2} \sim Ga(a,b), \quad \mu \sim N(\eta, \Lambda), \quad \Sigma^{-1} \sim Wi(\Omega, \nu) \tag{7}$$

where the mutually independent Gamma (Ga), Normal (N) and Wishart (Wi) prior distributions are chosen to facilitate computations (Davidian and Giltinan, 1995). The hyper-parameters $a, b, \eta, \Lambda, \Omega$ and ν were determined from previous studies and the literature (Perelson and Nelson, 1999; Ho et al., 1995; Perelson et al., 1996, 1997; Nowak and May, 2000). See Huang et al. (2006) for a detailed discussion of the Bayesian modeling approach, including the choice of the hyper-parameters, and the implementation of the Markov chain Monte Carlo (MCMC) procedures (Gamerman, 1997; Wakefield, 1996).

4. Results

4.1 Subject characteristics

Of the 31 subjects used in our analysis, the mean age was 40 years (SD=7); 94% were men; and 65% were white, 23% black, 10% Hispanic and 3% Asian. At baseline, 58% had prior nonnucleoside reverse transcriptase inhibitor (NNRTI) experience. Median baseline CD4 cell count was 196 cells/uL (interquartile range=120-308 cells/uL) and median baseline viral load was 38,019 copies/mL (interquartile range=19,498-181,970 copies/mL). Median time to the last viral load measurement while on protocol-defined treatment was 227 days (interquartile range=168-321 days). Median baseline IC_{50} values were 21.2 ng/mL and 38.9 ng/mL for APV and NFV, respectively. Among the 13 subjects with IC_{50} values at failure time, the median time to virologic failure was 157 days. Overall mean questionnaire adherence rate was 0.95 and 0.96 respectively for APV and NFV and the MEMS adherence rate for APV was 0.80. Fig. 1 shows the viral load ($\log_{10}$ transformed) and adherence rates over time based on questionnaire data for APV and NFV drugs and APV MEMS data (13 summary metrics) for one representative subject.

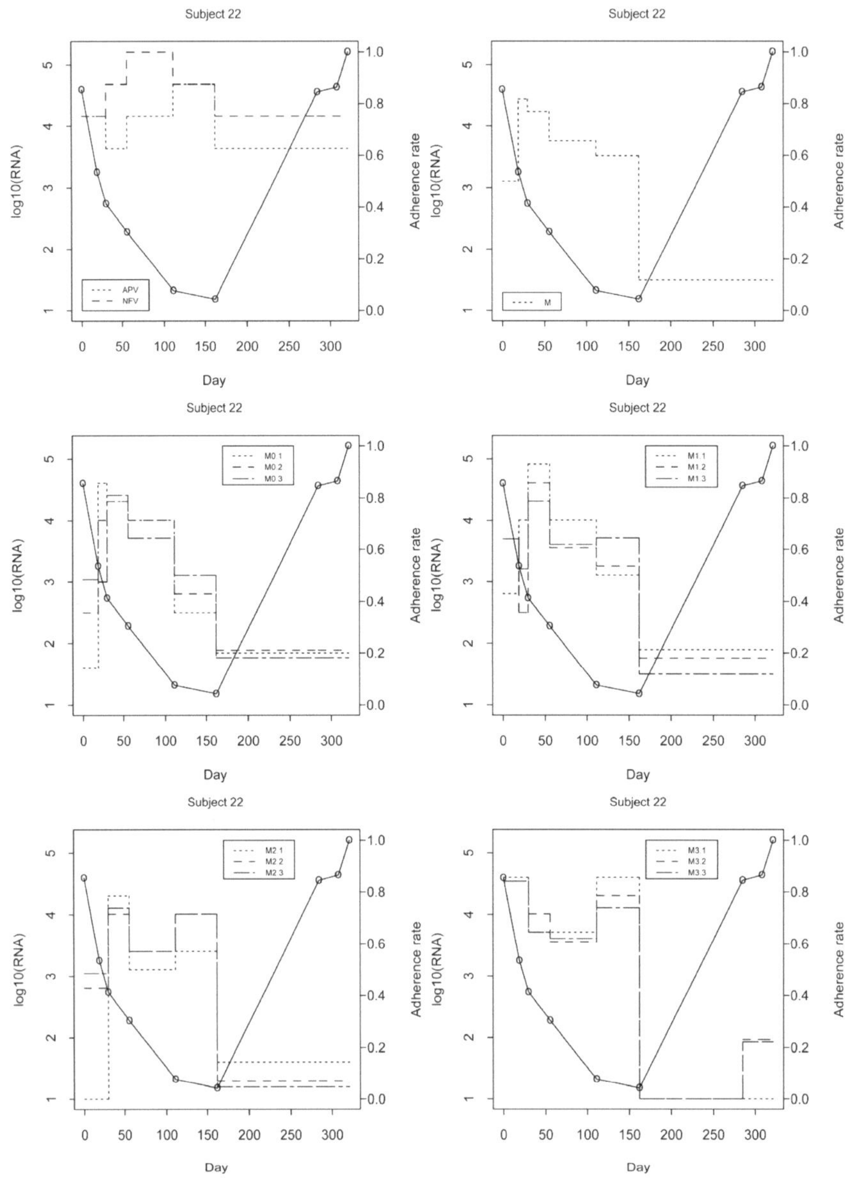

Fig. 1. The trajectories of viral load on $\log_{10}$ scale (solid curves) and adherence rates (stairsteps) over time based on questionnaire data for APV and NFV drugs (upper-left panel) and MEMS data summarized by the 13 models for APV drug (other panels) for one subject

We fit the viral dynamic model to the data from 31 subjects described previously using the proposed Bayesian approach. We incorporated the two clinical factors, drug adherence (questionnaire or MEMS) and drug susceptibility (phenotype IC_{50} values), into a function of treatment efficacy (3). For model fitting and the purpose of comparisons, we set up a control model as the one without using any adherence and drug susceptibility data which corresponds to setting $A(t)$ and $IC_{50}(t)$ to be 1 in Eq. (3), i.e., $\gamma(t) = 2/(\phi + 2)$. Other 14 models are specified based on the combination of drug susceptibility (IC_{50}) data and 14 different adherence summary metrics (1 questionnaire and 13 MEMS summary metrics listed in Table 1). Note that the abbreviation IM2.2, for example, denotes the model incorporating the data of drug resistance (I) and MEMS adherence rate (M2.2) summarized as an interval length of 2 weeks fixed to end 2 weeks prior to the next viral load measurement. For example, the MEMS adherence rate for a subject at study week 8 (day 56) was calculated over a 14 day interval from study days 29-42 and this value was used to represent adherence from the previous study visit to the study visit at day 56 for modeling fitting.

4.2 Model fitting

In order to assess how adherence rates, determined from 14 different scenarios, interact with drug susceptibility to contribute to virologic response, we fitted the models to all 14 scenarios as well as the control model and compared the fitting results. We found that, overall, the model with adherence rate determined from MEMS dosing events averaged over a 2 week assessment interval either 1 week prior to a viral load measurement (IM1.2) or 2 weeks prior to a viral load measurement (IM2.2) provided the best fits to the observed data, compared to the other 13 models for most subjects; the control model, lacking factors for subject-specific drug adherence and susceptibility, failed to fit viral load rebounds and

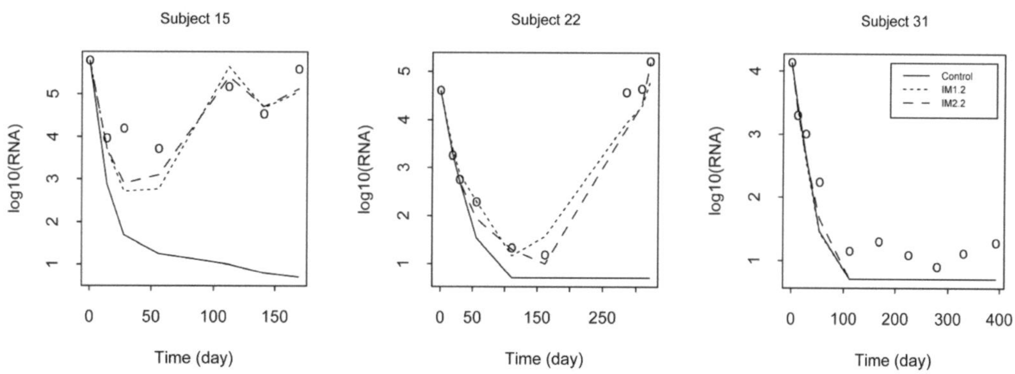

Fig. 2. The estimated viral trajectory for three representative subjects from the model fitting: (i) Control model (solid curves), (ii) IM1.2 (dotted curves) and (iii) IM2.2 (dashed curves). The observed values are indicated by circles.

fluctuations and provided the worst fitting results for the majority of subjects. For the purpose of illustration, the model fitting curves for three representative subjects from the control model (solid curves), the IM1.2 model (dotted curves), and the IM2.2 model (dashed curves) are displayed in Fig. 2.

4.3 Individual dynamics parameter estimates

Table 2 presents the results of estimated dynamic parameters for individual subjects and the sample summary statistics (minimum, median, mean, maximum, standard deviation (SD) and coefficient of variation (CV) for the model IM2.2 that provided the best fit to the observed data. We can see from Table 2 a relatively large between-subject variation in the

Subject	ϕ_i	c_i	δ_i	λ_i	d_{Ti}	N_i	$k_i \times 10^4$
1	0.002	3.144	0.105	68.830	0.041	126.353	2.083
2	0.002	3.366	0.203	193.493	0.021	763.481	0.800
3	0.002	3.065	0.228	103.261	0.051	516.932	1.363
4	0.001	3.963	0.294	67.549	0.110	709.988	0.738
5	0.002	2.499	1.238	171.962	0.142	9384.339	0.868
6	0.002	3.219	0.224	108.737	0.056	495.182	1.526
7	0.002	3.631	0.078	111.508	0.017	109.594	1.549
8	0.001	4.103	0.157	73.195	0.050	354.894	1.124
9	0.002	2.286	0.809	177.204	0.097	4070.423	1.112
10	0.002	2.620	1.058	208.394	0.091	6031.472	1.033
11	0.002	3.213	0.219	83.127	0.058	479.131	1.316
12	0.002	2.804	0.315	96.976	0.071	806.579	1.622
13	0.001	3.705	0.164	88.307	0.056	581.903	0.727
14	0.002	2.877	0.132	130.303	0.026	341.015	1.347
15	0.003	2.316	0.434	207.091	0.043	2197.731	1.064
16	0.003	1.753	0.924	160.891	0.120	4224.349	1.867
17	0.001	4.041	0.211	127.465	0.023	765.045	0.692
18	0.002	3.367	0.216	85.716	0.051	508.451	1.148
19	0.002	3.955	0.114	74.292	0.033	164.046	1.498
20	0.001	3.938	0.116	117.911	0.023	356.109	0.801
21	0.001	2.887	0.314	306.351	0.019	1636.315	0.486
22	0.003	2.003	0.569	100.966	0.067	1186.222	0.654
23	0.001	4.273	0.260	43.015	0.136	474.269	1.258
24	0.001	3.506	0.131	157.873	0.028	643.514	0.847
25	0.002	2.277	0.839	174.871	0.105	4912.339	1.189
26	0.001	3.847	0.340	54.983	0.135	714.569	1.116
27	0.003	2.730	0.218	103.326	0.042	411.427	1.690
28	0.002	3.510	0.073	133.204	0.015	106.627	1.366
29	0.002	3.751	0.186	108.477	0.026	435.276	1.111
30	0.002	3.760	0.162	96.575	0.031	354.927	1.192
31	0.002	3.415	0.144	112.288	0.034	392.298	1.140
Min	0.001	1.753	0.073	43.015	0.015	106.627	0.486
Med	0.002	3.367	0.218	108.737	0.050	516.932	1.140
Max	0.003	4.273	1.238	306.351	0.142	9384.339	2.083
Mean	0.0017	3.285	0.328	124.134	0.059	1427.574	1.172
SD	0.0006	0.647	0.305	55.726	0.039	2118.271	0.373
CV (%)	33.037	19.686	93.066	44.892	66.245	148.383	31.801

Table 2. The estimated dynamic parameters from the IM2.2 model for individual subjects, where Min, Med, Max, SD and CV=SD/Mean denote the minimum, median, maximum, standard deviation and coefficient of variation, respectively.

seven viral dynamic parameters was observed (CV ranges from 20% to 148%) among the 31 subjects. Generally speaking, the virologically successful subjects (maintaining plasma HIV-1 RNA levels of less than 200 copies/mL) have higher clearance rates of free virions (c), but smaller efficacy parameter estimates (ϕ), and lower death rates of infected cells (δ); these results show the similar patterns to those displayed in Figure 4 studied by Wu et al. (2005) The individual parameter estimates from both the IM2.2 and IM1.2 models are significantly correlated for all seven parameters, while the individual parameter estimates for the control model appear significantly different from those for the model IM2.2 for most of the seven parameters (data not shown here).

4.4 Effects of adherence rate determined by questionnaire vs. MEMS data

In order to assess how different adherence rates measured by questionnaires and MEMS contribute to the virologic response, we compared the fitting results of models with all 14 adherence scenarios and the control model. The mean of the sum of the squared deviations (SSD) was used to assess model fit and the SSD was calculated by $\sum_{j=1}^{m_i}(y_{ij}-\hat{y}_{ij})^2$ for each subject, where y_{ij} and $\hat{y}_{ij}$ are the observed and predicted values, respectively. The mean SSDs are plotted for all the models in Fig. 3, with the best fitting models having a smaller mean SSD, and sign test p-values from pairwise comparisons are reported in Table 3.

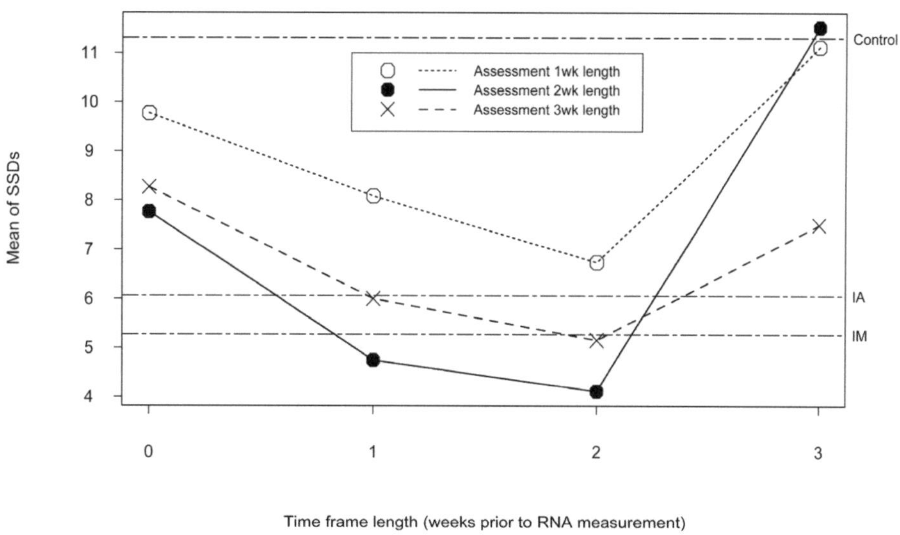

Fig. 3. Comparison of mean of SSDs for models from the 14 different determinants of adherence with drug resistance and the control model. The three horizontal lines represent mean of the SSDs for control, IA and IM models, respectively.

4.5 What MEMS assessment interval length is best?

The pattern in Fig. 3 shows that when the time frame for MEMS assessment is fixed, models with a 2 week MEMS assessment interval length generally outperform models with an assessment interval length of 1 or 3 weeks.

Model	Control	IA	IM	IM0.1	IM0.2	IM0.3	IM1.1	IM1.2	IM1.3	IM2.1	IM2.2	IM2.3	IM3.1	IM3.2
IA	<0.001													
IM	<0.001	0.106												
IM0.1	0.106	0.007	0.002											
IM0.2	0.019	0.209	0.007	0.020										
IM0.3	0.048	0.048	0.020	0.106	0.369									
IM1.1	0.001	0.590	0.020	0.106	0.209	0.858								
IM1.2	<0.001	0.048	0.029	0.002	0.007	0.007	0.007							
IM1.3	0.001	0.858	0.858	0.048	0.048	0.048	0.209	0.048						
IM2.1	<0.001	0.106	0.209	0.020	0.007	0.048	0.048	0.048	0.209					
IM2.2	<0.001	0.007	0.020	<0.001	0.001	<0.001	0.048	0.590	0.048	0.020				
IM2.3	<0.001	0.369	0.209	0.011	0.002	0.002	0.209	0.106	0.858	0.590	0.048			
IM3.1	0.106	0.007	<0.001	0.369	0.590	0.048	0.007	<0.001	0.007	0.001	0.002	0.002		
IM3.2	0.106	0.209	0.002	0.858	0.858	0.007	0.007	0.001	0.002	0.007	0.007	0.002	0.048	
IM3.3	0.001	0.858	0.020	0.048	0.020	0.369	0.209	0.007	0.369	0.369	0.001	0.020	0.002	0.020
MSSD	11.30	6.06	5.27	9.77	7.77	8.27	8.09	4.75	6.00	6.73	4.11	5.16	11.12	11.56

Table 3. Pairwise comparisons of sum of squared deviations (SSD) from individual subjects for 15 models. The p-values were obtained using the sign test and MSSD is the mean of SSD

4.6 What MEMS assessment time frame (delay effect of timing) is best?

As seen in Fig. 3, regardless of the assessment interval length, models which assess compliance 2 weeks prior to viral load generally outperform models which assess compliance immediately before viral load, 1 week before or 3 weeks before viral load measurement. Overall, the model with a MEMS assessment interval length of 2 weeks measured from 4 to 2 weeks prior to viral load measurement (IM2.2) was significantly a better predicator of viral load over time than any other models, with the exception of the IM1.2 model.

From Table 3, the means and standard deviations of the SSDs for the models based on IM1.2 (4.75 ± 5.38) and IM2.2 (4.11 ± 4.18) were significantly less than those of the other 13 models. We can see that that the IM1.2 and IM2.2 models were significantly better than the models based on the other 13 models ($p \le 0.001 \sim 0.048$), but they were not significantly different each other (p=0.590). The control model was significantly worse than those based on all other models ($p \le 0.001 \sim 0.020$) except for the 2 models (IM3.1 and IM3.2: p =0.106).

4.7 What adherence assessment method (questionnaire vs MEMS) is best?

Further, we compared the model fittings with all possible combinations of IC_{50} and the four determinants of adherence (A, M, M1.2 and M2.2). The mean of SSD for all the 10 models is plotted in Figure 4, and sign test p —values from pairwise comparisons are reported in Table 4. The results indicate that (i) the control model was significantly worse than those based on all other 9 models ($p \le 0.001 \sim 0.007$); (ii) the models IM1.2 and IM2.2 were significantly better than the other eight models ($p \le 0.001 \sim 0.048$); (iii) the models I, A, M, M1.2, M2.2, IA and IM do not provide significantly different results (p=0.048 ~ 0.858) except for two marginally significant results. In particular, the models IA and IM are not better than the model I (p=0.209, 0.590), and the models IM1.2 and IM2.2 are significantly better than the models I, M1.2 and M2.2 (p=0.007 ~ 0.048). Overall, adherence assessed by an optimal summary MEMS metric with the confounding resistance factor combinations (IM1.2 and IM2.2) was a better predictor of virologic response than adherence assessed by questionnaires, MEMS alone or two-factor combinations.

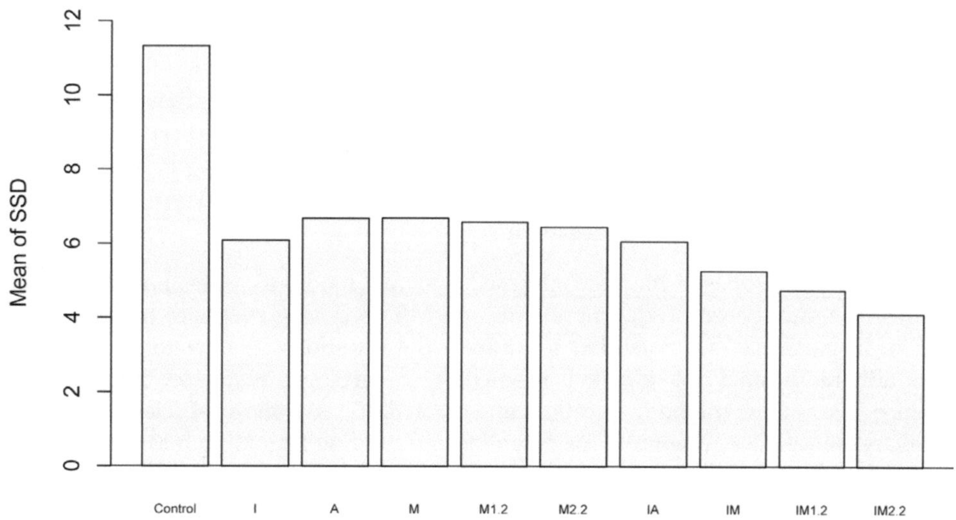

Fig. 4. Comparison of SSDs for the models from 9 different determinants of adherence and/or drug resistance as well as the control model

	Models	Control	I	A	M	M1.2	M2.2	IA	IM	IM1.2	IM2.2
	I	<0.001									
	A	0.007	0.106								
	M	0.007	0.106	0.858							
	M1.2	<0.001	0.106	0.590	0.858						
p	M2.2	<0.001	0.209	0.858	0.858	0.369					
	IA	<0.001	0.209	0.209	0.590	0.209	0.590				
	IM	<0.001	0.590	0.209	0.048	0.048	0.209	0.106			
	IM1.2	<0.001	0.048	0.002	0.002	0.020	0.048	0.048	0.026		
	IM2.2	<0.001	0.048	0.002	0.002	0.007	0.048	0.007	0.020	0.590	
SSD	Mean	11.30	6.09	6.68	6.69	6.68	6.45	6.06	5.27	4.75	4.11
	±SD	9.28	6.84	6.02	6.87	6.79	6.33	5.66	5.52	5.38	4.18

Table 4. Pairwise comparisons of sum of squared deviations (SSD) from individual subjects for 10 models. The p-values were obtained using the sign test.

5. Conclusion and discussion

Several studies investigated the association between virologic responses and adherence assessed by MEMS data only without considering other confounding factors such as drug resistance using standard modeling methods including Poisson regression (Knafl et al., 2004), logistic regression (Vrijens et al., 2005) and linear mixed-effects model (Liu et al., 2007). In this article, we developed a mechanism-based nonlinear time-varying differential equation model for long-term dynamics to (i) establish the relationship of virologic response (viral load trajectory) with drug adherence and drug resistance, (ii) to describe both suppression and resurgence of virus, (iii) to directly incorporate observed drug adherence and susceptibility into a function of treatment efficacy and (iv) to use a hierarchical Bayesian mixed-effects modeling approach that can not only combine prior information with current clinical data for estimating dynamic parameters, but also characterize inter-subject variability. Our modeling approach allows us to estimate time-varying antiretroviral efficacy during the entire course of a treatment regimen by incorporating the information of drug exposure and drug susceptibility. Thus, the results of estimated dynamic parameters based on this model should be more reliable and reasonable to interpret long-term HIV dynamics. Our models are simplified with the main goals of retaining crucial features of HIV dynamics and, at the same time, guaranteeing their applicability to typical clinical data, in particular, long-term viral load measurements.

We employed the proposed mechanism-based dynamic model to assess how to efficiently use adherence rates based on questionnaires and MEMS dosing events to predict virologic response. In particular, we intended to address the questions (i) how to summarize the MEMS adherence data for efficient prediction of virologic response, and (ii) which adherence assessment method, questionnaire or MEMS, is a more efficient predictor of virologic response after accounting for potential confounding factors such as drug resistance between subjects.

For the MEMS data, we found that the best summary metric for prediction of virologic response in terms of model fitting residuals (prediction error) is the adherence rate determined from MEMS dosing events averaged over a 2 week assessment interval, 1 week or 2 weeks prior to the next measured RNA observation (denoted by IM1.2 or IM2.2). The model fitting residuals from both models (IM2.2 and IM1.2) are significantly smaller than any other 13 models ($p \leq 0.001 \sim 0.048$), but they were not significantly different each other ($p=0.590$).

The model which used all available MEMS data between study visits to determine the adherence rate (the standard analysis) did not perform significantly better in terms of prediction of virologic response compared to the model with questionnaire adherence data ($p=0.106$).

We also compared the model fittings with all possible combinations of IC_{50} and the four determinants of adherence data (see Fig. 4). The results indicate that (i) the control model was significantly worse than those based on all other 9 models ($p \leq 0.001 \sim 0.007$); (ii) the models IM1.2 and IM2.2 were significantly better than the eight other models ($p \leq 0.001 \sim 0.048$); (iii) the models I, A, M, M1.2, M2.2, IA and IM do not provide significantly different results ($p=0.048 \sim 0.858$) except for two marginally significant results. In particular, the models IA and IM did not improve upon the model I, which indicates that adherence measured by questionnaire and MEMS dosing events averaged over study visit interval did not provide any additional information to drug susceptibility in predicting virologic response. However, the models IM1.2 and IM2.2 did outperform the models I, M1.2 and M2.2, which indicates that the combination of drug susceptibility and adherence assessed over 2 week interval measured from 1 or 2 weeks prior to a RNA measurement provided significant additional information compared to either drug susceptibility or adherence alone in predicting virologic response.

Although the analysis presented here used a simplified model, which appeared to perform well in capturing and explaining the observed patterns, and characterizing the biological mechanisms of HIV infection under relatively complex clinical situations, some limitations exist for the proposed modeling method. Firstly, our model is a simplified model and there are many possible variations (Perelson and Nelson, 1999; Nowak and May, 2000; Callaway and Perelson, 2002). We did not separately consider the compartments of short-lived productively infected cells, long-lived and latently infected cells.(Perelson et al., 1997). Instead we examined a pooled productively infected cell population. The virus compartment was not further decomposed into infectious virions and non-infectious virions as in the paper by Perelson *et al.* (1996). Thus, different mechanisms of RTI and PI drug effects were not modeled. In fact, we only considered PI drug effects in the drug efficacy model (3) since the RTI drugs have a different adherence-resistance relationship. Further studies will be conducted in considering both PI and RTI drug effects in the models. Secondly, the availability of IC_{50} data was limited to baseline and failure time, as is typical in clinical trials. Thus, we extrapolated the IC_{50} data linearly to the whole treatment period in our modeling. The linear extrapolation is the best approximation that we can get from the sparse IC_{50} data (Wu et al., 2005). The linear assumption might have some influence on the estimation results since the IC_{50} might have jumped to a higher level earlier before the failure time when we obtained the sample for drug resistance test. However, we expect that this assumption had little effect on the prediction of virologic response since we had relatively frequent monitoring (monthly in the later stage) of virologic failure in this study. Thirdly, a more complete model of antiretroviral treatment efficacy would ideally also consider the time-varying function of concentrations of drug in plasma (Huang et al., 2003). Unfortunately, the limited availability of drug concentration data prohibited our inclusion of PK parameters in our model. Lastly, as measurements of adherence may not reflect actual adherence profiles for individual patients, the data quality would affect our estimation results for viral dynamic parameters. For example, adherence data measured by questionnaires may not be accurate. More accurate measurements of the MEMS adherence data were used in this paper and it was found that the MEMS adherence data can provide a better prediction of virologic response compared with the questionnaire adherence data, when the MEMS data are summarized in an appropriate way. Further studies on these issues are definitely needed. Nevertheless, these limitations would not offset the major findings from our modeling approach, although further improvement may be warranted.

In summary, MEMS adherence data may not be correlated better to virologic response compared to questionnaire adherence data unless the MEMS cap data are summarized in an appropriate way where adherence was assessed over 2 week interval measured from 1 or 2 weeks prior to a RNA measurement in our case. Our study also shows that the mechanism-based dynamic model is powerful and effective to establish a relationship of antiviral response with drug exposure and drug susceptibility.

6. Acknowledgment

The author would like to thank the ACTG398 study team for allowing me to use the clinical data from their study. This research was partially supported by NIAID/NIH grant AI080338 and MSP/NSA grant H98230-09-1-0053.

7. References

Arnsten, J.; Demas, P. & Gourvetch, M.; et al. (February, 2001a). Adherence and viral load in HIV infected drug users: Comparison of self-report and medication event monitors (MEMS). 8th CROI. Chicago, USA

Arnsten, J. H.; Demas, P. A.; Farzadegan, H.; et al. (2001b). Antiretroviral therapy adherence and viral suppression in HIV-infected drug users: comparison of self-report and electronic monitoring. *Clinical Infectious Diseases*, Vol.33, pp.1417-1423

Bangsberg, D. R.; Hecht, F. M.; Charlebois, E. D.; et al. (March, 2000). Adherence to protease inhibitors, HIV-1 viral load, and development of drug resistance in an indigent population. *AIDS,* Vol.14, No.4, pp.357-366

Bangsberg, D. R. (2006). Less than 95% adherence to nonnucleoside reverse-transcriptase inhibitor therapy can lead to viral suppression. *Clinical Infectious Diseases*, Vol.43, pp.939–941

Berg, K. M. & Arnsten, J. H. (2006). Practical and conceptual challenges in measuring antiretroviral adherence. *J Acquir Immune Defic Syndr.*, Vol.43, pp.S79-S87

Bova, C. A.; Fennie, K. P.; Knafl, G. J.; et al. (2005). Use of electronic monitoring devices to measure antiretroviral adherence: practical considerations. *AIDS and Behavior*, Vol.9, pp.103-110

Callaway, D. S. & Perelson, A. S. (2002). HIV-1 infection and low steady state viral loads. *Bull. Math. Biol.*, Vol.64, pp.29–64

Centers for Disease Control and Prevention (CDC). (2009). *HIV/AIDS Surveillance Report*, pp.1-44, Atlanta, GA, USA

Davidian, M. & Giltinan, D. M. (Eds). (1005). *Nonlinear Models for Repeated Measurement Data*. Chapman & Hall, London

Ding, A. A. & Wu, H. (2001). Assessing antiviral potency of anti-HIV therapies *in vivo* by comparing viral decay rates in viral dynamic models. *Biostatistics*. Vol.2, pp.13-29

Dixit, N. M.; Markowitz, M.; Ho DD; et al. (2004). Estimates of intracellular delay and average drug efficacy from viral load data of HIV-infected individuals under antiretroviral therapy. *Antiviral Therapy*. Vol.9, pp.237-246

Fennie, K. P.; Bova, C. A. & Williams, A. B. (2006). Adjusting and censoring electronic monitoring device data. Implications for study outcomes. *J Acquir Immune Defic Syndr.*, Vol.43, pp.S88-S95

Fletcher, C. V.; Testa, M. A.; Brundage, R. C.; et al. (2005). Four measures of antiretroviral medication adherence and virologic response in AIDS clinical trials group study 359. *J Acquir Immune Defic Syndr.* , Vol.40, pp.301-306

Gamerman, D. (1997). *Markov Chain Monte Carlo: Stochastic Simulation for Bayesian Inference*. Chapman & Hall, London

Hammer, S. M.; Vaida, F.; Bennett, K. K.; et al. (2002). Dual vs single protease inhibitor therapy following antiretroviral treatment failure: a randomized trial. *JAMA*, Vol.288, pp.169–180

Han, C.; Chaloner, K. & Perelson, A. S. (2002). Bayesian analysis of a population HIV dynamic model. *Case Studies in Bayesian Statistics, Vol. 6*. Springer-Verlag, New York

Haubrich, R. H.; Little, S. J.; Currier, J. S.; et al. (1999). The value of patient-reported adherence to antiretroviral therapy in predicting virologic and immunologic response. *AIDS*, Vol.13, pp.1099-1107

Ho, D. D.; Neumann, A. U.; Perelson, A. S.; et al. (1995). Rapid turnover of plasma virions and CD4 lymphocytes in HIV-1 infection. *Nature*, Vol.373, pp.123–126

Huang, Y.; Rosenkranz, S. L. & Wu, H. (2003). Modeling HIV dynamics and antiviral responses with consideration of time-varying drug exposures, sensitivities and adherence. *Math. Biosci.*, Vol.184, pp.165–86

Huang, Y.; Liu, D. & Wu, H. (2006). Hierarchical Bayesian methods for estimation of parameters in a longitudinal HIV dynamic system. *Biometrics*, Vol.62, pp.413-423

Huang, Y., Wu, H. & Acosta, P. E. (2010). Hierarchical Bayesian inference for HIV dynamic differential equation models incorporating multiple treatment factors. *Biometrical Journal*, Vol.52, No.4, pp.470–486

Ickovics, J. R. & Meisler, A. W. (1997). Adherence in AIDS clinical trial: a framework for clinical research and clinical care. *J Clin Epidemiol.*, Vol., pp.385–391

Kastrissios, H.; Suarez, J. R.; Katzenstein, D.; et al. (1998). Characterizing patterns of drug-taking behavior with a multiple drug regimen in an AIDS clinical trial. *AIDS*, Vol.12, pp.2295–2303

Knafl, G. J.; Fennie, K. P.; Bova, C.; et al. (2004). Electronic monitoring device event modeling on an individual-subject basis using adaptive Poisson regression. *Statistics in Medicine*, Vol.23, pp.783-801

Levine, A. J.; Hinkin, C. H.; Marion, S.; et al. (2006). Adherence to antiretroviral medications in HIV: differences in data collected via self-report and electronic monitoring. *Health Psychol.* , Vol.25, pp.329-35

Llabre, M. M.; Weaver, K. E.; Duran, R. E.; et al.(2006). A measurement model of medication adherence to highly active antiretroviral therapy and its relation to viral load in HIV-positive adults. *AIDS Patient Care STDS.*, Vol.20, pp.701-711

Liu, H.; Golin, C. E.; Miller, L. G.; et al. (2001). A comparison study of multiple measures of adherence to HIV protease inhibitors. *Ann Intern Med.* , Vol.134, pp.968-77

Liu, H.; Miller, L. G.; Hays, R. D.; et al. (2006). Repeated measures longitudinal analyses of HIV virologic response as a function of percent adherence, dose timing, genotypic sensitivity, and other factors. *J Acquir Immune Defic Syndr.* , Vol.41, pp.315-322

Liu, H.; Miller, L. G.; Golin, C.E.; et al. (2007). Repeated measures analyses of dose timing of antiretroviral medication and its relationship to HIV virologic outcomes. *Statistics in Medicine*, Vol.26, pp.991-1007

Markowitz, M.; Louie, M.; Hurley, A.; et al. (2003). A novel antiviral intervention results in more accurate assessment of human immunodeficiency virus type 1 replication dynamics and T-cell decay in vivo. *Journal of Virology*, Vol.77, pp.5037–5038

Molla, A.; Korneyeva, M.; Gao, Q.; et al. (1996). Ordered accumulation of mutations in HIV protease confers resistance to ritonavir. *Nat Med.*, Vol.2, pp.760-766

Nowak, M. A. & May, R.M. (Eds). (2000). *Virus Dynamics: Mathematical Principles of Immunology and Virology*. Oxford University Press, Oxford

Notermans, D. W.; Goudsmit, J.; Danner, S.A.; et al. (1998). Rate of HIV-1 decline following antiretroviral therapy is related to viral load at baseline and drug regimen. *J Acquir Immune Defic Syndr.*, Vol.12, pp.1483-1490

Palella, F. J.; Delaney, K. M; Moorman, A. C.; et al. (1998). Declining morbidity and mortality among patients with advanced human immunodeficiency virus infection. *The New England Journal of Medicine*, Vol.338, No.13, pp. 853-860, ISSN 0028-4793

Paterson, D. L.; Swindells, S.; Mohr, J.; et al. (2000). Adherence to protease inhibitor therapy and outcomes in patients with HIV infection. *J Intern Med.*, Vol.133, pp.21-30

Pearson, C. R.; Simoni, J. M.; Hoff, P.; et al. (2007). Assessing antiretroviral adherence via electronic drug monitoring and self-report: an examination of key methodological issues. *AIDS and Behavior*, Vol.11, pp.161-173

Perelson, A. S.; Neumann, A. U.; Markowitz, M.; et al. (1996). HIV-1 dynamics in vivo: virion clearance rate, infected cell life-span, and viral generation time. *Science*, Vol.271, pp.1582–1586

Perelson, A. S.; Essunger, P.; Cao, Y.; et al. (1997). Decay characteristics of HIV-1-infected compartments during combination therapy. *Nature*, Vol.387, pp.188–191

Perelson, A. S. & Nelson, P. W. (1999). Mathematical analysis of HIV-1 dynamics in vivo. *SIAM Review*, Vol.41, pp.3-44

Pfister, M.; Labbé, L.; Hammer, S. M.; et al. (2003). Population Pharmacokinetics and Pharmacodynamics of Efavirenz, Nelfinavir, and Indinavir: Adult AIDS Clinical Trial Group Study 398. *Antimicrob Agents Chemoter.*, Vol.47, pp130-137

Sheiner, L. B. (1985). Modeling pharmacodynamics: parametric and nonparametric approaches. In: Rowland M, et al, eds. *Variability in Drug Therapy: Description, Estimation, and Control*. pp.139-152, Raven Press, New York.

Vrijens, B. & Goetghebeur, E. (1997). Comparing compliance patterns between randomized treatments. *Control Clin Trials.* , Vol.18, pp.187-203

Vrijens, B.; Goetghebeur, E.; de Klerk, E.; et al. (2005). Modelling the association between adherence and viral load in HIV-infected patients. *Statistics in Medicine*, Vol.24, pp.2719-2731

Wakefield, J. C. (1996). The Bayesian approach to population Pharmacokinetic models. *Journal of the American Statistical Association*, Vol.91, pp.61–76

Wu, H. & Ding, A. A. (1999). Population HIV-1 dynamics in vivo: applicable models and inferential tools for virological data from AIDS clinical trials. *Biometrics*, Vol.55, pp.410-418

Wu, H.; Kuritzkes, D. R.; McClernon, D. R.; et al. (1999). Characterization of viral dynamics in Human Immunodeficiency Virus Type 1-infected patients treated with combination antiretroviral therapy: relationships to host factors, cellular restoration and virological endpoints. *Journal of Infectious Diseases*, Vol.179, pp.799–807

Wu, H.; Huang, Y.; Acosta E. P.; et al. (2005). Modeling long-term HIV dynamics and antiretroviral response: effects of drug potency, pharmacokinetics, adherence and drug resistance. *J Acquir Immune Defic Syndr.*, Vol.39, pp.272-283

Part 2

Developing New Antivirals

5

Use of Animal Models for Anti-HIV Drug Development

Zandrea Ambrose
University of Pittsburgh, USA

1. Introduction

Animal models serve as important tools for preclinical testing of therapeutic regimens against human immunodeficiency virus (HIV-1), the primary etiologic agent that causes acquired immunodeficiency syndrome (AIDS). Infection and treatment of patients often cannot be controlled in clinical studies. In addition, performing certain procedures and sampling cannot be routinely performed in humans with ease and may be unethical. There are many different primate and murine models of HIV/AIDS, each with their advantages and disadvantages. Some models are appropriate in certain contexts but not others. Knowing how the different models work and their limitations will help guide the researcher to select the appropriate model to answer a specific question. Information gained from the use of preclinical testing of antiretroviral therapies will help identify and improve preventive, therapeutic, and eradication strategies against HIV/AIDS in humans.

2. HIV-1 infection of nonhuman primates or humanized mice: Which is the better model to use?

An animal model for human disease should mimic the infection of humans as closely as possible. The disease course in the model should be similar to or more accelerated than in humans. In the case of HIV-1, an animal model that progresses to AIDS over the period of many years will cost time and money in preclinical studies. The use of animals instead of humans usually means certain procedures can be performed more easily and/or ethically. For example, removing vital organs to study pathogenesis, drug penetration, immunity, or virology cannot be performed in humans but can be done after necropsy of an animal. Moreover, unlike in humans, the exact virus, timing of infection, and timing of treatment can be controlled in a model.

HIV-1 does not efficiently replicate in most animals, including nonhuman primates. This is due to differences in host cell factors present in different species that are required for infection or due to innate immunity that appears to have evolved in mammals to ward off infections. Thus, either modification to HIV-1 or to the animal must be made for significant viral replication to occur. This is important for assessing the efficacy of experimental interventions for inhibiting the virus rather than spontaneous control by the host immune system.

2.1 Nonhuman primate models

Nonhuman primates are genetically and anatomically most similar to humans and would be the obvious choice for an animal model to study HIV-1. While HIV-1 is believed to have arisen from cross-species transmission of simian immunodeficiency virus (SIV) strains from chimpanzees and gorillas to humans (Keele et al., 2006; Van Heuverswyn et al., 2006), these animals are not routinely used for HIV research. These great apes are both endangered and very large. And although HIV-1 has been used in the past to infect chimpanzees in captivity, it does not cause significant disease for more than a decade (Novembre et al., 1997). Thus, this is an impractical model for testing treatments and vaccines against the virus.

Macaques, a genus of Old World monkeys, are routinely bred at primate centers and have been extensively investigated as HIV models. HIV-1 inoculation of macaques does not lead to productive infection, mainly due to restriction by simian innate immune factors, such as APOBEC3G and TRIM5α, that target HIV-1 (Mariani et al., 2003; Stremlau et al., 2004). SIV is a primate lentivirus that is similar to HIV-1 and highly homologous to HIV type 2 (HIV-2), which was isolated from rhesus macaques at a primate facility (Daniel et al., 1985; Kanki et al., 1985). SIV infection of macaques is believed to have been another cross-species transmission during captivity from infected African primates (Hirsch et al., 1989), leading to pathogenesis similar to AIDS but in a more accelerated time frame as compared to HIV-1 infection of humans. In addition, adaptive immune responses against SIV in macaques are similar to anti-HIV-1 responses seen in humans (Sato and Johnson, 2007; Valentine and Watkins, 2008). The most widely used species of macaques for HIV/AIDS models are rhesus (*Macaca mulatta*), cynomolgus (*M. fasicularis*), and pigtailed (*M. nemestrina*).

While SIV shares high structural and sequence identity to HIV-1, the differences are significant enough to limit the design of both vaccines and therapy against the human virus. Therefore, HIV-1 sequences have been added into the SIV genome to make chimeric viruses, called SHIVs, which can still replicate well within macaques (Fig. 1). The first examples of SHIVs were SIV strains that encoded HIV-1 envelope in place of SIV envelope, such that vaccines or drugs could target this entry protein (Li et al., 1992; Luciw et al., 1995; Reimann et al., 1996; Shibata et al., 1991). More recently, the reverse transcriptase (RT) coding region of SIVs have been replaced with that of HIV-1 to produce RT-SHIV that can be targeted by RT inhibitors (Ambrose et al., 2004; Uberla et al., 1995). Both types of SHIVs have been shown to infect macaques after mucosal exposure, simulating sexual transmission (Lu et al., 1996; Turville et al., 2008). Simian-tropic HIV-1 (stHIV-1) viruses have been made that contain minimal SIV sequences (capsid and Vif coding regions) to circumvent restriction from APOBEC3G and TRIM5α, but they suffered significant decreases in replication in the host compared to SIV or the previously described SHIVs, likely due to differences in the accessory proteins of HIV-1 as compared to SIV (Hatziioannou et al., 2009; Igarashi et al., 2007).

Baboons and other species of Old World monkeys have also been used as nonhuman primate models for studying HIV infection and AIDS. Baboons could be productively infected with HIV-2 but showed little pathogenesis (Barnett et al., 1994). African green monkeys and sooty mangabeys are naturally infected with SIV but do not experience disease despite very high levels of viremia. These animals are studied for their differences to Asian macaques to understand chronic, pathogenic SIV/HIV infection (Paiardini et al., 2009).

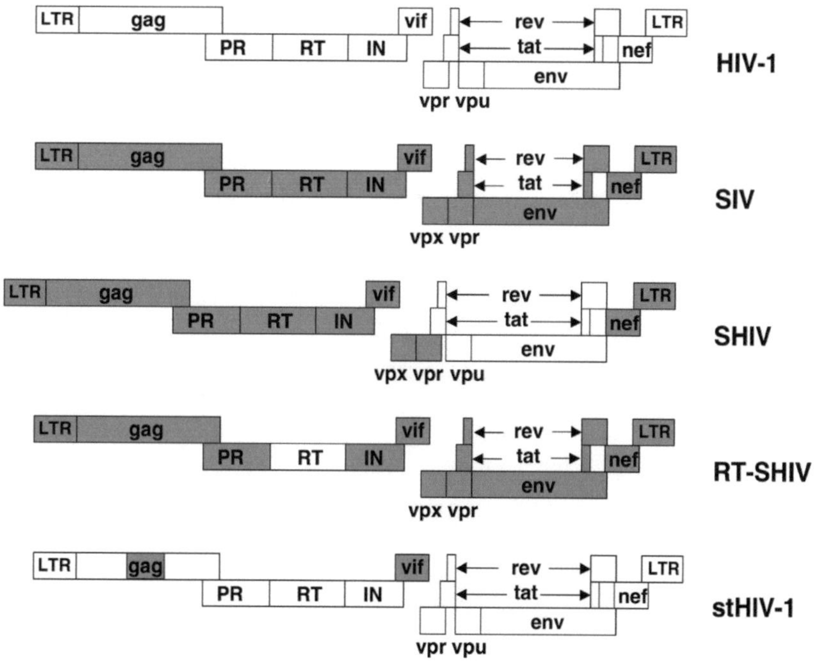

Fig. 1. Diagram of the genomes of HIV-1, SIV, and chimeric viruses used in macaques. White color denotes HIV-1 sequences, while gray shading denotes SIV sequences.

2.2 Humanized mouse models

The strengths of murine models for biomedical research are the small size of mice and their relatively low cost, making it feasible to have increased numbers of animals in experiments for greater statistical power. However, HIV-1 encounters multiple barriers in the infection of mouse cells, beginning with the inability of the virus to use the murine CD4 receptor and co-receptors. To overcome these issues, scientists reconstituted a partial human immune system in severe combined immunodeficient (SCID) mice lacking lymphocytes by engrafting them with human peripheral blood lymphocytes or human fetal thymus and liver (Mosier et al., 1988; Namikawa et al., 1990). However, while peripheral T cell subsets could be reconstituted temporarily in these SCID-hu mice, they were not detected to a great extent in tissues. In addition, other human immune cells did not develop and only transient HIV-1 replication could be detected in vivo.

Due to the limitations of SCID-hu mice, new advances in humanized murine models have been made to better reconstitute a human immune system and to lead to sustained HIV-1 replication. First, the addition of the SCID mutation into the nonobese diabetic strain (NOD/SCID), which lacks the IL-2 receptor γ-chain, resulted in mice without T, B, and NK cells. With the implantation of human $CD34^+$ hematopoietic stem cells into these mice, they developed human lymphocytes and dendritic cells in the blood and in multiple lymphoid tissues. Thus, HIV-1 infection could be sustained at high levels for more than 40 days (Watanabe et al., 2007). Similarly, transplantation of human fetal bone marrow (containing $CD34^+$ cells), liver, and thymus (BLT) into NOD/SCID mice could also generate functional human T, B, and dendritic cells in both the periphery and tissues. These animals could stably maintain HIV-1 replication after intrarectal or intravaginal challenge (Denton et al., 2008; Sun et al., 2007). However, NOD/SCID mice develop thymic lymphomas, resulting in a limited lifespan (Shultz et al., 1995).

Another humanized mouse model utilizes Rag2$^{-/-}\gamma C^{-/-}$ double knockout mice, which also lack T, B, and NK cells. These mice can also be reconstituted with CD34^{+} hematopoietic stem cells, leading to development of human T, B, and dendritic cells in the blood and different lymphoid tissues (Traggiai et al., 2004). The animals could be infected with HIV-1 and had detectable viremia for more than 27 weeks (Baenziger et al., 2006). Like the BLT model, Rag2$^{-/-}\gamma C^{-/-}$ mice also had CD4^{+} target cells in mucosal tissues and could be infected intrarectally or intravaginally (Berges et al., 2008).

Macaques		Humanized CD34^{+} reconstituted mice	
Advantages	**Disadvantages**	**Advantages**	**Disadvantages**
Similar viral pathogenesis to humans	Genetically different than humans	Target cells are human	Lack of macro-phages (Rag2/$\gamma C^{-/-}$) and robust anti-retroviral immunity
Similar antiviral immune responses to humans	Requires SIV or SHIV	Can use different HIV-1 strains	Small tissue/blood samples
Long-term viral persistence during suppressive anti-retroviral therapy	Expensive and requires trained veterinary staff	Can create genetic-ally identical animals with cells from same donor	Requires access to donor tissues and ability to perform transplants
Access to large tissue/blood samples	Large size requiring more drugs	Less overall cost	Anatomically diff-erent than humans
Longer lifespan		Small size allows the use of less drugs	Limited lifespan, especially BLT

Table 1. Advantages and disadvantages to simian and murine models of HIV/AIDS

2.3 What virus should be used with which model?

With a wide array of simian and murine models of HIV/AIDS, it is difficult to know which one to use to answer a scientific question. Each model has its advantages and disadvantages (Table 1). Depending on the question, one has to weigh the pros and cons that may affect the results in deciding which model and which virus to employ. For example, macaques are more anatomically similar to humans and studying drug penetration into tissues or inhibition of virus in tissues, such as microbicides, may be more relevant in the monkey model. However, at this time HIV-1 replication is very limited in simians, necessitating the use of SIV or SHIVs. Therefore, drugs targeting viral proteins or virus-host cell protein interactions may be limited with these viruses and may require the use of HIV-1 in mice. Although mice are smaller and cheaper than monkeys, humanized murine models require significant expertise and human donors for tissue implantation and stem cell reconstitution that may not be more cost-effective for the investigator. The rest of the chapter will discuss the use of both simian and murine models for preclinical studies of anti-HIV therapies.

3. Therapy for HIV-1 prevention in animal models

As there is no cure for HIV-1 yet, efforts have been made to develop and evaluate compounds that would prevent HIV-1 infection prior to or immediately after exposure to the virus. These differ from vaccines in that they are not designed to elicit antiviral immunity in advance of exposure, but rather would inhibit the virus before, during, or just after exposure to HIV-1 to avoid systemic infection. Pre-exposure prophylaxis would be initiated in high-risk individuals likely to be exposed to HIV-1, whereas post-exposure prophylaxis would be used in individuals who were believed to be recently exposed to the virus. Animal models have been used rather extensively over the past decade in this area of research with generally positive results. Unlike in clinical trials, the timing and adherence of treatment and the timing of virus challenge can be controlled in the model.

3.1 Pre-exposure prophylaxis

The majority of prevention therapy studies have focused on pre-exposure prophylaxis, or microbicides, against mucosal transmission of virus. This is particularly relevant in areas of the world where people, especially women, often are unable to control their partners' use of condoms during sexual intercourse. Thus, a compound that can be applied mucosally or taken orally could inhibit HIV-1 infection either by targeting the virus or targeting viral interaction with host cell factors necessary for viral replication.

3.1.1 Toxicity of mucosal drug application

Generally, compounds that inhibit HIV-1 are discovered and characterized *in vitro*. Before going to clinical trials for efficacy testing, tolerability and toxicity studies in animals or people are often performed. In the case of topically applied microbicides, this entails determining whether a drug causes disruption of the mucosal epithelial layer that forms an intact barrier against incoming pathogens. The need for toxicity testing was made dramatically clear in the case of nonoxynol-9 (N-9), which was halted in clinical trials as a potential anti-HIV topical microbicide due to toxic effects that made users more susceptible to HIV-1 infection. N-9, a nonionic detergent present in some contraceptive gels, was shown long ago to inhibit viral replication *in vitro* (Hicks et al., 1985). Several clinical studies of N-9 use in women during vaginal sexual intercourse suggested that it slightly increased the risk for HIV-1 seroconversion (Wilkinson et al., 2002). There were discrepancies on whether or not N-9 caused toxicity in the female genital tract, which may have been due to poor adherence and inappropriate application of the product. A careful study in the pigtailed macaque model showed that N-9 caused genital tissue damage (Patton et al., 1999).

The female genital tract consists of stratified squamous epithelial cells (vagina and ectocervix) and simple columnar epithelium (endocervix), while the GI tract consists only of a single layer of columnar epithelial cells. Trials of N-9 for rectal use showed that histological abnormalities occurred in almost 90% of the subjects (Tabet et al., 1999) and caused rapid exfoliation of the rectal epithelium (Phillips et al., 2000). Similar results were also observed in pigtailed macaques (Patton et al., 2002), suggesting that safety testing is necessary for microbicides prior to initiating clinical studies to prevent enhanced HIV-1 transmission.

Inflammation and toxicity markers and their correlation, or lack thereof, with complete protection from transmission are still incompletely defined. Administration of a foreign compound is likely to induce innate immune responses. This is also the initial response of the body in countering HIV-1 immediately following exposure. Maintaining normal, intact tissue and normal microflora at mucosal sites during use of a topical microbicide will continue to be a challenge. And the use of oral drugs that can penetrate tissues also will need to be evaluated for safety and lack of mucosal toxicity.

3.1.2 Therapeutic prevention studies

Many compounds have been tested as pre-exposure prophylaxis in animal models prior to intravaginal, intrarectal, or oral exposure of virus. Such preventive drugs can be nonspecific to HIV-1 or specific antiretroviral compounds. Intravaginal or intrarectal transmission of HIV-1 occurs during sexual contact, while oral transmission may contribute to infection of infants during vaginal delivery. While both macaque and humanized mouse models have been useful for mucosal viral transmission, HIV-1 can only be used to infect humanized mice. Macaques can be infected effectively with chimeric SHIV viruses containing HIV-1 envelope or RT. And the anatomy of nonhuman primates, including the gastrointestinal and genital tracts, is more similar to that of humans.

The majority of such pre-exposure prophylaxis studies have been performed with various levels of success in female macaques for the prevention of vaginal transmission. Compounds tested in macaque models have aimed to interfere with nonspecific viral attachment (Ambrose et al., 2008; Boadi et al., 2005; Kenney et al., 2011; Kim et al., 2006; Lagenaur et al., 2011; Li et al., 2009; Manson et al., 2000; Tevi-Benissan et al., 2000; Tsai et al., 2004; Wyand et al., 1999), specific interactions of envelope with receptor/co-receptors (Kish-Catalone et al., 2007; Lederman et al., 2004; Mascola et al., 2000; Parren et al., 2001; Veazey et al., 2008; Veazey et al., 2010; Veazey et al., 2003a; Veazey et al., 2005a; Veazey et al., 2009; Veazey et al., 2003b; Veazey et al., 2005b), and reverse transcription (Kenney et al., 2011; Parikh et al., 2009; Stolte-Leeb et al., 2011; Turville et al., 2008). Another study investigated hormone treatment, which leads to thickening of the vaginal epithelium, to prevent vaginal transmission of SIV in macaques (Smith et al., 2000b). More recently, the humanized mouse model has been used to prevent intravaginal transmission, using drugs targeting RT (Denton et al., 2008; Denton et al., 2011), integrase (Neff et al., 2011a), the CCR5 co-receptor (Neff et al., 2011a; Neff et al., 2010), and viral protein expression (Wheeler et al., 2011).

Fewer studies have evaluated compounds that prevent intrarectal or oral transmission of HIV-1 or SHIVs. The FDA-approved RT inhibitor tenofovir was successful in preventing intrarectal transmission of SIV in macaques (Cranage et al., 2008) and of HIV-1 in humanized mice (Denton et al., 2010). Also, a novel RT inhibitor (Singer et al., 2011) and a nonspecific envelope attachment inhibitor (Tsai et al., 2003) were used to prevent intrarectal transmission of SHIVs in macaques. For prevention of oral viral transmission, only macaque models have been used. First, neutralizing antibodies were shown to be protective in neonates (Baba et al., 2000). More recently, subcutanously administered tenofovir was found to be somewhat protective against oral SIV challenge (Van Rompay et al., 2006; Van Rompay et al., 2001) while an oral tenofovir solution was ineffective (Van Rompay et al., 2006; Van Rompay et al., 2002b).

While most of these studies have focused on topical gels and novel compounds, oral FDA-approved antiretroviral compounds have been investigated recently as pre-exposure prophylaxis. Tenofovir prevents HIV-1 replication, it is already approved for use in humans in the oral formulation, and high drug concentrations can be achieved in the male and female genital tracts (Kwara et al., 2008; Vourvahis et al., 2008). The use of a gel may not provide complete coverage of the mucosal surface, possibly leading to breakthrough infections. The CAPRISA 004 clinical trial recently showed a 39% overall reduction in HIV-1 incidence in women using a vaginal tenofovir gel (Abdool Karim et al., 2010). The iPrEx and TDF2 trials showed that oral tenofovir in combination with another RT inhibitor, emtracitabine (FTC), reduced transmission in men who have sex with men (Grant et al., 2010) or in heterosexual men and women (Roehr, 2011) by 44% and 63%, respectively. It is unclear whether the greater efficacy in the latter studies as compared to the CAPRISA 004 study was due to oral administration of drug or use of two drugs instead of tenofovir alone. In macaques, intermittent dosing (2 hours before and 24 hours after challenge) of tenofovir alone or with FTC was equally as effective as daily dosing during weekly repeated low-dose rectal challenges (Garcia-Lerma et al., 2008). Less frequent doses would reduce cost to the user and would not require strict daily adherence. However, breakthrough infections in 2 of 6 animals resulted in drug resistant viruses, which could potentially compromise future therapy.

Interestingly, with the exception of tenofovir or tenofovir/FTC, no other microbicides have been successful in the clinic. It remains to be seen whether or not this is due to a specific property of tenofovir or RT inhibitors in general. Tenofovir acts specifically on viral reverse transcription, whereas most other microbicides tested clinically were nonspecific entry inhibitors. Also, tenofovir is the only drug that has been tested with repeated low-dose SIV oral, intravaginal, and intrarectal challenges in macaques (Garcia-Lerma et al., 2008; Parikh et al., 2009; Van Rompay et al., 2006). A nonspecific virus inactivating compound was tested in repeated high-dose intravaginal challenges 10-47 weeks apart, in which 90% of the animals were protected after the initial challenge (Ambrose et al., 2008). However, nearly all the animals became infected after the second challenge. It is unclear if noninfectious virus at the site of transmission elicits a detrimental immune response, inflammation, and/or an increase in target cells that can cause a subject to become more sensitized to infection.

Until recently, mucosal challenge of SIV or SHIV required high doses of virus to ensure that all or most of the control animals become infected. More and more investigators are using repeated low-dose challenges in animal studies to recapitulate more realistic levels of virus detected in semen of untreated HIV+ men. Semen viral RNA levels are often similar to or lower than in the blood (Gupta et al., 1997; Liuzzi et al., 1996), but are significantly lower than those of laboratory stocks used in high-dose challenges (Marthas et al., 2001). Also, high-risk individuals may be exposed multiple times prior to becoming infected. A direct comparison of a high-dose challenge and repeated low-dose rectal challenges in a small study on oral tenofovir pre-exposure prophylaxis showed that the low-dose model was actually somewhat more stringent (Subbarao et al., 2007). The disadvantage of the low-dose model is that multiple challenges are required to infect untreated control monkeys, and this number varies significantly among animals. This can affect statistics and often leads to longer experiments, which can increase study costs.

3.2 Post-exposure prophylaxis

Most post-exposure prophylaxis research has focused on entry and reverse transcription inhibitors that target the earliest steps of HIV-1 replication. Tenofovir was the first successful drug used for post-exposure treatment in the macaque model against intravenous challenge of SIV (Tsai et al., 1995). Animals did not become infected when daily tenofovir treatment was initiated 4 or 24 hours post-challenge, continuing for 4 weeks. A similar study with AZT did not show protection 3 hours after intravenous SIV inoculation (Fazely et al., 1991). Later, vaginal transmission was largely prevented in macaques after tenofovir treatment began 12 or 36 hours post-challenge but not after 72 hours (Otten et al., 2000).

The other post-exposure prophylaxis method used in the macaque model has been passive transfer of neutralizing antibodies targeting HIV-1 envelope. Antibody transfer into macaques 6 hours post-infection with SHIV showed 75% protection, which declined to 50% after 24 hours (Nishimura et al., 2003). Multiple monoclonal antibodies were more successful than an individual antibody. Complete protection was also seen after antibody infusion 1 hour after oral SHIV challenge of neonates, which decreased after 12 or 24 hours (Ferrantelli et al., 2004).

While these post-exposure prophylaxis studies showed promise, highly pathogenic viruses may be more difficult to control. One study showed that a combination of neutralizing antibodies given to neonates at 1 hour and 8 days post-challenge led to 100% protection in animals infected with a SHIV, but did not protect animals from a more pathogenic virus (Hofmann-Lehmann et al., 2001). This same highly pathogenic virus also failed to be controlled by triple therapy of AZT, 3TC, and the protease inhibitor indinavir when initiated 4 hours after intravenous infection and continued for 14-28 days (Bourry et al., 2009; Le Grand et al., 2000). These studies noted that although most of the animals became infected, plasma viremia was reduced compared to the control animals, suggesting a partial protective effect of the treatment regimens.

3.3 Mother-to-child transmission prevention

Mother-to-child transmission (MTCT) of HIV-1 occurs via three mechanisms: *in utero* via virus transfer across the placenta, intrapartum presumably by oral inoculation of the infected mother's blood, and breastfeeding. An early clinical trial showed that AZT therapy of HIV-infected women during pregnancy and of infants in the first 6 weeks after birth led to a 67.5% reduction in MTCT (Connor et al., 1994).

In resource-rich nations, combination therapy is now the standard of care for pregnant women. However, the cost of multiple drugs and/or multiple doses of drugs poses a challenge in resource-limited countries. Thus, studies were conducted in which single doses of nevirapine were administered to women during labor (and sometimes to the infant) to prevent MTCT. Nevirapine, a non-nucleoside RT inhibitor, has less toxicity than AZT and has a long half-life (Musoke et al., 1999). Single-dose nevirapine treatment effectively reduced HIV-1 MTCT to a similar degree as multiple doses of AZT (Guay et al., 1999). Unfortunately, it was revealed that single-dose nevirapine caused the development of drug-resistant virus in the mothers and in infants that subsequently became infected (Eshleman et al., 2001), which could be present at low frequencies for long periods of time (Flys et al., 2005; Palmer et al., 2006). Such drug resistance compromised subsequent treatment in the mothers (Jourdain et al., 2004).

Few studies on MTCT have been performed in animal models. One study using a pregnant macaque model of MTCT showed that short-term combination therapy could successfully prevent *in utero* transmission of HIV-2 to the fetus/infant (Ho et al., 2000). SIV transmission in nonhuman primates via breastfeeding has been demonstrated and used to study tenofovir pharmacokinetics in breast milk (Van Rompay et al., 2005). However, this model has not be used in any therapeutic prevention studies. Oral inoculation macaque models have been used to study pre-exposure and post-exposure prophylaxis, as discussed above.

It appears that the first few hours after virus exposure is critical for using therapy to stop infection. This is important to minimize the spread of virus to new target cells. While most research has focused on a single inhibitor or class of inhibitors, it remains to be seen if drug combinations will afford more time to an exposed individual to prevent fulminant infection. Treatment of adults and infants, even when initiated immediately after exposure, may be ineffective if they have been exposed to drug-resistant or highly pathogenic viruses. This could be alleviated with combination therapy. Also, post-exposure treatment has generally been administered daily for 4 weeks. To save money and to avoid prolonged side effects from the drugs, can the duration of therapy be shortened and remain effective? Finally, will breakthrough infections result in selection of drug-resistant viruses, which could lead to virologic failure during subsequent antiretroviral treatment?

4. Animal models for new suppressive antiretrovirals, combinations, and deliveries

Animal models for antiretroviral research can be used to test novel compounds for their toxic properties, pharmacokinetics and bioavailability, and antiretroviral efficacy.

4.1 Toxicity, pharmacokinetics, tissue distribution

While it is impossible to document or list all antiretroviral pharmacokinetics and toxicity research in animals here, a few examples of early and new studies should be noted. Nucleoside analogs that inhibit reverse transcription, such as ddC (Kelley et al., 1987) and d4T (Keller et al., 1995), were tested in mice and monkeys for toxicity and pharmacokinetics. The short-term and long-term effects of tenofovir in newborn/infant macaques showed bone and kidney toxicities (Van Rompay et al., 2004). Also, non-nucleoside RT inhibitors, such as efavirenz, were tested in animals for pharmacokinetics (Balani et al., 1999). Investigators also developed drugs to the other HIV-1 enzymes: protease and integrase. While many of the protease inhibitors had poor efficacy against SIV, their pharmacokinetics could be assessed in animals, such as that of nelfinavir (Kaldor et al., 1997). Many integrase inhibitors were screened by Merck, leading to testing of many potential new compounds for good bioavailability in nonhuman primates and mice (Gardelli et al., 2007; Pace et al., 2007). Even HIV-1 entry inhibitors, such as SCH-D, which would later be named vicriviroc, were tested in mice and monkeys for general pharmacokinetics (Tagat et al., 2004). Also, maraviroc was studied for intrapartum pharmacokinetics and dynamics in pregnant macaques as a potential method to prevent MTCT (Winters et al., 2010).

4.2 Efficacy in viral inhibition

The virus and model used to test antiretroviral drug efficacy are dependent on the drug target. For example, due to sequence differences in the Gag protein, the maturation inhibitor bevirimat does not inhibit SIV (Zhou et al., 2004). Therefore, proof of concept *in vivo* studies were performed in a humanized mouse model to show drug inhibition against HIV-1 (Stoddart et al., 2007). Similarly, testing of a CCR5 inhibitor like maraviroc is best used with HIV-1 envelope. Therefore, nonhuman primate studies were performed with SHIV virus containing a CCR5-tropic envelope (Veazey et al., 2003a).

Many novel antiretroviral small molecule inhibitors have been characterized for efficacy against HIV, SIV, or SHIV in animal models, many leading to FDA approval or to more improved versions of the compounds (reviewed in Ambrose and KewalRamani, 2008; Van Rompay, 2010). For example, PMEA, a drug related to tenofovir, was found to inhibit SIV infection effectively in macaques (Balzarini et al., 1991). Unfortunately, PMEA was very toxic *in vivo*, which lead to the development of the related and less-toxic compound tenofovir (previously called PMPA), which has been studied extensively in monkeys for viral inhibition (Balzarini et al., 1991; Lifson et al., 2003; Smith et al., 2000a; Tsai et al., 1998). Another RT inhibitor, stavudine, was tested for antiretroviral properties in HIV-2-infected macaques (Watson et al., 1997). And after many years of screening compounds *in vitro*, a precursor to the first FDA-approved integrase inhibitor, raltegravir, was shown to be effective in viral inhibition in the macaque model (Hazuda et al., 2004).

While many exciting novel antiretroviral inhibitors are currently under investigation in *in vitro* models, general efficacy testing is not always performed in an animal model prior to clinical studies. This is due to the high costs associated with these experiments, particularly in macaques and humanized mice. The major advantage of an animal model is the ability to perform procedures that may exacerbate disease or that are highly invasive. These may not be ethical or easy to perform in humans. For example, treatment interruptions or intentional induction of drug resistance is likely to be harmful to an HIV-infected individual. However, understanding the effects of these procedures can lead to a better understanding of the development of drug resistance and its effects on subsequent treatment regimens. Also, obtaining organs, longitudinal blood or tissue samples, and specific time points after infection or therapy initiation cannot be acquired easily in people.

4.3 Drug resistance

Drug resistance in HIV-infected individuals arises from inadequate therapy, which could be the result of ineffective prescribed therapy or nonadherence. While most data on HIV-1 drug resistance have been obtained from clinical studies, the macaque model has been used to address various questions on the development and consequences of drug-resistant virus.

Because nucleoside analogs such as tenofovir and FTC inhibit SIV and have good pharmacokinetics in macaques, mutations to these drugs have been studied in the monkey model. The primary resistance mutation to FTC has been studied for its effects on *in vivo* viral virulence and fitness (Van Rompay et al., 2002a). Similarly, mutations conferring resistance to tenofovir were studied in SIV for their emergence and suppression *in vivo* during tenofovir monotherapy (Van Rompay et al., 2007). Resistant viruses were identified in macaques with breakthrough infections after intermittent tenofovir/FTC pre-exposure prophylaxis with intrarectal challenge (Garcia-Lerma et al., 2008). And FTC- and tenofovir-resistant SHIV mutants were created and tested for their mucosal transmissibility (Cong et al., 2011), presumably to determine the effects of tenofovir and FTC pre-exposure prophylaxis on transmitted drug-resistant virus.

RT-SHIVs were created to study non-nucleoside RT inhibitors, such as efavirenz, that are specific to HIV-1 but not to HIV-2 or SIV. Efavirenz monotherapy leads to the emergence of common resistance mutations that are seen in patients (Ambrose et al., 2007; Hofman et al., 2004). Efavirenz combined with tenofovir and FTC is a commonly prescribed combination therapy for HIV-infected individuals and was shown to be effective in reducing RT-SHIV plasma viremia in two species of macaques (Ambrose et al., 2007; North et al., 2005). Prior efavirenz resistance was shown to compromise combination therapy in one animal, leading to accumulation of FTC-resistant mutations in the virus and, ultimately, failure of therapy (Ambrose et al., 2007). This was similar to results described earlier in the single-dose nevirapine trials for prevention of MTCT. In addition, the RT-SHIV model allowed the study of viral subpopulation dynamics in animals, including those of drug-resistant viral variants (Shao et al., 2009).

While resistance to clinically used antiretrovirals, such as FTC, tenofovir, and efavirenz, are well documented, compounds for pre-exposure prophylaxis have also been evaluated *in vivo* for the ability to select for drug-resistant viruses. As stated earlier, breakthrough infections after FTC and tenofovir prophylaxis was demonstrated in macaques (Garcia-Lerma et al., 2008). Similarly, mutations in the SHIV envelope were observed in virus from a macaque after ineffective use of the topical entry inhibitor PSC-RANTES that conferred little or no resistance to the compound (Dudley et al., 2009). Monitoring of potential drug-resistant virus is critical in preclinical and clinical studies with new inhibitors, as resistance may negatively impact efficacy of future treatment regimens.

4.4 New delivery methods

One complication of HIV-1 infection is the presence of large numbers of infected cells within different tissues. Although discussed more in the next section, CD4+ target cells are present within lymphoid tissues, the brain, and multiple mucosal tissues. Drug penetration into these tissues is likely to be lower than in the blood, allowing viral replication to continue within tissues. Research on better drug delivery methods into different tissues has been ongoing. This will be especially important for methods to target drugs into mucosal tissues during pre-exposure prophylaxis and also persisting viral reservoirs.

While there may be many novel delivery methods in the pipeline, only a few have been tested *in vivo* to specifically prevent transmission of or reduce replication of HIV-1/2. One novel delivery method of antiretrovirals to tissues is the formation and administration of drug nanocomplexes. A protease inhibitor, indinavir, was formed into nanoparticles and delivered to HIV-2-infected macaques, leading to significantly increased lymph node lymphocyte drug concentrations as compared to animals given the drug orally (Kinman et al., 2003). Nanoparticles are often cleared from the blood and tissues by phagocytic cells, such as macrophages. As macrophages are infected by HIV-1, these cells have been proposed as a target for drug delivery and phagocytosis of drug by infected cells may be beneficial. A single intravenous dose of indinavir-containing nanoparticles in mice with HIV+ brain macrophages led to drug levels in the brain for up to 14 days and reduced virus replication in the brain (Dou et al., 2009). Nevertheless, optimization of nanocomplexes by coating their surfaces with polyethylene glycol resulted in sustained levels in the blood of mice and less clearing by macrophages (Levchenko et al., 2002).

Another newly developed technology is the silencing of protein expression by small interfering RNAs (siRNA). siRNA can be designed to target specific mRNA in cells for degradation, leading to loss of protein expression (Hammond et al., 2000; Zamore et al., 2000). Because siRNA can be designed specifically to silence almost any RNA, they have been proposed for treatment of various diseases, including HIV-1 infection. However, targeting siRNA to specific cell types, to infected cells, and into tissues has been challenging, as they do not easily cross the plasma membrane and are quickly degraded by nucleases. Therefore, different delivery methods have been explored for more optimal targeting of siRNA to HIV-infected cells. For example, siRNA were bound to an antibody fragment that recognized HIV-1 envelope. These antibody-siRNA molecules were able to specifically target and enter envelope-expressing cells in mice (Song et al., 2005). And many techniques for introducing siRNA into nanoparticles have been tested for better pharmacokinetics, but these have been mainly preclinical studies not involving HIV-1 (reviewed in Yuan et al., 2011).

More recently, another method of delivering siRNA has been tested in both humanized mouse models to inhibit HIV-1 infection. RNA aptamer-siRNA chimeras were generated such that the aptamer portion would selectively bind to a cell surface molecule, delivering the siRNA to target cells (McNamara et al., 2006). RNA aptamers are oligonucleotides that are designed to bind tightly to specific proteins (Ellington and Szostak, 1990; Tuerk and Gold, 1990). One group used a mixture of chimeric RNAs with a CD4-binding aptamer and with siRNA targeting mRNA encoding the HIV-1 co-receptor CCR5 and viral proteins as a topical vaginal microbicide in BLT mice (Wheeler et al., 2011). The drug was able reduce CCR5 expression *in vivo* and resulted in a significant reduction of virus transmission. Another group used chimeric RNAs with HIV-1 envelope-binding aptamers and siRNA targeting multiple HIV-1 mRNA (Neff et al., 2011b). They were injected into HIV-1-infected Rag2$^{-/-}\gamma$C$^{-/-}$ humanized mice, leading to a significant reduction of both plasma viremia and CD4+ cell depletion.

The development of novel drugs and drug delivery methods is important for HIV-1 research. First, toxicity and adverse side effects of existing antiretrovirals are not trivial and should be improved to promote better adherence. Second, a lack of adherence will lead to drug resistance, which can affect multiple available treatment regimens. Third, improved prevention strategies will be necessary in the absence of a cure and in curbing the spread of HIV-1 infection among high-risk individuals. Lastly, as discussed below, targeting of new drugs to tissues to eliminate infected cells is an exciting possibility only recently realized.

5. Animal models for targeting persisting viral reservoirs

There is no cure for HIV-1. While HIV-infected individuals can suppress plasma viremia to undetectable levels with effective therapy, infected cells remain in the body and virus will return to the blood if therapy is halted or drug-resistance arises. The cells and tissues that harbor proviral DNA are considered viral reservoirs and are not completely characterized. Animal models allow investigators to more easily evaluate where infected cells are located and how to eradicate them than in humans.

5.1 Evaluating viral reservoirs during antiretroviral therapy

Because antiretroviral drugs were designed to target HIV-1, some of them are inefficient or unable to suppress SIV replication. In an animal model, antiretroviral suppression should be as good as what is observed in humans on combination antiretroviral therapy. Standard assays detect down to 50 copies of viral RNA per milliliter of plasma, but even with typical three drug regimens it has been difficult to completely inhibit plasma viremia in some macaques to undetectable levels (Ambrose et al., 2007; Dinoso et al., 2009; Lugli et al., 2011; North et al., 2005). The ability to achieve complete suppression generally correlates with the level of plasma viremia prior to treatment, such that higher viral loads are more difficult to completely suppress (Kearney et al., 2011). In mouse models, combination therapy has only been evaluated in humanized Rag2$^{-/-}\gamma$C$^{-/-}$ mice, which also showed incomplete viral suppression (Choudhary et al., 2009; Sango et al., 2010). These results may be due to reduced efficacy against SIV proteins and/or different drug pharmacokinetics in macaques or mice as compared to humans.

In identifying and characterizing persistent viral reservoirs in an animal model, complete and sustained suppression is necessary. Recent reports suggest that ongoing viral replication does not occur during suppressive therapy in humans, based on a lack of viral evolution (Bailey et al., 2006; Kieffer et al., 2004; Nottet et al., 2009; Persaud et al., 2007). This was also observed in RT-SHIV-infected monkeys with sustained plasma virus suppression (Kearney et al., 2011). Continued virus replication in the presence of incomplete suppression will lead to infection of new target cells and re-seeding of reservoirs, which will interfere with identification of the actual reservoir that was established prior to initiation of therapy. This is especially important when looking at the reduction of infected cells by virus eradication therapies, as discussed below.

Despite the lack of complete suppression in many animals, the macaque model has been used to try to identify and characterize viral reservoirs. In an SIV model with FTC and tenofovir therapy, it was shown that resting CD4+ T lymphocytes from lymph nodes but not thymocytes contribute to the reservoir (Shen et al., 2003). While viral DNA was detected in multiple tissues of RT-SHIV-infected animals with and without triple therapy, very little or no viral RNA was detected in these tissues during complete suppression (North et al., 2010; Ambrose et al., unpublished results). Lymphoid and gastrointestinal tissues showed the highest level of viral DNA in virally suppressed animals, suggesting that they consist of the majority of the viral reservoir. In a model of neuropathogenic AIDS, although viremia in plasma and cerebral spinal fluid was significantly reduced by therapy, levels of viral DNA in the brains of these animals were not significantly different than the untreated controls, suggesting that virally infected cells in the central nervous system can contribute to the reservoir (Zink et al., 2010).

5.2 Preliminary studies using animal models for eradication strategies

To target persisting HIV-infected cells with therapeutic drugs for their eradication, one needs to know where the reservoirs are located and what types of cells are infected. While more research needs to be performed to address the type and location of infected CD4+ cells that persist and if these vary at different anatomical locations, investigators are already testing novel therapies to selectively target infected cells.

The majority of these strategies aim to stimulate latently infected, resting CD4+ cells during suppressive antiretroviral therapy. The purpose is to promote replication of virus in those cells without causing global immune activation and without leading to spread of infection to new cells. Histone deacetylase (HDAC) inhibitors and phorbol esters that stimulate protein kinase C (PKC) have received attention for their ability to activate latent HIV-1 expression *in vitro* (Colin and Van Lint, 2009). Clinical studies showed little or no decrease in latently infected cells or vDNA in most subjects by administration of a FDA-approved HDAC inhibitor, valproic acid, in the presence of suppressive ART (Archin et al., 2008; Sagot-Lerolle et al., 2008; Siliciano et al., 2007). This is most likely to be a result of incorrect HDAC(s) targeting and/or inadequate drug concentrations (Huber et al., 2011; Keedy et al., 2009).

Animal models will be useful to test efficacy and mechanisms of action of potential therapies to eliminate infected cells from the body. Very recently a few studies have described the use of novel strategies *in vivo* and *ex vivo* to target viral reservoirs. Lipid nanoparticles containing the PKC activator bryostatin minimally induced proviral expression from infected CD4+ cells isolated from SCID-hu mice with thymus/liver implants (Kovochich et al., 2011). Also, a gold-based compound, auranofin, was used to treat SIV-infected macaques already receiving triple therapy (Lewis et al., 2011). After a month of treatment, PBMC proviral DNA levels decreased in the animals and plasma viral RNA was reduced after interruption of treatment.

While new eradication treatments are promising for reducing or eliminating viral reservoirs, there are many issues and remaining questions that need to be addressed. First, an assumption is that latently infected cells will die after they are activated. However, to date this has not been demonstrated in animals or in people. And it remains to be seen if there are strategies that can selectively activate HIV- or SIV-infected cells but not uninfected cells. Second, it is important to identify models or treatment options that can achieve complete, sustained virus suppression as is observed in patients. If this is achieved, methods to measure decreases in viral reservoirs will need to be optimized, including assays to measure a single copy of plasma viral RNA, a single infected cell, and spliced vs. unspliced viral RNA.

Finally, there are two caveats to the mouse and macaque models for studying persisting viral reservoirs. While mice can be rather effectively repopulated with a largely functional immune system, their anatomy is largely different than that of humans. Identification of reservoirs in mice will need to be confirmed with what is already known in humans. And although monkeys are more similar anatomically to humans, HIV-1 replication is not maintained in these animals. It remains to be seen whether transcriptional activation of SIV is similar to or different than that of HIV-1. Compounds designed to target activation of the HIV-1 LTR may not work or may work differently against SIV LTRs. Characterization of the various models for investigation of virus reservoirs should, therefore, continue.

6. Conclusion

This chapter has highlighted the use of macaque and mouse models for antiretroviral therapies. These animal models have improved greatly since the development of SHIVs and the ability to reconstitute a functional human immune system in mice. Refinement of these models is ongoing to make them more closely resemble humans with regards to infection, pathogenesis, and antiretroviral immunity. For example, macaque models can be improved by increased understanding of macaque cell proteins that inhibit HIV-1 infection as well as the genetic differences between HIV-1 and SIV, particularly the accessory proteins that appear to significantly contribute to pathogenesis. Not only will these findings make a better animal model, but virus-host cell protein interactions characterized by these studies may also lead to new therapeutic targets. Also, alterations of the current humanized mouse models to improve tissue immune cell reconstitution and anti-HIV adaptive immune responses will better recapitulate HIV-1 infection of humans.

While much work has been accomplished in HIV-1 research, questions remain for pre- and post-exposure prophylaxis, antiretroviral pharmacokinetics and efficacy, drug resistance, new drug delivery technologies, and methods for virus eradication. Using the models described here can help answer many of these questions, if used appropriately. Animal models continue to improve therapeutics against HIV-1 and they will be critical for addressing these important issues, bridging basic research together with clinical trials for HIV-1 prevention, treatment, and eradication.

7. References

Abdool Karim, Q., Abdool Karim, S.S., Frohlich, J.A., Grobler, A.C., Baxter, C., Mansoor, L.E., Kharsany, A.B., Sibeko, S., Mlisana, K.P., Omar, Z., *et al.* (2010). Effectiveness and safety of tenofovir gel, an antiretroviral microbicide, for the prevention of HIV infection in women. *Science*, Vol.329, No.5996, pp. 1168-1174.

Ambrose, Z., Boltz, V., Palmer, S., Coffin, J.M., Hughes, S.H., and Kewalramani, V.N. (2004). In vitro characterization of a simian immunodeficiency virus-human immunodeficiency virus (HIV) chimera expressing HIV type 1 reverse transcriptase to study antiviral resistance in pigtail macaques. *Journal of Virology*, Vol.78, No.24, pp. 13553-13561.

Ambrose, Z., Compton, L., Piatak, M., Jr., Lu, D., Alvord, W.G., Lubomirski, M.S., Hildreth, J.E., Lifson, J.D., Miller, C.J., and KewalRamani, V.N. (2008). Incomplete protection against simian immunodeficiency virus vaginal transmission in rhesus macaques by a topical antiviral agent revealed by repeat challenges. *Journal of Virology*, Vol.82, No.13, pp. 6591-6599.

Ambrose, Z., and KewalRamani, V.N. (2008). Of mice and monkeys: new advances in animal models to study HIV-1 therapy and prophylaxis. *Future HIV Therapy*, Vol.2, No.4, pp. 363-373.

Ambrose, Z., Palmer, S., Boltz, V.F., Kearney, M., Larsen, K., Polacino, P., Flanary, L., Oswald, K., Piatak, M., Smedley, J., *et al.* (2007). Suppression of viremia and evolution of human immunodeficiency virus type 1 drug resistance in a macaque model for antiretroviral therapy. *Journal of Virology*, Vol.81, No.22, pp. 12145-12155.

Archin, N.M., Eron, J.J., Palmer, S., Hartmann-Duff, A., Martinson, J.A., Wiegand, A., Bandarenko, N., Schmitz, J.L., Bosch, R.J., Landay, A.L., *et al.* (2008). Valproic acid without intensified antiviral therapy has limited impact on persistent HIV infection of resting CD4+ T cells. *AIDS*, Vol.22, No.10, pp. 1131-1135.

Baba, T.W., Liska, V., Hofmann-Lehmann, R., Vlasak, J., Xu, W., Ayehunie, S., Cavacini, L.A., Posner, M.R., Katinger, H., Stiegler, G., *et al.* (2000). Human neutralizing monoclonal antibodies of the IgG1 subtype protect against mucosal simian-human immunodeficiency virus infection. *Nature Medicine*, Vol.6, No.2, pp. 200-206.

Baenziger, S., Tussiwand, R., Schlaepfer, E., Mazzucchelli, L., Heikenwalder, M., Kurrer, M.O., Behnke, S., Frey, J., Oxenius, A., Joller, H., *et al.* (2006). Disseminated and sustained HIV infection in CD34+ cord blood cell-transplanted Rag2-/-gamma c-/- mice. *Proceedings of the National Academy of Sciences USA*, Vol.103, No.43, pp. 15951-15956.

Bailey, J.R., Sedaghat, A.R., Kieffer, T., Brennan, T., Lee, P.K., Wind-Rotolo, M., Haggerty, C.M., Kamireddi, A.R., Liu, Y., Lee, J., *et al.* (2006). Residual human immunodeficiency virus type 1 viremia in some patients on antiretroviral therapy is dominated by a small number of invariant clones rarely found in circulating CD4+ T cells. *Journal of Virology*, Vol.80, No.13, pp. 6441-6457.

Balani, S.K., Kauffman, L.R., deLuna, F.A., and Lin, J.H. (1999). Nonlinear pharmacokinetics of efavirenz (DMP-266), a potent HIV-1 reverse transcriptase inhibitor, in rats and monkeys. *Drug Metabolism and Disposition: the Biological Fate of Chemicals*, Vol.27, No.1, pp. 41-45.

Balzarini, J., Naesens, L., Slachmuylders, J., Niphuis, H., Rosenberg, I., Holy, A., Schellekens, H., and De Clercq, E. (1991). 9-(2-Phosphonylmethoxyethyl)adenine (PMEA) effectively inhibits retrovirus replication in vitro and simian immunodeficiency virus infection in rhesus monkeys. *AIDS*, Vol.5, No.1, pp. 21-28.

Barnett, S.W., Murthy, K.K., Herndier, B.G., and Levy, J.A. (1994). An AIDS-like condition induced in baboons by HIV-2. *Science*, Vol.266, No.5185, pp. 642-646.

Berges, B.K., Akkina, S.R., Folkvord, J.M., Connick, E., and Akkina, R. (2008). Mucosal transmission of R5 and X4 tropic HIV-1 via vaginal and rectal routes in humanized Rag2-/- gammac -/- (RAG-hu) mice. *Virology*, Vol.373, No.2, pp. 342-351.

Boadi, T., Schneider, E., Chung, S., Tsai, L., Gettie, A., Ratterree, M., Blanchard, J., Neurath, A.R., and Cheng-Mayer, C. (2005). Cellulose acetate 1,2-benzenedicarboxylate protects against challenge with pathogenic X4 and R5 simian/human immunodeficiency virus. *AIDS*, Vol.19, No.15, pp. 1587-1594.

Bourry, O., Brochard, P., Souquiere, S., Makuwa, M., Calvo, J., Dereudre-Bosquet, N., Martinon, F., Benech, H., Kazanji, M., and Le Grand, R. (2009). Prevention of vaginal simian immunodeficiency virus transmission in macaques by postexposure prophylaxis with zidovudine, lamivudine and indinavir. *AIDS*, Vol.23, No.4, pp. 447-454.

Choudhary, S.K., Rezk, N.L., Ince, W.L., Cheema, M., Zhang, L., Su, L., Swanstrom, R., Kashuba, A.D., and Margolis, D.M. (2009). Suppression of human immunodeficiency virus type 1 (HIV-1) viremia with reverse transcriptase and integrase inhibitors, CD4+ T-cell recovery, and viral rebound upon interruption of therapy in a new model for HIV treatment in the humanized Rag2-/-{gamma}c-/- mouse. *Journal of Virology*, Vol.83, No.16, pp. 8254-8258.

Colin, L., and Van Lint, C. (2009). Molecular control of HIV-1 postintegration latency: implications for the development of new therapeutic strategies. *Retrovirology*, Vol.6, p. 111.

Cong, M.E., Youngpairoj, A.S., Aung, W., Sharma, S., Mitchell, J., Dobard, C., Heneine, W., and Garcia-Lerma, J.G. (2011). Generation and mucosal transmissibility of emtricitabine- and tenofovir-resistant SHIV162P3 mutants in macaques. *Virology*, Vol.412, No.2, pp. 435-440.

Connor, E.M., Sperling, R.S., Gelber, R., Kiselev, P., Scott, G., O'Sullivan, M.J., VanDyke, R., Bey, M., Shearer, W., Jacobson, R.L., *et al.* (1994). Reduction of maternal-infant transmission of human immunodeficiency virus type 1 with zidovudine treatment. Pediatric AIDS Clinical Trials Group Protocol 076 Study Group. *New England Journal of Medicine*, Vol.331, No.18, pp. 1173-1180.

Cranage, M., Sharpe, S., Herrera, C., Cope, A., Dennis, M., Berry, N., Ham, C., Heeney, J., Rezk, N., Kashuba, A., *et al.* (2008). Prevention of SIV rectal transmission and priming of T cell responses in macaques after local pre-exposure application of tenofovir gel. *PLoS Medicine*, Vol.5, No.8, pp. e157.

Daniel, M.D., Letvin, N.L., King, N.W., Kannagi, M., Sehgal, P.K., Hunt, R.D., Kanki, P.J., Essex, M., and Desrosiers, R.C. (1985). Isolation of T-cell tropic HTLV-III-like retrovirus from macaques. *Science*, Vol.228, No.4704, pp. 1201-1204.

Denton, P.W., Estes, J.D., Sun, Z., Othieno, F.A., Wei, B.L., Wege, A.K., Powell, D.A., Payne, D., Haase, A.T., and Garcia, J.V. (2008). Antiretroviral pre-exposure prophylaxis prevents vaginal transmission of HIV-1 in humanized BLT mice. *PLoS Medicine*, Vol.5, No.1, p. e16.

Denton, P.W., Krisko, J.F., Powell, D.A., Mathias, M., Kwak, Y.T., Martinez-Torres, F., Zou, W., Payne, D.A., Estes, J.D., and Garcia, J.V. (2010). Systemic administration of antiretrovirals prior to exposure prevents rectal and intravenous HIV-1 transmission in humanized BLT mice. *PLoS One*, Vol.5, No.1, p. e8829.

Denton, P.W., Othieno, F., Martinez-Torres, F., Zou, W., Krisko, J.F., Fleming, E., Zein, S., Powell, D.A., Wahl, A., Kwak, Y.T., *et al.* (2011). One Percent Tenofovir Applied Topically to Humanized BLT Mice and Used According to the CAPRISA 004 Experimental Design Demonstrates Partial Protection from Vaginal HIV Infection, Validating the BLT Model for Evaluation of New Microbicide Candidates. *Journal of Virology*, Vol.85, No.15, pp. 7582-7593.

Dinoso, J.B., Rabi, S.A., Blankson, J.N., Gama, L., Mankowski, J.L., Siliciano, R.F., Zink, M.C., and Clements, J.E. (2009). A simian immunodeficiency virus-infected macaque model to study viral reservoirs that persist during highly active antiretroviral therapy. *Journal of Virology*, Vol.83, No.18, pp. 9247-9257.

Dou, H., Grotepas, C.B., McMillan, J.M., Destache, C.J., Chaubal, M., Werling, J., Kipp, J., Rabinow, B., and Gendelman, H.E. (2009). Macrophage delivery of nanoformulated antiretroviral drug to the brain in a murine model of neuroAIDS. *Journal of Immunology*, Vol.183, No.1, pp. 661-669.

Dudley, D.M., Wentzel, J.L., Lalonde, M.S., Veazey, R.S., and Arts, E.J. (2009). Selection of a simian-human immunodeficiency virus strain resistant to a vaginal microbicide in macaques. *Journal of Virology*, Vol.83, No.10, pp. 5067-5076.

Ellington, A.D., and Szostak, J.W. (1990). In vitro selection of RNA molecules that bind specific ligands. Nature *346*,6287, 818-822.

Eshleman, S.H., Mracna, M., Guay, L.A., Deseyve, M., Cunningham, S., Mirochnick, M., Musoke, P., Fleming, T., Glenn Fowler, M., Mofenson, L.M., *et al.* (2001). Selection and fading of resistance mutations in women and infants receiving nevirapine to prevent HIV-1 vertical transmission (HIVNET 012). *AIDS*, Vol.15, No.15, pp. 1951-1957.

Fazely, F., Haseltine, W.A., Rodger, R.F., and Ruprecht, R.M. (1991). Postexposure chemoprophylaxis with ZDV or ZDV combined with interferon-alpha: failure after inoculating rhesus monkeys with a high dose of SIV. *Journal of Acquired Immune Deficiency Syndromes*, Vol.4, No.11, pp. 1093-1097.

Ferrantelli, F., Rasmussen, R.A., Buckley, K.A., Li, P.L., Wang, T., Montefiori, D.C., Katinger, H., Stiegler, G., Anderson, D.C., McClure, H.M., *et al.* (2004). Complete protection of neonatal rhesus macaques against oral exposure to pathogenic simian-human immunodeficiency virus by human anti-HIV monoclonal antibodies. *Journal of Infectious Diseases*, Vol.189, No.12, pp. 2167-2173.

Flys, T., Nissley, D.V., Claasen, C.W., Jones, D., Shi, C., Guay, L.A., Musoke, P., Mmiro, F., Strathern, J.N., Jackson, J.B., *et al.* (2005). Sensitive drug-resistance assays reveal long-term persistence of HIV-1 variants with the K103N nevirapine (NVP) resistance mutation in some women and infants after the administration of single-dose NVP: HIVNET 012. *Journal of Infectious Diseases*, Vol.192, No.1, pp. 24-29.

Garcia-Lerma, J.G., Otten, R.A., Qari, S.H., Jackson, E., Cong, M.E., Masciotra, S., Luo, W., Kim, C., Adams, D.R., Monsour, M., *et al.* (2008). Prevention of rectal SHIV transmission in macaques by daily or intermittent prophylaxis with emtricitabine and tenofovir. *PLoS Medicine*, Vol.5, No.2, p. e28.

Gardelli, C., Nizi, E., Muraglia, E., Crescenzi, B., Ferrara, M., Orvieto, F., Pace, P., Pescatore, G., Poma, M., Ferreira Mdel, R., *et al.* (2007). Discovery and synthesis of HIV integrase inhibitors: development of potent and orally bioavailable N-methyl pyrimidones. *Journal of Medicinal Chemistry*, Vol.50, No.20, pp. 4953-4975.

Grant, R.M., Lama, J.R., Anderson, P.L., McMahan, V., Liu, A.Y., Vargas, L., Goicochea, P., Casapia, M., Guanira-Carranza, J.V., Ramirez-Cardich, M.E., *et al.* (2010). Preexposure chemoprophylaxis for HIV prevention in men who have sex with men. *New England Journal of Medicine*, Vol.363, No.27, pp. 2587-2599.

Guay, L.A., Musoke, P., Fleming, T., Bagenda, D., Allen, M., Nakabiito, C., Sherman, J., Bakaki, P., Ducar, C., Deseyve, M., *et al.* (1999). Intrapartum and neonatal single-dose nevirapine compared with zidovudine for prevention of mother-to-child transmission of HIV-1 in Kampala, Uganda: HIVNET 012 randomised trial. *The Lancet*, Vol.354, No.9181, pp. 795-802.

Gupta, P., Mellors, J., Kingsley, L., Riddler, S., Singh, M.K., Schreiber, S., Cronin, M., and Rinaldo, C.R. (1997). High viral load in semen of human immunodeficiency virus type 1-infected men at all stages of disease and its reduction by therapy with protease and nonnucleoside reverse transcriptase inhibitors. *Journal of Virology*, Vol.71, No.8, pp. 6271-6275.

Hammond, S.M., Bernstein, E., Beach, D., and Hannon, G.J. (2000). An RNA-directed nuclease mediates post-transcriptional gene silencing in Drosophila cells. *Nature*, Vol.404, No.6775, pp. 293-296.

Hatziioannou, T., Ambrose, Z., Chung, N.P., Piatak, M., Jr., Yuan, F., Trubey, C.M., Coalter, V., Kiser, R., Schneider, D., Smedley, J., *et al.* (2009). A macaque model of HIV-1 infection. *Proceedings of the National Academy of Sciences USA*, Vol.106, No.11, pp. 4425-4429.

Hazuda, D.J., Young, S.D., Guare, J.P., Anthony, N.J., Gomez, R.P., Wai, J.S., Vacca, J.P., Handt, L., Motzel, S.L., Klein, H.J., *et al.* (2004). Integrase inhibitors and cellular immunity suppress retroviral replication in rhesus macaques. *Science*, Vol.305, No.5683, pp. 528-532.

Hicks, D.R., Martin, L.S., Getchell, J.P., Heath, J.L., Francis, D.P., McDougal, J.S., Curran, J.W., and Voeller, B. (1985). Inactivation of HTLV-III/LAV-infected cultures of normal human lymphocytes by nonoxynol-9 in vitro. *The Lancet*, Vol.2, No.8469-70, pp. 1422-1423.

Hirsch, V.M., Olmsted, R.A., Murphey-Corb, M., Purcell, R.H., and Johnson, P.R. (1989). An African primate lentivirus (SIVsm) closely related to HIV-2. *Nature*, Vol.339, No.6223, pp. 389-392.

Ho, R.J., Larsen, K., Bui, T., Wang, X.Y., Herz, A.M., Sherbert, C., Finn, E., Nosbisch, C., Schmidt, A., Anderson, D., *et al.* (2000). Suppression of maternal virus load with zidovudine, didanosine, and indinavir combination therapy prevents mother-to-fetus HIV transmission in macaques. *Journal of Acquired Immune Deficiency Syndromes*, Vol.25, No.2, pp. 140-149.

Hofman, M.J., Higgins, J., Matthews, T.B., Pedersen, N.C., Tan, C., Schinazi, R.F., and North, T.W. (2004). Efavirenz therapy in rhesus macaques infected with a chimera of simian immunodeficiency virus containing reverse transcriptase from human immunodeficiency virus type 1. *Antimicrobial Agents and Chemotherapy*, Vol.48, No.9, pp. 3483-3490.

Hofmann-Lehmann, R., Vlasak, J., Rasmussen, R.A., Smith, B.A., Baba, T.W., Liska, V., Ferrantelli, F., Montefiori, D.C., McClure, H.M., Anderson, D.C., *et al.* (2001). Postnatal passive immunization of neonatal macaques with a triple combination of human monoclonal antibodies against oral simian-human immunodeficiency virus challenge. *Journal of Virology*, Vol.75, No.16, pp. 7470-7480.

Huber, K., Doyon, G., Plaks, J., Fyne, E., Mellors, J.W., and Sluis-Cremer, N. (2011). Inhibitors of Histone Deacetylases: correlation between isoform specificity and HIV type 1 (HIV-1) from latently infected cells. *Journal of Biological Chemistry*, Vol.286, No.25, pp. 22211-22218.

Igarashi, T., Iyengar, R., Byrum, R.A., Buckler-White, A., Dewar, R.L., Buckler, C.E., Lane, H.C., Kamada, K., Adachi, A., and Martin, M.A. (2007). Human immunodeficiency virus type 1 derivative with 7% simian immunodeficiency virus genetic content is able to establish infections in pig-tailed macaques. *Journal of Virology*, Vol.81, No.20, pp. 11549-11552.

Jourdain, G., Ngo-Giang-Huong, N., Le Coeur, S., Bowonwatanuwong, C., Kantipong, P., Leechanachai, P., Ariyadej, S., Leenasirimakul, P., Hammer, S., and Lallemant, M. (2004). Intrapartum exposure to nevirapine and subsequent maternal responses to nevirapine-based antiretroviral therapy. *New England Journal of Medicine*, Vol.351, No.3, pp. 229-240.

Kaldor, S.W., Kalish, V.J., Davies, J.F., 2nd, Shetty, B.V., Fritz, J.E., Appelt, K., Burgess, J.A., Campanale, K.M., Chirgadze, N.Y., Clawson, D.K., *et al.* (1997). Viracept (nelfinavir mesylate, AG1343): a potent, orally bioavailable inhibitor of HIV-1 protease. *Journal of Medicinal Chemistry*, Vol.40, No.24, pp. 3979-3985.

Kanki, P.J., McLane, M.F., King, N.W., Jr., Letvin, N.L., Hunt, R.D., Sehgal, P., Daniel, M.D., Desrosiers, R.C., and Essex, M. (1985). Serologic identification and characterization of a macaque T-lymphotropic retrovirus closely related to HTLV-III. *Science*, Vol.228, No.4704, pp. 1199-1201.

Kearney, M., Spindler, J., Shao, W., Maldarelli, F., Palmer, S., Hu, S.L., Lifson, J.D., KewalRamani, V.N., Mellors, J.W., Coffin, J.M., *et al.* (2011). Genetic diversity of simian immunodeficiency virus encoding HIV-1 reverse transcriptase persists in macaques despite antiretroviral therapy. *Journal of Virology*, Vol.85, No.2, pp. 1067-1076.

Keedy, K.S., Archin, N.M., Gates, A.T., Espeseth, A., Hazuda, D.J., and Margolis, D.M. (2009). A limited group of class I histone deacetylases acts to repress human immunodeficiency virus type 1 expression. *Journal of Virology*, Vol.83, No.10, pp. 4749-4756.

Keele, B.F., Van Heuverswyn, F., Li, Y., Bailes, E., Takehisa, J., Santiago, M.L., Bibollet-Ruche, F., Chen, Y., Wain, L.V., Liegeois, F., *et al.* (2006). Chimpanzee reservoirs of pandemic and nonpandemic HIV-1. *Science*, Vol.313, No.5786, pp. 523-526.

Keller, R.D., Nosbisch, C., and Unadkat, J.D. (1995). Pharmacokinetics of stavudine (2',3'-didehydro-3'-deoxythymidine) in the neonatal macaque (*Macaca nemestrina*). *Antimicrobial Agents and Chemotherapy*, Vol.39, No.12, pp. 2829-2831.

Kelley, J.A., Litterst, C.L., Roth, J.S., Vistica, D.T., Poplack, D.G., Cooney, D.A., Nadkarni, M., Balis, F.M., Broder, S., and Johns, D.G. (1987). The disposition and metabolism of 2',3'-dideoxycytidine, an in vitro inhibitor of human T-lymphotrophic virus type III infectivity, in mice and monkeys. *Drug Metabolism and Disposition: the Biological Fate of Chemicals*, Vol.15, No.5, pp. 595-601.

Kenney, J., Aravantinou, M., Singer, R., Hsu, M., Rodriguez, A., Kizima, L., Abraham, C.J., Menon, R., Seidor, S., Chudolij, A., *et al.* (2011). An antiretroviral/zinc combination gel provides 24 hours of complete protection against vaginal SHIV infection in macaques. *PLoS One*, vol.6, no.1, p. e15835.

Kieffer, T.L., Finucane, M.M., Nettles, R.E., Quinn, T.C., Broman, K.W., Ray, S.C., Persaud, D., and Siliciano, R.F. (2004). Genotypic analysis of HIV-1 drug resistance at the limit of detection: virus production without evolution in treated adults with undetectable HIV loads. *Journal of Infectious Diseases*, Vol.189, No.8, pp. 1452-1465.

Kim, C.N., Adams, D.R., Bashirian, S., Butera, S., Folks, T.M., and Otten, R.A. (2006). Repetitive exposures with simian/human immunodeficiency viruses: strategy to study HIV pre-clinical interventions in non-human primates. *Journal of Medical Primatology*, Vol.35, No.4-5, pp. 210-216.

Kinman, L., Brodie, S.J., Tsai, C.C., Bui, T., Larsen, K., Schmidt, A., Anderson, D., Morton, W.R., Hu, S.L., and Ho, R.J. (2003). Lipid-drug association enhanced HIV-1 protease inhibitor indinavir localization in lymphoid tissues and viral load reduction: a proof of concept study in HIV-2287-infected macaques. *Journal of Acquired Immune Deficiency Syndromes*, Vol.34, No.4, pp. 387-397.

Kish-Catalone, T., Pal, R., Parrish, J., Rose, N., Hocker, L., Hudacik, L., Reitz, M., Gallo, R., and Devico, A. (2007). Evaluation of -2 RANTES vaginal microbicide formulations in a nonhuman primate simian/human immunodeficiency virus (SHIV) challenge model. *AIDS Research and Human Retroviruses*, Vol.23, No.1, pp. 33-42.

Kovochich, M., Marsden, M.D., and Zack, J.A. (2011). Activation of latent HIV using drug-loaded nanoparticles. *PLoS One*, Vol.6, No.4, p. e18270.

Kwara, A., Delong, A., Rezk, N., Hogan, J., Burtwell, H., Chapman, S., Moreira, C.C., Kurpewski, J., Ingersoll, J., Caliendo, A.M., *et al.* (2008). Antiretroviral drug concentrations and HIV RNA in the genital tract of HIV-infected women receiving long-term highly active antiretroviral therapy. *Clinical Infectious Diseases*, Vol.46, No.5, pp. 719-725.

Lagenaur, L.A., Sanders-Beer, B.E., Brichacek, B., Pal, R., Liu, X., Liu, Y., Yu, R., Venzon, D., Lee, P.P., and Hamer, D.H. (2011). Prevention of vaginal SHIV transmission in macaques by a live recombinant Lactobacillus. *Mucosal Immunology*, July 6, epub ahead of print.

Le Grand, R., Vaslin, B., Larghero, J., Neidez, O., Thiebot, H., Sellier, P., Clayette, P., Dereuddre-Bosquet, N., and Dormont, D. (2000). Post-exposure prophylaxis with highly active antiretroviral therapy could not protect macaques from infection with SIV/HIV chimera. *AIDS*, Vol.14, No.12, pp. 1864-1866.

Lederman, M.M., Veazey, R.S., Offord, R., Mosier, D.E., Dufour, J., Mefford, M., Piatak, M., Jr., Lifson, J.D., Salkowitz, J.R., Rodriguez, B., *et al.* (2004). Prevention of vaginal SHIV transmission in rhesus macaques through inhibition of CCR5. *Science*, Vol.306, No.5695, pp. 485-487.

Levchenko, T.S., Rammohan, R., Lukyanov, A.N., Whiteman, K.R., and Torchilin, V.P. (2002). Liposome clearance in mice: the effect of a separate and combined presence of surface charge and polymer coating. *International Journal of Pharmaceutics*, Vol.240, No.1-2, pp. 95-102.

Lewis, M.G., Dafonseca, S., Chomont, N., Palamara, A.T., Tardugno, M., Mai, A., Collins, M., Wagner, W.L., Yalley-Ogunro, J., Greenhouse, J., *et al.* (2011). Gold drug auranofin restricts the viral reservoir in the monkey AIDS model and induces containment of viral load following ART suspension. *AIDS*, Vol.25, No.11, pp. 1347-1356.

Li, J., Lord, C.I., Haseltine, W., Letvin, N.L., and Sodroski, J. (1992). Infection of cynomolgus monkeys with a chimeric HIV-1/SIVmac virus that expresses the HIV-1 envelope glycoproteins. *Journal of Acquired Immune Deficiency Syndromes*, Vol.5, No.7, pp. 639-646.

Li, Q., Estes, J.D., Schlievert, P.M., Duan, L., Brosnahan, A.J., Southern, P.J., Reilly, C.S., Peterson, M.L., Schultz-Darken, N., Brunner, K.G., *et al.* (2009). Glycerol monolaurate prevents mucosal SIV transmission. *Nature*, Vol.458, No.7241, pp. 1034-1038.

Lifson, J.D., Piatak, M., Jr., Cline, A.N., Rossio, J.L., Purcell, J., Pandrea, I., Bischofberger, N., Blanchard, J., and Veazey, R.S. (2003). Transient early post-inoculation anti-retroviral treatment facilitates controlled infection with sparing of CD4+ T cells in gut-associated lymphoid tissues in SIVmac239-infected rhesus macaques, but not resistance to rechallenge. *Journal of Medical Primatology*, Vol.32, No.4-5, pp. 201-210.

Liuzzi, G., Chirianni, A., Clementi, M., Bagnarelli, P., Valenza, A., Cataldo, P.T., and Piazza, M. (1996). Analysis of HIV-1 load in blood, semen and saliva: evidence for different viral compartments in a cross-sectional and longitudinal study. *AIDS*, Vol.10, No.14, pp. F51-56.

Lu, Y., Brosio, P., Lafaile, M., Li, J., Collman, R.G., Sodroski, J., and Miller, C.J. (1996). Vaginal transmission of chimeric simian/human immunodeficiency viruses in rhesus macaques. *Journal of Virology*, Vol.70, No.5, pp. 3045-3050.

Luciw, P.A., Pratt-Lowe, E., Shaw, K.E., Levy, J.A., and Cheng-Mayer, C. (1995). Persistent infection of rhesus macaques with T-cell-line-tropic and macrophage-tropic clones of simian/human immunodeficiency viruses (SHIV). *Proceedings of the National Academy of Sciences USA*, Vol.92, No.16, pp. 7490-7494.

Lugli, E., Mueller, Y.M., Lewis, M.G., Villinger, F., Katsikis, P.D., and Roederer, M. (2011). Interleukin-15 delays suppression and fails to promote immune reconstitution in virally suppressed chronically SIV-infected macaques. *Blood*, July 14, epub ahead of print.

Manson, K.H., Wyand, M.S., Miller, C., and Neurath, A.R. (2000). Effect of a cellulose acetate phthalate topical cream on vaginal transmission of simian immunodeficiency virus in rhesus monkeys. *Antimicrobial Agents and Chemotherapy*, Vol.44, No.11, pp. 3199-3202.

Mariani, R., Chen, D., Schrofelbauer, B., Navarro, F., Konig, R., Bollman, B., Munk, C., Nymark-McMahon, H., and Landau, N.R. (2003). Species-specific exclusion of APOBEC3G from HIV-1 virions by Vif. *Cell*, Vol.114, No.1, pp. 21-31.

Marthas, M.L., Lu, D., Penedo, M.C., Hendrickx, A.G., and Miller, C.J. (2001). Titration of an SIVmac251 stock by vaginal inoculation of Indian and Chinese origin rhesus macaques: transmission efficiency, viral loads, and antibody responses. *AIDS Research and Human Retroviruses*, Vol.17, No.15, pp. 1455-1466.

Mascola, J.R., Stiegler, G., VanCott, T.C., Katinger, H., Carpenter, C.B., Hanson, C.E., Beary, H., Hayes, D., Frankel, S.S., Birx, D.L., *et al.* (2000). Protection of macaques against vaginal transmission of a pathogenic HIV-1/SIV chimeric virus by passive infusion of neutralizing antibodies. *Nature Medicine*, Vol.6, No.2, pp. 207-210.

McNamara, J.O., 2nd, Andrechek, E.R., Wang, Y., Viles, K.D., Rempel, R.E., Gilboa, E., Sullenger, B.A., and Giangrande, P.H. (2006). Cell type-specific delivery of siRNAs with aptamer-siRNA chimeras. *Nature Biotechnology*, Vol.24, No.8, pp. 1005-1015.

Mosier, D.E., Gulizia, R.J., Baird, S.M., and Wilson, D.B. (1988). Transfer of a functional human immune system to mice with severe combined immunodeficiency. *Nature*, Vol.335, No.6187, pp. 256-259.

Musoke, P., Guay, L.A., Bagenda, D., Mirochnick, M., Nakabiito, C., Fleming, T., Elliott, T., Horton, S., Dransfield, K., Pav, J.W., *et al.* (1999). A phase I/II study of the safety and pharmacokinetics of nevirapine in HIV-1-infected pregnant Ugandan women and their neonates (HIVNET 006). *AIDS*, Vol.13, No.4, pp. 479-486.

Namikawa, R., Weilbaecher, K.N., Kaneshima, H., Yee, E.J., and McCune, J.M. (1990). Long-term human hematopoiesis in the SCID-hu mouse. *Journal of Experimental Medicine*, Vol.172, No.4, pp. 1055-1063.

Neff, C.P., Kurisu, T., Ndolo, T., Fox, K., and Akkina, R. (2011a). A Topical Microbicide Gel Formulation of CCR5 Antagonist Maraviroc Prevents HIV-1 Vaginal Transmission in Humanized RAG-hu Mice. *PLoS One*, Vol.6, No.6, p. e20209.

Neff, C.P., Ndolo, T., Tandon, A., Habu, Y., and Akkina, R. (2010). Oral pre-exposure prophylaxis by anti-retrovirals raltegravir and maraviroc protects against HIV-1 vaginal transmission in a humanized mouse model. *PLoS One*, Vol.5, No.12, p. e15257.

Neff, C.P., Zhou, J., Remling, L., Kuruvilla, J., Zhang, J., Li, H., Smith, D.D., Swiderski, P., Rossi, J.J., and Akkina, R. (2011b). An aptamer-siRNA chimera suppresses HIV-1 viral loads and protects from helper CD4(+) T cell decline in humanized mice. *Science Translational Medicine*, Vol.3, No.66, p. 66ra66.

Nishimura, Y., Igarashi, T., Haigwood, N.L., Sadjadpour, R., Donau, O.K., Buckler, C., Plishka, R.J., Buckler-White, A., and Martin, M.A. (2003). Transfer of neutralizing IgG to macaques 6 h but not 24 h after SHIV infection confers sterilizing protection: implications for HIV-1 vaccine development. *Proceedings of the National Academy of Sciences USA*, Vol.100, No.25, pp. 15131-15136.

North, T.W., Higgins, J., Deere, J.D., Hayes, T.L., Villalobos, A., Adamson, L., Shacklett, B.L., Schinazi, R.F., and Luciw, P.A. (2010). Viral sanctuaries during highly active antiretroviral therapy in a nonhuman primate model for AIDS. *Journal of Virology*, Vol.84, No.6, pp. 2913-2922.

North, T.W., Van Rompay, K.K., Higgins, J., Matthews, T.B., Wadford, D.A., Pedersen, N.C., and Schinazi, R.F. (2005). Suppression of virus load by highly active antiretroviral therapy in rhesus macaques infected with a recombinant simian immunodeficiency virus containing reverse transcriptase from human immunodeficiency virus type 1. *Journal of Virology*, Vol.79, No.12, pp. 7349-7354.

Nottet, H.S., van Dijk, S.J., Fanoy, E.B., Goedegebuure, I.W., de Jong, D., Vrisekoop, N., van Baarle, D., Boltz, V., Palmer, S., Borleffs, J.C., *et al.* (2009). HIV-1 can persist in aged memory CD4+ T lymphocytes with minimal signs of evolution after 8.3 years of effective highly active antiretroviral therapy. *Journal of Acquired Immune Deficiency Syndromes*, Vol.50, No.4, pp. 345-353.

Novembre, F.J., Saucier, M., Anderson, D.C., Klumpp, S.A., O'Neil, S.P., Brown, C.R., 2nd, Hart, C.E., Guenthner, P.C., Swenson, R.B., and McClure, H.M. (1997). Development of AIDS in a chimpanzee infected with human immunodeficiency virus type 1. *Journal of Virology*, Vol.71, No.5, pp. 4086-4091.

Otten, R.A., Smith, D.K., Adams, D.R., Pullium, J.K., Jackson, E., Kim, C.N., Jaffe, H., Janssen, R., Butera, S., and Folks, T.M. (2000). Efficacy of postexposure prophylaxis after intravaginal exposure of pig-tailed macaques to a human-derived retrovirus (human immunodeficiency virus type 2). *Journal of Virology*, Vol.74, No.20, pp. 9771-9775.

Pace, P., Di Francesco, M.E., Gardelli, C., Harper, S., Muraglia, E., Nizi, E., Orvieto, F., Petrocchi, A., Poma, M., Rowley, M., *et al.* (2007). Dihydroxypyrimidine-4-carboxamides as novel potent and selective HIV integrase inhibitors. *Journal of Medicinal Chemistry*, Vol.50, No.9, pp. 2225-2239.

Paiardini, M., Pandrea, I., Apetrei, C., and Silvestri, G. (2009). Lessons learned from the natural hosts of HIV-related viruses. *Annual Review of Medicine*, Vol.60, pp. 485-495.

Palmer, S., Boltz, V., Martinson, N., Maldarelli, F., Gray, G., McIntyre, J., Mellors, J., Morris, L., and Coffin, J. (2006). Persistence of nevirapine-resistant HIV-1 in women after single-dose nevirapine therapy for prevention of maternal-to-fetal HIV-1 transmission. *Proceedings of the National Academy of Sciences USA*, Vol.103, No.18, pp. 7094-7099.

Parikh, U.M., Dobard, C., Sharma, S., Cong, M.E., Jia, H., Martin, A., Pau, C.P., Hanson, D.L., Guenthner, P., Smith, J., *et al.* (2009). Complete protection from repeated vaginal simian-human immunodeficiency virus exposures in macaques by a topical gel containing tenofovir alone or with emtricitabine. *Journal of Virology*, Vol.83, No.20, pp. 10358-10365.

Parren, P.W., Marx, P.A., Hessell, A.J., Luckay, A., Harouse, J., Cheng-Mayer, C., Moore, J.P., and Burton, D.R. (2001). Antibody protects macaques against vaginal challenge with a pathogenic R5 simian/human immunodeficiency virus at serum levels giving complete neutralization in vitro. *Journal of Virology*, Vol.75, No.17, pp. 8340-8347.

Patton, D.L., Cosgrove Sweeney, Y.T., Rabe, L.K., and Hillier, S.L. (2002). Rectal applications of nonoxynol-9 cause tissue disruption in a monkey model. *Sexually Transmitted Diseases*, Vol.29, No.10, pp. 581-587.

Patton, D.L., Kidder, G.G., Sweeney, Y.C., Rabe, L.K., and Hillier, S.L. (1999). Effects of multiple applications of benzalkonium chloride and nonoxynol 9 on the vaginal epithelium in the pigtailed macaque (*Macaca nemestrina*). *American Journal of Obstetrics and Gynecology*, Vol.180, No.5, pp. 1080-1087.

Persaud, D., Ray, S.C., Kajdas, J., Ahonkhai, A., Siberry, G.K., Ferguson, K., Ziemniak, C., Quinn, T.C., Casazza, J.P., Zeichner, S., *et al.* (2007). Slow human immunodeficiency virus type 1 evolution in viral reservoirs in infants treated with effective antiretroviral therapy. *AIDS Research and Human Retroviruses*, Vol.23, No.3, pp. 381-390.

Phillips, D.M., Taylor, C.L., Zacharopoulos, V.R., and Maguire, R.A. (2000). Nonoxynol-9 causes rapid exfoliation of sheets of rectal epithelium. *Contraception*, Vol.62, No.3, pp. 149-154.

Reimann, K.A., Li, J.T., Veazey, R., Halloran, M., Park, I.W., Karlsson, G.B., Sodroski, J., and Letvin, N.L. (1996). A chimeric simian/human immunodeficiency virus expressing a primary patient human immunodeficiency virus type 1 isolate env causes an AIDS-like disease after in vivo passage in rhesus monkeys. *Journal of Virology*, Vol.70, No.10, pp. 6922-6928.

Roehr, B. (2011). Tenofovir works as pre-exposure prophylaxis against HIV, two studies confirm. *BMJ*, Vol.343, p. d4540.

Sagot-Lerolle, N., Lamine, A., Chaix, M.L., Boufassa, F., Aboulker, J.P., Costagliola, D., Goujard, C., Pallier, C., Delfraissy, J.F., and Lambotte, O. (2008). Prolonged valproic acid treatment does not reduce the size of latent HIV reservoir. *AIDS*, Vol.22, No.10, pp. 1125-1129.

Sango, K., Joseph, A., Patel, M., Osiecki, K., Dutta, M., and Goldstein, H. (2010). Highly active antiretroviral therapy potently suppresses HIV infection in humanized Rag2-/-gammac-/- mice. *AIDS Research and Human Retroviruses*, Vol.26, No.7, pp. 735-746.

Sato, S., and Johnson, W. (2007). Antibody-mediated neutralization and simian immunodeficiency virus models of HIV/AIDS. *Current HIV Research*, Vol.5, No.6, pp. 594-607.

Shao, W., Kearney, M., Maldarelli, F., Mellors, J.W., Stephens, R., Lifson, J.D., KewalRamani, V.N., Ambrose, Z., Coffin, J.M., and Palmer, S. (2009). RT-SHIV subpopulation dynamics during anti-HIV-1 therapy. *Retrovirology*, Vol.6, p. 101.

Shen, A., Zink, M.C., Mankowski, J.L., Chadwick, K., Margolick, J.B., Carruth, L.M., Li, M., Clements, J.E., and Siliciano, R.F. (2003). Resting CD4+ T lymphocytes but not thymocytes provide a latent viral reservoir in a simian immunodeficiency virus-Macaca nemestrina model of human immunodeficiency virus type 1-infected patients on highly active antiretroviral therapy. *Journal of Virology*, Vol.77, No.8, pp. 4938-4949.

Shibata, R., Kawamura, M., Sakai, H., Hayami, M., Ishimoto, A., and Adachi, A. (1991). Generation of a chimeric human and simian immunodeficiency virus infectious to monkey peripheral blood mononuclear cells. *Journal of Virology*, Vol.65, No.7, pp. 3514-3520.

Shultz, L.D., Schweitzer, P.A., Christianson, S.W., Gott, B., Schweitzer, I.B., Tennent, B., McKenna, S., Mobraaten, L., Rajan, T.V., Greiner, D.L., *et al.* (1995). Multiple defects in innate and adaptive immunologic function in NOD/LtSz-scid mice. *Journal of Immunology*, Vol.154, No.1, pp. 180-191.

Siliciano, J.D., Lai, J., Callender, M., Pitt, E., Zhang, H., Margolick, J.B., Gallant, J.E., Cofrancesco, J., Jr., Moore, R.D., Gange, S.J., *et al.* (2007). Stability of the latent reservoir for HIV-1 in patients receiving valproic acid. *Journal of Infectious Diseases*, Vol.195, No.6, pp. 833-836.

Singer, R., Derby, N., Rodriguez, A., Kizima, L., Kenney, J., Aravantinou, M., Chudolij, A., Gettie, A., Blanchard, J., Lifson, J.D., *et al.* (2011). The nonnucleoside reverse transcriptase inhibitor MIV-150 in carrageenan gel prevents rectal transmission of simian/human immunodeficiency virus infection in macaques. *Journal of Virology*, Vol.85, No.11, pp. 5504-5512.

Smith, M.S., Foresman, L., Lopez, G.J., Tsay, J., Wodarz, D., Lifson, J.D., Page, A., Wang, C., Li, Z., Adany, I., *et al.* (2000a). Lasting effects of transient postinoculation tenofovir

[9-R-(2-Phosphonomethoxypropyl)adenine] treatment on SHIV(KU2) infection of rhesus macaques. *Virology*, Vol.277, No.2, pp. 306-315.

Smith, S.M., Baskin, G.B., and Marx, P.A. (2000b). Estrogen protects against vaginal transmission of simian immunodeficiency virus. *Journal of Infectious Diseases*, Vol.182, No.3, pp. 708-715.

Song, E., Zhu, P., Lee, S.K., Chowdhury, D., Kussman, S., Dykxhoorn, D.M., Feng, Y., Palliser, D., Weiner, D.B., Shankar, P., *et al.* (2005). Antibody mediated in vivo delivery of small interfering RNAs via cell-surface receptors. *Nature Biotechnology*, Vol.23, No.6, pp. 709-717.

Stoddart, C.A., Joshi, P., Sloan, B., Bare, J.C., Smith, P.C., Allaway, G.P., Wild, C.T., and Martin, D.E. (2007). Potent activity of the HIV-1 maturation inhibitor bevirimat in SCID-hu Thy/Liv mice. *PLoS One*, Vol.2, No.11, p. e1251.

Stolte-Leeb, N., Loddo, R., Antimisiaris, S., Schultheiss, T., Sauermann, U., Franz, M., Mourtas, S., Parsy, C., Storer, R., La Colla, P., *et al.* (2011). Topical non-nucleoside reverse transcriptase inhibitor MC 1220 partially prevents vaginal RT-SHIV infection of macaques. *AIDS Research and Human Retroviruses*, Vol.27, No.9, pp. 933-43.

Stremlau, M., Owens, C.M., Perron, M.J., Kiessling, M., Autissier, P., and Sodroski, J. (2004). The cytoplasmic body component TRIM5alpha restricts HIV-1 infection in Old World monkeys. *Nature*, Vol.427, No.6977, pp. 848-853.

Subbarao, S., Ramos, A., Kim, C., Adams, D., Monsour, M., Butera, S., Folks, T., and Otten, R.A. (2007). Direct stringency comparison of two macaque models (single-high vs. repeat-low) for mucosal HIV transmission using an identical anti-HIV chemoprophylaxis intervention. *Journal of Medical Primatology*, Vol.36, No.4-5, pp. 238-243.

Sun, Z., Denton, P.W., Estes, J.D., Othieno, F.A., Wei, B.L., Wege, A.K., Melkus, M.W., Padgett-Thomas, A., Zupancic, M., Haase, A.T., *et al.* (2007). Intrarectal transmission, systemic infection, and CD4+ T cell depletion in humanized mice infected with HIV-1. *Journal of Experimental Medicine*, Vol.204, No.4, pp. 705-714.

Tabet, S.R., Surawicz, C., Horton, S., Paradise, M., Coletti, A.S., Gross, M., Fleming, T.R., Buchbinder, S., Haggitt, R.C., Levine, H., *et al.* (1999). Safety and toxicity of nonoxynol-9 gel as a rectal microbicide. *Sexually Transmitted Diseases*, Vol.26, No.10, pp. 564-571.

Tagat, J.R., McCombie, S.W., Nazareno, D., Labroli, M.A., Xiao, Y., Steensma, R.W., Strizki, J.M., Baroudy, B.M., Cox, K., Lachowicz, J., *et al.* (2004). Piperazine-based CCR5 antagonists as HIV-1 inhibitors. IV. Discovery of 1-[(4,6-dimethyl-5-pyrimidinyl)carbonyl]- 4-[4-[2-methoxy-1(R)-4-(trifluoromethyl)phenyl]ethyl-3(S)-methyl-1-piperaz inyl]- 4-methylpiperidine (Sch-417690/Sch-D), a potent, highly selective, and orally bioavailable CCR5 antagonist. *Journal of Medicinal Chemistry*, Vol.47, No.10, pp. 2405-2408.

Tevi-Benissan, C., Makuva, M., Morelli, A., Georges-Courbot, M.C., Matta, M., Georges, A., and Belec, L. (2000). Protection of cynomolgus macaque against cervicovaginal transmission of SIVmac251 by the spermicide benzalkonium chloride. *Journal of Acquired Immune Deficiency Syndromes*, Vol.24, No.2, pp. 147-153.

Traggiai, E., Chicha, L., Mazzucchelli, L., Bronz, L., Piffaretti, J.C., Lanzavecchia, A., and Manz, M.G. (2004). Development of a human adaptive immune system in cord blood cell-transplanted mice. *Science*, Vol.304, No.5667, pp. 104-107.

Tsai, C.C., Emau, P., Follis, K.E., Beck, T.W., Benveniste, R.E., Bischofberger, N., Lifson, J.D., and Morton, W.R. (1998). Effectiveness of postinoculation (R)-9-(2-

phosphonylmethoxypropyl) adenine treatment for prevention of persistent simian immunodeficiency virus SIVmne infection depends critically on timing of initiation and duration of treatment. *Journal of Virology*, Vol.72, No.5, pp. 4265-4273.

Tsai, C.C., Emau, P., Jiang, Y., Agy, M.B., Shattock, R.J., Schmidt, A., Morton, W.R., Gustafson, K.R., and Boyd, M.R. (2004). Cyanovirin-N inhibits AIDS virus infections in vaginal transmission models. *AIDS Research and Human Retroviruses*, Vol.20, No.1, pp. 11-18.

Tsai, C.C., Emau, P., Jiang, Y., Tian, B., Morton, W.R., Gustafson, K.R., and Boyd, M.R. (2003). Cyanovirin-N gel as a topical microbicide prevents rectal transmission of SHIV89.6P in macaques. *AIDS Research and Human Retroviruses*, Vol.19, No.7, pp. 535-541.

Tsai, C.C., Follis, K.E., Sabo, A., Beck, T.W., Grant, R.F., Bischofberger, N., Benveniste, R.E., and Black, R. (1995). Prevention of SIV infection in macaques by (R)-9-(2-phosphonylmethoxypropyl)adenine. *Science*, Vol.270, No.5239, pp. 1197-1199.

Tuerk, C., and Gold, L. (1990). Systematic evolution of ligands by exponential enrichment: RNA ligands to bacteriophage T4 DNA polymerase. *Science*, Vol.249, No.4968, pp. 505-510.

Turville, S.G., Aravantinou, M., Miller, T., Kenney, J., Teitelbaum, A., Hu, L., Chudolij, A., Zydowsky, T.M., Piatak, M., Jr., Bess, J.W., Jr., *et al.* (2008). Efficacy of Carraguard-based microbicides in vivo despite variable in vitro activity. *PLoS One*, Vol.3, No.9, pp. e3162.

Uberla, K., Stahl-Hennig, C., Bottiger, D., Matz-Rensing, K., Kaup, F.J., Li, J., Haseltine, W.A., Fleckenstein, B., Hunsmann, G., Oberg, B., *et al.* (1995). Animal model for the therapy of acquired immunodeficiency syndrome with reverse transcriptase inhibitors. *Proceedings of the National Academy of Sciences USA*, Vol.92, No.18, pp. 8210-8214.

Valentine, L.E., and Watkins, D.I. (2008). Relevance of studying T cell responses in SIV-infected rhesus macaques. *Trends in Microbiology*, Vol.16, No.12, pp. 605-611.

Van Heuverswyn, F., Li, Y., Neel, C., Bailes, E., Keele, B.F., Liu, W., Loul, S., Butel, C., Liegeois, F., Bienvenue, Y., *et al.* (2006). Human immunodeficiency viruses: SIV infection in wild gorillas. *Nature*, Vol.444, No.7116, p. 164.

Van Rompay, K.K. (2010). Evaluation of antiretrovirals in animal models of HIV infection. *Antiviral Research*, Vol.85, No.1, pp. 159-175.

Van Rompay, K.K., Brignolo, L.L., Meyer, D.J., Jerome, C., Tarara, R., Spinner, A., Hamilton, M., Hirst, L.L., Bennett, D.R., Canfield, D.R., *et al.* (2004). Biological effects of short-term or prolonged administration of 9-[2-(phosphonomethoxy)propyl]adenine (tenofovir) to newborn and infant rhesus macaques. *Antimicrobial Agents and Chemotherapy*, Vol.48, No.5, pp. 1469-1487.

Van Rompay, K.K., Hamilton, M., Kearney, B., and Bischofberger, N. (2005). Pharmacokinetics of tenofovir in breast milk of lactating rhesus macaques. *Antimicrobial Agents and Chemotherapy*, Vol.49, No.5, pp. 2093-2094.

Van Rompay, K.K., Johnson, J.A., Blackwood, E.J., Singh, R.P., Lipscomb, J., Matthews, T.B., Marthas, M.L., Pedersen, N.C., Bischofberger, N., Heneine, W., *et al.* (2007). Sequential emergence and clinical implications of viral mutants with K70E and K65R mutation in reverse transcriptase during prolonged tenofovir monotherapy in rhesus macaques with chronic RT-SHIV infection. *Retrovirology*, Vol.4, p. 25.

Van Rompay, K.K., Kearney, B.P., Sexton, J.J., Colon, R., Lawson, J.R., Blackwood, E.J., Lee, W.A., Bischofberger, N., and Marthas, M.L. (2006). Evaluation of oral tenofovir disoproxil fumarate and topical tenofovir GS-7340 to protect infant macaques against repeated oral challenges with virulent simian immunodeficiency virus. *Journal of Acquired Immune Deficiency Syndromes*, Vol.43, No.1, pp. 6-14.

Van Rompay, K.K., Matthews, T.B., Higgins, J., Canfield, D.R., Tarara, R.P., Wainberg, M.A., Schinazi, R.F., Pedersen, N.C., and North, T.W. (2002a). Virulence and reduced fitness of simian immunodeficiency virus with the M184V mutation in reverse transcriptase. *Journal of Virology*, Vol.76, No.12, pp. 6083-6092.

Van Rompay, K.K., McChesney, M.B., Aguirre, N.L., Schmidt, K.A., Bischofberger, N., and Marthas, M.L. (2001). Two low doses of tenofovir protect newborn macaques against oral simian immunodeficiency virus infection. *Journal of Infectious Diseases*, Vol.184, No.4, pp. 429-438.

Van Rompay, K.K., Schmidt, K.A., Lawson, J.R., Singh, R., Bischofberger, N., and Marthas, M.L. (2002b). Topical administration of low-dose tenofovir disoproxil fumarate to protect infant macaques against multiple oral exposures of low doses of simian immunodeficiency virus. *Journal of Infectious Diseases*, Vol.186, No.10, pp. 1508-1513.

Veazey, R.S., Ketas, T.A., Klasse, P.J., Davison, D.K., Singletary, M., Green, L.C., Greenberg, M.L., and Moore, J.P. (2008). Tropism-independent protection of macaques against vaginal transmission of three SHIVs by the HIV-1 fusion inhibitor T-1249. *Proceedings of the National Academy of Sciences USA*, Vol.105, No.30, pp. 10531-10536.

Veazey, R.S., Ketas, T.J., Dufour, J., Moroney-Rasmussen, T., Green, L.C., Klasse, P.J., and Moore, J.P. (2010). Protection of rhesus macaques from vaginal infection by vaginally delivered maraviroc, an inhibitor of HIV-1 entry via the CCR5 co-receptor. *Journal of Infectious Diseases*, Vol.202, No.5, pp. 739-744.

Veazey, R.S., Klasse, P.J., Ketas, T.J., Reeves, J.D., Piatak, M., Jr., Kunstman, K., Kuhmann, S.E., Marx, P.A., Lifson, J.D., Dufour, J., *et al.* (2003a). Use of a small molecule CCR5 inhibitor in macaques to treat simian immunodeficiency virus infection or prevent simian-human immunodeficiency virus infection. *Journal of Experimental Medicine*, Vol.198, No.10, pp. 1551-1562.

Veazey, R.S., Klasse, P.J., Schader, S.M., Hu, Q., Ketas, T.J., Lu, M., Marx, P.A., Dufour, J., Colonno, R.J., Shattock, R.J., *et al.* (2005a). Protection of macaques from vaginal SHIV challenge by vaginally delivered inhibitors of virus-cell fusion. *Nature*, Vol.438, No.7064, pp. 99-102.

Veazey, R.S., Ling, B., Green, L.C., Ribka, E.P., Lifson, J.D., Piatak, M., Jr., Lederman, M.M., Mosier, D., Offord, R., and Hartley, O. (2009). Topically applied recombinant chemokine analogues fully protect macaques from vaginal simian-human immunodeficiency virus challenge. *Journal of Infectious Diseases*, Vol.199, No.10, pp. 1525-1527.

Veazey, R.S., Shattock, R.J., Pope, M., Kirijan, J.C., Jones, J., Hu, Q., Ketas, T., Marx, P.A., Klasse, P.J., Burton, D.R., *et al.* (2003b). Prevention of virus transmission to macaque monkeys by a vaginally applied monoclonal antibody to HIV-1 gp120. *Nature* Medicine, Vol.9, No.3, pp. 343-346.

Veazey, R.S., Springer, M.S., Marx, P.A., Dufour, J., Klasse, P.J., and Moore, J.P. (2005b). Protection of macaques from vaginal SHIV challenge by an orally delivered CCR5 inhibitor. *Nature Medicine*, Vol.11, No.12, pp. 1293-1294.

Vourvahis, M., Tappouni, H.L., Patterson, K.B., Chen, Y.C., Rezk, N.L., Fiscus, S.A., Kearney, B.P., Rooney, J.F., Hui, J., Cohen, M.S., *et al.* (2008). The pharmacokinetics and viral activity of tenofovir in the male genital tract. *Journal of Acquired Immune Deficiency Syndromes*, Vol.47, No.3, pp. 329-333.

Watanabe, S., Terashima, K., Ohta, S., Horibata, S., Yajima, M., Shiozawa, Y., Dewan, M.Z., Yu, Z., Ito, M., Morio, T., *et al.* (2007). Hematopoietic stem cell-engrafted NOD/SCID/IL2Rgamma null mice develop human lymphoid systems and induce long-lasting HIV-1 infection with specific humoral immune responses. *Blood*, Vol.109, No.1, pp. 212-218.

Watson, A., McClure, J., Ranchalis, J., Scheibel, M., Schmidt, A., Kennedy, B., Morton, W.R., Haigwood, N.L., and Hu, S.L. (1997). Early postinfection antiviral treatment reduces viral load and prevents CD4+ cell decline in HIV type 2-infected macaques. *AIDS Research and Human Retroviruses*, Vol.13, No.16, pp. 1375-1381.

Wheeler, L.A., Trifonova, R., Vrbanac, V., Basar, E., McKernan, S., Xu, Z., Seung, E., Deruaz, M., Dudek, T., Einarsson, J.I., *et al.* (2011). Inhibition of HIV transmission in human cervicovaginal explants and humanized mice using CD4 aptamer-siRNA chimeras. *Journal of Clinical Investigation*, Vol.121, No.6, pp. 2401-2412.

Wilkinson, D., Tholandi, M., Ramjee, G., and Rutherford, G.W. (2002). Nonoxynol-9 spermicide for prevention of vaginally acquired HIV and other sexually transmitted infections: systematic review and meta-analysis of randomised controlled trials including more than 5000 women. *The Lancet*, Vol.2, No.10, pp. 613-617.

Winters, M.A., Van Rompay, K.K., Kashuba, A.D., Shulman, N.S., and Holodniy, M. (2010). Maternal-fetal pharmacokinetics and dynamics of a single intrapartum dose of maraviroc in rhesus macaques. *Antimicrobial Agents and Chemotherapy*, Vol.54, No.10, pp. 4059-4063.

Wyand, M.S., Manson, K.H., Miller, C.J., and Neurath, A.R. (1999). Effect of 3-hydroxyphthaloyl-beta-lactoglobulin on vaginal transmission of simian immunodeficiency virus in rhesus monkeys. *Antimicrobial Agents and Chemotherapy*, Vol.43, No.4, pp. 978-980.

Yuan, X., Naguib, S., and Wu, Z. (2011). Recent advances of siRNA delivery by nanoparticles. *Expert Opinion on Drug Delivery*, Vol.8, No.4, pp. 521-536.

Zamore, P.D., Tuschl, T., Sharp, P.A., and Bartel, D.P. (2000). RNAi: double-stranded RNA directs the ATP-dependent cleavage of mRNA at 21 to 23 nucleotide intervals. *Cell*, Vol.101, No.1, pp. 25-33.

Zhou, J., Chen, C.H., and Aiken, C. (2004). The sequence of the CA-SP1 junction accounts for the differential sensitivity of HIV-1 and SIV to the small molecule maturation inhibitor 3-O-{3',3'-dimethylsuccinyl}-betulinic acid. *Retrovirology*, Vol.1, p. 15.

Zink, M.C., Brice, A.K., Kelly, K.M., Queen, S.E., Gama, L., Li, M., Adams, R.J., Bartizal, C., Varrone, J., Rabi, S.A., *et al.* (2010). Simian immunodeficiency virus-infected macaques treated with highly active antiretroviral therapy have reduced central nervous system viral replication and inflammation but persistence of viral DNA. *Journal of Infectious Diseases*, Vol.202, No.1, pp. 161-170.

6

Discovery of Novel Antiviral Agents Directed Against the Influenza A Virus Nucleoprotein

Yoko Aida, Yutaka Sasaki and Kyoji Hagiwara
Viral Infectious Diseases Unit, RIKEN, 2-1 Hirosawa, Wako, Saitama, Japan

1. Introduction

The influenza virus types A, B, and C belong to the family *Orthomyxoviridae*. Influenza B and C viruses are predominantly human pathogens, whereas influenza A virus spreads not only in humans but also in many animals, including birds and pigs. This characteristic of influenza A viruses is a major cause of influenza pandemics in humans. Influenza A viruses are responsible for periodic widespread epidemics, or pandemics, which have taken the form of respiratory diseases with cold-like symptoms, but also sometimes serious disease with high mortality rates (Webster et al., 1992). Four outbreaks of influenza occurred in the last and current centuries: Spanish influenza (H1N1) in 1918, Asian influenza (H2N2) in 1957, Hong Kong influenza (H3N2) in 1968, and H1N1 influenza in 2009. Recently, an influenza pandemic was caused by swine influenza (H1N1) in 2009, and according to the European Centre for Disease Prevention and Control, so far this global pandemic brought on 1.2 million infections and took the lives of more than fourteen thousand people. A strong sense of fear pervaded, but many lessons were learned from this pandemic. For example, this pandemic illustrated once again that the available vaccines against influenza virus were not completely effective for the prevention of influenza outbreaks, due to the extraordinarily rapid mutation rate that influenza viruses possess (Steinhauer & Holland, 1987). In addition, we did not have enough efficient antiviral drugs to cover all of the people infected (Stiver, 2004). On the other hand, there had been avian influenza (H5N1) infections in humans several years ago in Southeast Asia (Tran et al., 2004), and, importantly, that virus caused a high mortality rate. Putting it all together, in the face of the persistent threat of human influenza A infections, and moreover, the possibility of outbreaks of an avian influenza (H5N1) pandemic (Ungchusak et al., 2005; Wang et al., 2008), there is much concern about the shortage of effective anti-influenza virus agents, and for this reason, the development of novel anti-influenza virus agents is being strongly demanded.

Influenza A virus is a negative-stranded RNA virus with an eight-segmented genome that encodes 12 different proteins, including polymerase basic (PB)1, PB1-F2, an N-terminally truncated version of the polypeptide (N40), the translation of which is directed by PB1 codon 40, PB2, polymerase acidic protein (PA), hemagglutinin (HA), nucleoprotein (NP), neuraminidase (NA), matrix protein (M)1, M2, nonstructural protein (NS)1 and NS2 (Wise et al., 2009) (Fig. 1b). Nine of these proteins are incorporated into the virion. The influenza virus particles, which are ~100 nm in diameter, form by budding from the plasma membrane of infected cells (Fig. 1a). On the surface of the virion, there are two main antigenic determinants, the spike glycoproteins HA and NA. There are considerable antigenic variations among influenza viruses consisting of 16 different types of HA (H1-H16) and 9 different types of NA (N1-N9) (Fouchier et al., 2005; Hinshaw et al., 1982; Kawaoka et al., 1990; Rohm et al., 1996; World Health Organization, 1980). In addition, another viral protein is inserted in the viral membrane: M2, a low-abundance ion channel involved in uncoating and HA maturation (Fig. 1b). Underlying the membrane is the matrix or M1 protein, the major structural component of the virion, which is thought to act as an adaptor between the lipid envelope and the ribonucleoprotein (RNP) complexes and is probably the mediator of virus budding (Gómez-Puertas et al., 2000). Inside the shell of M1 lie the viral RNP complexes (vRNPs), which comprise the genomic RNA segments in association with a trimeric RNA polymerase (PB1, PB2 and PA subunits) and the stoichiometric quantities of NP (Fig. 1c). Also found in the virion are small quantities of the NEP and NS2 proteins.

The surface proteins HA, NA, and M2 are the targets of vaccines and anti-viral drugs. Two classes of drugs including adamantanes (amantadine and rimantadine) and NA inhibitors (oseltamivir, zanamivir, peramivir, and laninamivir) are available for the treatment of the influenza infection (Kubo et al., 2010; Vanvoris et al., 1981; Wingfiel et al., 1969; Yamashita, 2011). Because the adamantanes exert several toxic effects on the central nervous system (Bryson et al., 1980; Keyser et al., 2000) and also because of the emergence of resistant variants (Bright et al., 2005, 2006), the use of these drugs is limited. Currently, the NA inhibitors are used widely for drug therapies to treat influenza patients because of high inhibitory effects and little toxicity. However, resistant strains, and especially oseltamivir-resistant strains, have also been reported in recent years (Besselaar et al., 2008; Dharan et al., 2009; Hauge et al., 2009; Hurt et al., 2009). The fact that available drugs target only two steps of the viral life cycle, along with the appearance of oseltamivir-resistant influenza strains, strongly highlights the need for treatment alternatives or novel antiviral drugs targeting other proteins besides M2 or NA.

In contrast to the surface proteins, after entry into the cytoplasm, the vRNPs are imported into the nucleus for the production of viral messenger RNAs. RNA polymerases, such as PB1, PB2, and PA, transcribe and replicate the virus genome, while NP encapsidates the virus genome to form an RNP complex for the purposes of transcription and packaging. Thus, influenza virus transcription and replication are initiated after transport to the nucleus of vRNPs. A promising target for blocking influenza A viruses is the NP, which is expressed in the early stage of infection and plays important roles in numerous steps of viral replication. NP preserves viral genomic RNA (vRNA) stability and contains many functional domains in its sequence, such as a nuclear localization signal (NLS), an RNA binding site, an NP-NP binding site, and a PB2 binding domain. In addition, NP is relatively well conserved compared with viral surface spike protein. Here, we summarize current knowledge about influenza therapy, the functions of NP involved in the nuclear-import step of influenza virus replication, and how this could facilitate the discovery of a new small molecule involved in influenza replication.

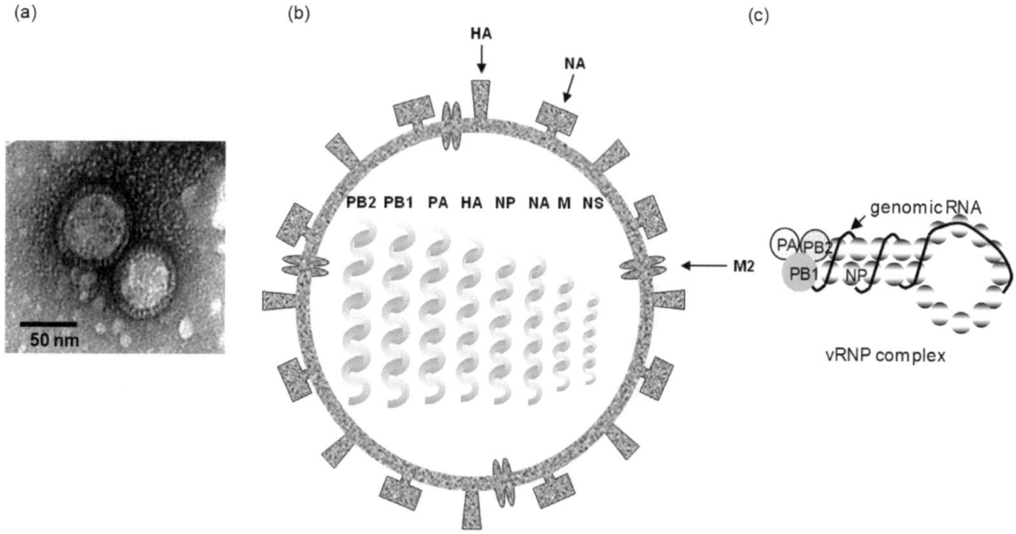

(a) Influenza virus particles (A/WSN/33) were isolated by sucrose density gradient ultracentrifugation, and purified particles were observed by electron microscope with uranyl acetate-staining. (b) Model of influenza virus particle. The particle contains eight segments that make up the RNA genome. There were three major proteins (HA, NA, and M2) on the surface of the viron. (c) Diagram of the viral ribonucleoprotein (vRNP). The vRNA is associated with NP, PB2, PB1, and PA, which are composed of vRNPs.

Fig. 1. Electron microscopy and model of influenza virus particles.

2. Viral life cycle

Influenza A virus is one of the rare RNA viruses that replicate in the nucleus. The design of effective anti-influenza virus therapeutics is based on detailed knowledge of the biology of the virus. Fig. 2 shows the viral life cycle of the influenza virus. Generally, the influenza virus is adsorbed to the host cell through the binding of HA glycoproteins with sialic acid groups as receptors on the host cell, which are distributed on membrane-bound proteins and lipids. Then, the influenza virus is taken up into host cells through receptor-mediated endocytosis (Matlin et al., 1981). In the acidic environment of the endosome, HA changes to the active form and promotes fusion of the viral envelope with the endosomal membrane (Stegmann et al., 1987; White et al., 1982). The acidification of the endosome is necessary not only for the membrane fusion of HA but also the activation of the M2 ion channel. The activation of the M2 ion channel leads to proton entry into the virions, which causes uncoating of the vRNPs (Bui et al., 1996; Pinto et al., 1992). All vRNA are associated with the NP, which is bound at a distance of 24 nucleotides (Compans et al., 1972; Ortega et al., 2000). It is also suggested that vRNA is associated with trimeric RNA polymerase, which are composed of vRNPs (Klumpp et al., 1997). Influenza virus transcription and replication are initiated after the transport of vRNPs into the nucleus. After uncoating, the vRNPs are transported into the nucleus through importin α/β transport systems, where they undergo transcription and replication (Herz et al., 1981; Martin & Helenius, 1991). Transcription of vRNA requires capped RNA primers snartched from cellular pre-mRNAs and premature poly(A) termination of transcripts (Bouloy et al., 1978; Plotch et al., 1979; Robertson et al.,

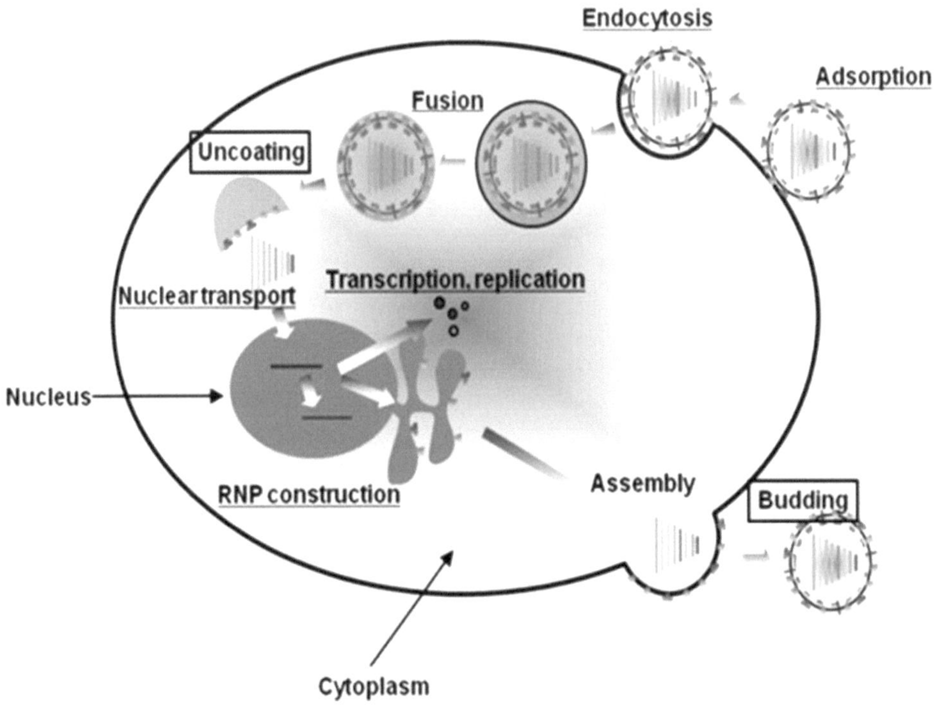

The crucial steps in Influenza virus multiplication are: 1) attachment of the virus to its target cell; 2) entry of the virus via receptor-mediated endocytosis; 3) fusion of endosome and viral membranes; 4) the RNPs release into the cytoplasm and 5) transport into nucleus; 6) virus transcription and replication in nucleus; 7) the RNPs construction; 8) virion assembly and 9) viral budding. Anti-influenza drugs target two different steps in the viral life-cycle; these steps are shown in boxes.

Fig. 2. Model of the life cycle of the influenza virus.

1981). In contrast, the replication of vRNA is performed in a primer-independent manner (Nagata et al., 2008). The newly synthesized vRNPs are exported from the nucleus to the cytoplasm in association with the viral proteins M1 and NS2 and the cellular protein chromosome region maintenance 1 (CRM1) (Cros & Palese, 2003; Neumann et al., 2004). These vRNPs are incorporated into budding virions. The vRNA is specifically packaged in preference to other cellular RNAs and the different vRNAs are present in an equimolar ratio within a population of virions (Palese, 1977). A mechanism for the specific packaging of vRNA is mediated by *cis*-acting packaging signals in the vRNAs. Specific packaging signals exist in the UTRs and coding regions at both the 5′ and 3′ ends of the vRNAs (de Wit et al., 2006; Fujii et al., 2003; Liang et al., 2008; Muramoto et al., 2006; Noda et al., 2006; Ozawa et al., 2007). The structure of eight separate segments is associated with inter-segment interactions (Muramoto et al., 2006). However, it remains uncertain whether there are specific interactions among the eight RNPs within the virions. The M1 and M2 proteins play central roles in the assembly and budding process. The M1 protein is associated with the cytoplasmic tail of HA and NA. This binding allows for M1 to associate with lipid raft membrane domains, triggering a conformational change that enables M1 polymerization at the site of virus budding (Barman et al., 2004; Gómez-Puertas et al., 2000; Ruigrok et al., 2001). The M2 protein is required for the membrane scission of the budding virions. M2 binds to cholesterol and this allows M2 to alter membrane curvature at the site of virus budding (Rossman et al., 2010a, 2010b). Bud formation and bud release are the last steps of the viral life cycle. NA is responsible for cleaving terminal sialic acid residues from the ends of glycoconjugates on both the virus particle and the host cell in order to facilitate virus release (Air & Laver, 1989).

3. Influenza therapy

The life-cycle of influenza virus is a major target for drug development. Accordingly, significant efforts have been made recently to identify molecules that inhibit the different stages of the influenza virus life cycle. As shown in Fig. 2, the current treatments for influenza infections target two steps of the replication cycle: uncoating and budding. Six drugs are currently available (Table 1): the adamantanes and neuraminidase inhibitors, including amantadine, rimantadine, zanamivir, oseltamivir, peramivir, and laninamivir (Kubo et al., 2010; Vanvoris et al., 1981; Wingfiel et al., 1969, Yamashita, 2011). The adamantanes block the function of the M2 ion channel, preventing acidification-triggered uncoating. The adamantanes were the first effective drugs licensed for influenza treatment (Davies et al., 1964; Dolin et al., 1982; Wang et al., 1993). Despite a degree of treatment effectiveness, however, both drugs induced significant adverse effects in the central nervous system, as well as the emergence of drug-resistant mutants (Bright et al., 2005, 2006; Bryson et al., 1980; Keyser et al., 2000). Recently, the vast majority of circulating seasonal influenza strains has been adamantanes-resistant (Bright et al., 2005, 2006). Neuraminidase inhibitors inhibit the release of virions by competitively inhibiting viral NA. Currently, zanamivir and oseltamivir are widely used to treat acute uncomplicated illness due to influenza A and B. Zanamivir mimics the natural substrate, which fits into the active site pocket of NA (Varghese et al., 1992, 1995; von Itzstein et al., 1993). Oseltamivir was developed through the modification of the sialic acid analogue framework (Kim et al., 1997). Many reports have shown that both drugs are highly efficient in the treatment of influenza (Cooper et al., 2003; Hayden et al., 1997; Monto et al., 1999; Nicholson et al., 2000). In recent years, peramivir and laninamivir, which also target NA, have been licensed as anti-influenza drugs (Kubo et al., 2010; Yamashita, 2011). For oseltamivir, the appearance of drug-resistant mutants has significantly increased in many countries (Besselaar et al., 2008; Dharan et al., 2009; Hauge et al., 2009; Hurt et al., 2009). The oseltamivir-resistant H275Y virus also displays reduced susceptibility to peramivir *in vitro* (Nguyen et al., 2010). On the other hand, no zanamivir-resistant virus has emerged at present. However, because zanamivir requires treatment by the intravenous route, it is not commonly used in clinical treatment.

As mentioned above, in addition to the fact that available drugs target only two steps of the viral life cycle, this appearance of oseltamivir-resistant influenza strains strongly highlights the need for treatment alternatives or novel antiviral drugs targeting other proteins besides M2 or NA. Potential targets for blocking influenza A virus replication are influenza virus RNA polymerases and NP, which is required to form the RNPs. Recently, favipiravir, a novel therapeutic drug targeting viral replication and translation, has been identified (Furuta et al., 2005). Favipiravir, developed by Furuta *et al.* at Toyama Chemical Co., Ltd., inhibits the replication and translation of influenza viruses in a GTP-competitive manner. In addition to these drugs, a few novel antiviral compounds, mycalamide analogs (Hagiwara et al., 2010), nucleozin (Kao et al., 2010) and nucleozin analog FA-2 (Su et al., 2010), were recently reported as influenza inhibitors targeting NP. Moreover, another anti-influenza compound, 367, has been identified that targets the PB1 protein and influenza RNA-dependent RNA polymerase activity (Su et al., 2010). These observations suggest that the drug targeting of components of the RNPs, such as PA, PB1, PB2, and NP, may provide a new strategy for influenza therapy.

Classification	Generic Name	Commercial Name
M2 Channel Inhibitor	Amantadine	Symmetrel
	Rimantadine	Flumadine
Neuraminidase Inhibitor	Oseltamivir	Tamiflu
	Zanamivir	Relenza
	Peramivir	Rapiacta
	Laninamivir	Inamivir

Table 1. Available drugs against influenza virus infection.

4. NP of influenza A virus

4.1. Function of NP

The influenza virus NP, which is encoded by the fifth genome segment, is expressed in the early stage of infection. It is the major component of the RNP and contains many functional domains in its sequence, such as a NLS, an RNA binding site, an NP-NP binding site, and a PB2 binding domain (Albo et al., 1995; Biswas et al., 1998; Cros et al., 2005; Davey et al., 1985; Elton et al., 1999; Ketha & Atreya, 2008; Kobayashi et al., 1994; Neumann et al., 1997; Ozawa et al., 2007; Wang et al., 1997; Weber et al., 1998; Ye et al., 2006). The major functional domains of NP are summarized in Fig. 3. Thus, NP plays important roles in numerous stages of viral replication, such as in the nuclear transport of NP and RNPs, replication and transcription of genomic RNA, and nuclear export and packaging of RNPs. In addition to these, some domains that are important for the maintenance of three-dimensional structure, such as the tail-loop structure, pocket structure, and regulation of particle formation, as well as domains that are important for interactions with host proteins, have been reported (Fig. 3) (Digard et al., 1999; Momose et al., 2001; Ng et al., 2008, 2009; Noton et al., 2009; Wang et al., 1997; Ye et al., 2006). Moreover, phylogenetic analysis of viral strains isolated from different hosts revealed that the NP gene is relatively well conserved (Shu et al., 1993), especially in the functional domains (Heiny et al., 2007; Li et al., 2009; Ng et al., 2009). Thus, all of these functional domains could be considered potential targets for antiviral agents.

4.2 Structure of NP

The crystal structure of NP of influenza A virus H1N1 (Ye et al., 2006) is shown in Fig. 4. The N-terminal truncated NP derived from H1N1 forms trimers through NP-NP interactions using a tail-loop structure constructed from the segment at amino acid positions 402-428 (Fig. 3 & 4) and pocket structures constructed from segments at amino acid positions 160-167, 321-334, and 340-349 (Fig. 3, Ye et al., 2006).

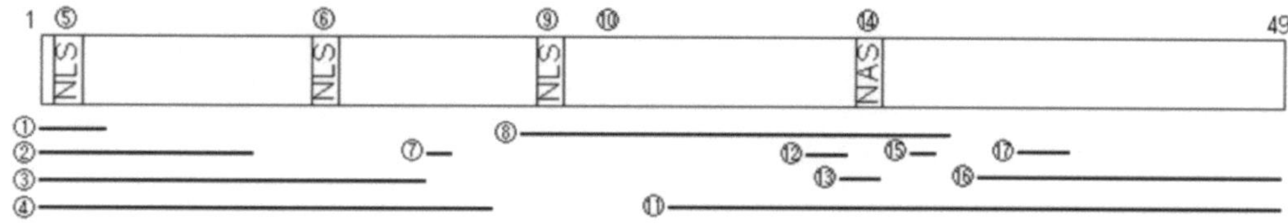

Position	Function	Reference
①1-20:	RAF-2p48 interaction	Momose et al., 2001
②1-73:	NPI-1/NPI-3 interaction	Wang et al., 1997
③1-160:	PB2 interaction	Biswas et al., 1998
④1-180:	RNA interaction	Albo et al., 1995; Kobayashi et al., 1994
⑤3-13:	unconventional nuclear localization signal	Cros et al., 2005; Neumann et al., 1997; Ozawa et al., 2007; Wang et al., 1997
⑥90-121:	overlapping bipartite nuclear localization signal	Ketha & Atreya, 2008
⑦160-167:	pocket for tail loop	Ng et al., 2008, 2009; Ye et al., 2006
⑧189-354:	NP-NP interaction	Elton et al., 1999; Ye et al., 2006
⑨198-216:	bipartite nuclear localization signal	Ozawa et al., 2007; Weber et al., 1998
⑩239:	regulation site of particle formation	Sarah et al., 2009
⑪256-498:	PB2 interaction	Biswas et al., 1998
⑫321-334:	pocket for tail loop	Ng et al., 2008, 2009; Ye et al., 2006
⑬327-345:	F-actin interaction	Digard et al., 1999
⑭339-345:	nuclear accumulation signal	Davey et al., 1985
⑮340-349:	pocket for tail loop	Ng et al., 2008, 2009; Ye et al., 2006
⑯371-498:	NP-NP interaction	Elton et al., 1999; Ye et al., 2006
⑰402-428:	tail loop	Ng et al., 2008, 2009; Ye et al., 2006

NLS, nuclear localization signal; NAS, nuclear accumulation signal

Fig. 3. Summary of NP functions.

The nucleoprotein has been proven to bind non-specifically to RNA at one in every 24 nucleotides (Compans et al., 1972; Ortega et al., 2000), and indeed, the protein has been shown to have an RNA-binding groove between the head and body domains. This groove is located exterior to the nucleoprotein oligomers. The surface of the groove is occupied by several basic residues, such as R65, R150, R152, R156, R174, R175, R195, R199, R213, R214, R221, R236, R355, K357, R361, and R391 (Ye et al., 2006), which can interact with nucleotides. These distributed basic residues are highly conserved, and therefore it is likely that the compounds targeting these regions can inhibit viral multiplication.

The crystal structure of NP derived from H5N1 has also been reported. It forms a different trimer compared with H1N1; however, the tail-loop interactions were identical (Ng et al., 2008). Both papers suggest that the tail-loop binding pocket is a good target for the development of anti-influenza virus drugs.

5. Nuclear transport of NP

Most RNA viruses that lack a DNA phase replicate in the cytoplasm (Cros & Palese, 2003). However, several negative-stranded RNA viruses, such as influenza, Thogoto, and Borna disease viruses, replicate their RNAs in the nucleus, taking advantage of the host cell's

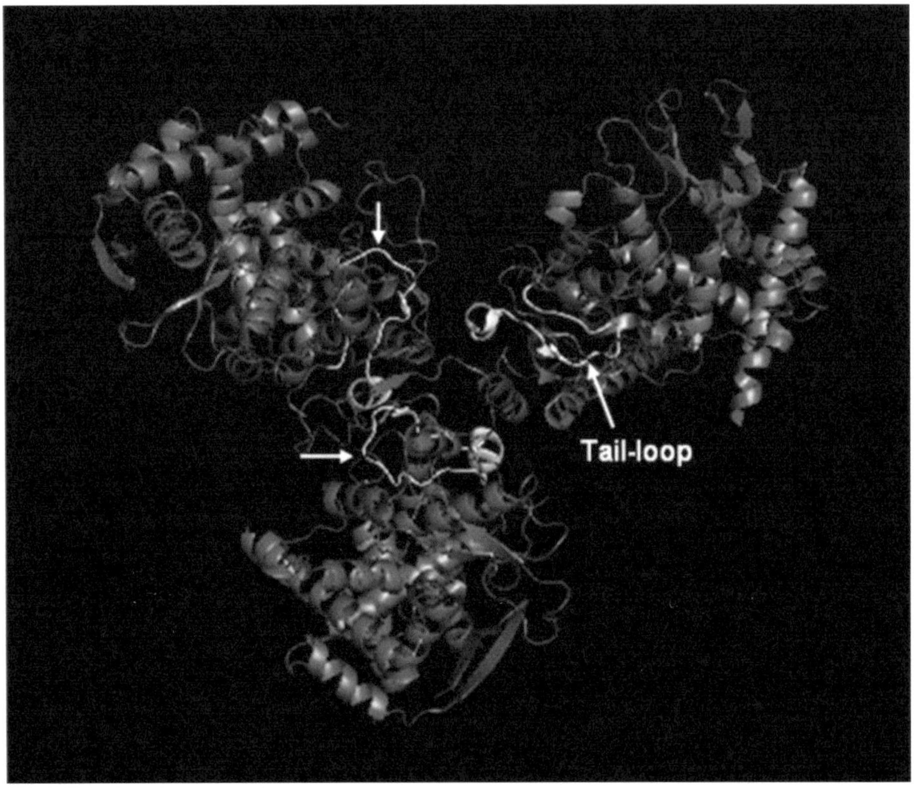

The NP trimer was constructed according to NP-NP interactions using pocket structure (amino acid positions 160-167, 327-334 and 340-349) and tail-loop structure (amino acid positions 402-428). The positions of the three tail loops are highlighted in white and indicated by arrows. This structure is based on the available structural information for NP (PDB code: 2IQH).

Fig. 4. Crystal structure of influenza virus NP trimer analyzed by X-ray.

nuclear machinery. The cell nucleus is separated from the cytoplasm by a double-layer membrane contiguous with the ER called the nuclear envelope (Terry et al., 2007). This nuclear envelope is composed of two lipid bilayers, the outer and inner nuclear membranes (Gruenbaum et al., 2005). Viruses that replicate their genome in the host cell nucleus have evolved strategies for moving viral components across this membrane barrier. These membranes are separated by a lumen and joined at nuclear pore complexes (NPCs) (Fahrenkrog & Aebi, 2003) that serve as gates for traffic crossing the nuclear envelope. Entrance into and exit from the nucleus occurs via these NPCs, which are > 60 MDa macromolecular structures that form channels spanning the nuclear envelope (Cronshaw et al., 2002; Rout et al., 2000). Each NPC is equipped to facilitate both the import and export of proteins and RNAs (Dworetzky & Feldherr, 1988).

The movement of ions, metabolites and other small molecules through the NPC occurs via passive diffusion, but the translocation of cargos larger than ~40 kDa generally requires specific signals known as NLSs. The nuclear import of basic NLS-bearing proteins is mediated by specific soluble factors, including importin-α (Impα) (Goldfarb et al., 2004), importin-β (Impβ) (Harel & Forbes, 2004), small GTPase Ran/TC4 (Quimby & Dasso, 2003), and NTF2 (Stewart, 2000). Impα functions as an adaptor molecule, binding Impβ via its amino-terminally located Impβ-binding (IBB) domain and binding an NLS-bearing protein via its two central region-located NLS-binding sites (Herold et al., 1998; Kobe, 1999) (Fig. 5). Impβ is the transport receptor that carries the Impα-NLS complex from the cytoplasm to the nuclear side of the NPC. Once the heterotrimer consisting of Impα, Impβ, and the NLS-bearing protein reaches the nuclear face of the NPC, the GTP-bound form of Ran binds directly to Impβ, releasing Impα and the NLS-bearing protein into the nucleoplasm. Ran, which is found in its GDP-bound form in the cytoplasm and in its GTP-bound form in the nucleus, is a major determinant of the directionality of transport across the nuclear membrane.

A challenge faced by influenza virus is that of the trafficking of viral components into the nucleus through the NPC (Fig. 5). The genomic RNAs of influenza virus associate with proteins to form large complexes called vRNPs, which exceed the size limit for passive diffusion through the NPCs. The vRNPs is believed to be 10–20 nm wide (Compans et al., 1972). The vRNA, coated by NPs (1NP for each 24 nucleotides) (Compans et al., 1972; Ortega et al., 2000), forms a loop (Fig. 1C & 6). The trimeric polymerase complex, PB1, PB2, and PA, binds to the partially complementary ends of the vRNA, giving rise to a complex panhandle structure (Martin-Benito et al., 2001).

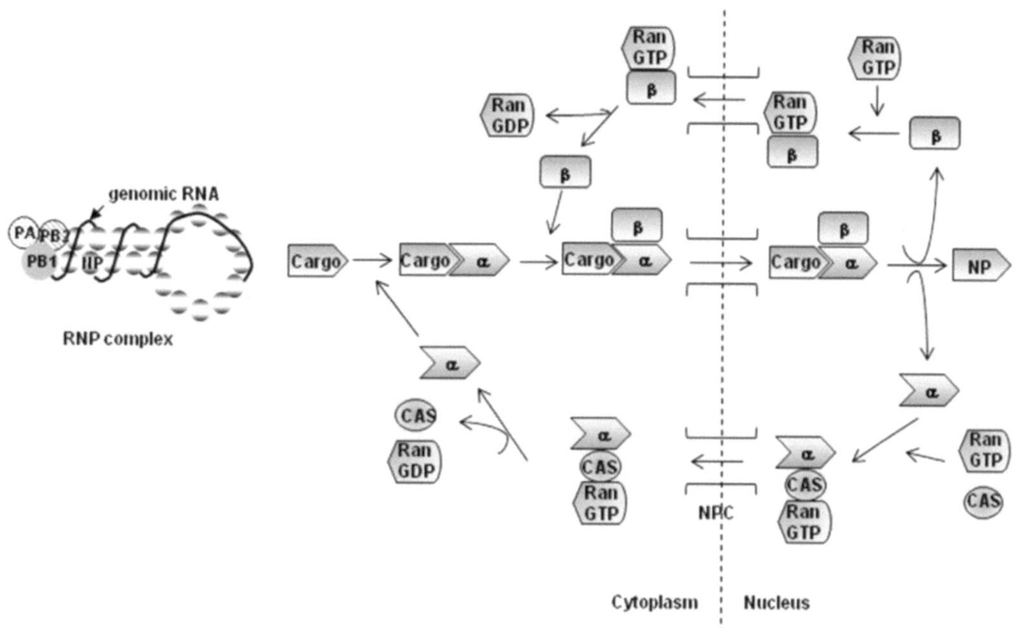

NPC, nuclear pore complex

Fig. 5. Model of the nuclear transport through classical importin α/β import pathway and influenza virus.

To ensure efficient transport across the nuclear membrane, influenza virus uses NLSs exposed on PB2, PB1, PA and NP. These signals recruit cellular import complexes, which are responsible for the translocation of the vRNPs through the NPC. Although all of the proteins of the vRNPs carry NLSs (Akkina et al., 1987; Jones et al., 1986; Nieto et al., 1994), the NP was shown to be sufficient to mediate the nuclear import of viral RNAs (O'Neill et al., 1995). As shown in Fig. 3, a more detailed analysis revealed the presence of three NLSs on the NP (Neumann et al., 1997; Wang et al., 1997), including an unconventional NLS at the very N-terminus, located between amino acids 3 and 13. A second NLS resides in the central part of the NP, located between amino acids 198 and 216. This bipartite signal appears to be weaker than the unconventional N-terminal NLS (Weber et al., 1998). Of these NLSs, the unconventional, N-terminal NLS of the NP is indispensable for the nuclear transport of NP and vRNPs (Cross et al., 2005; O'Neill et al., 1995). Alanine-substituted mutants of this unconventional NLS of the NP have shown that the amino acids at position 7 and 8 are critical for nuclear localization (Neumann et al., 1997). Furthermore, the mutation of amino acids at position 7 and 8 of NP leads to a reduction of viral growth compared with wild-type virus (Ozawa et al., 2007).

The transport of vRNPs of influenza A virus into the nucleus is performed through the classical nuclear import pathway, the impα/β transport system shown in Fig. 5. As an adaptor, impα binds with the NLSs of viral proteins and then NLS-impα binds to the receptor on impβ, through the IBB domain on impα (Cross et al., 2005; O'Neill et al., 1995). This NLS-bearing protein/receptor complex is imported into the nucleus. The impα family comprises six members in humans. Based on structural similarity, the impα family is grouped into three subfamilies, impα1/Rch1 (Rch1), impα3/Qip1 (Qip1), and impα5/NPI-1 (NPI-1) (Goldfarb et al., 2004). Interestingly, NP binds to several types of human impα, including Rch1, Qip1, and NPI-1, and regulates not only the nuclear transport of vRNPs but also host cell tropism and the growth of influenza virus (Gabriel et al., 2011). Therefore, NP functions as the main regulator of vRNPs trafficking and is a potentially useful target for the development of novel compounds that inhibit influenza A virus replication.

6. Screening of anti-viral drugs for NP

Recently, we demonstrated that NP is a novel target for the development of new antiviral drugs against the influenza virus using screening of NP-binding compounds by photo-cross-linked chemical arrays. Chemical arrays represent one of the most promising and high-throughput approaches for screening ligands against proteins of interest (Kanoh et al., 2006), and several successful results from chemical arrays have been reported (Koehler et al., 2003; Kuruvilla et al., 2002; Miyazaki et al., 2008). The screening protocol using chemical array was shown in Fig. 6. Approximately 25,000 small-molecules have been developed at RIKEN were fixed on a glass plate by photo-cross linker. To firstly identify inhibitors of NP, a large-scale chemical array approach of 6,800 compounds from an RIKEN NPDepo chemical library was used that detected specific interactions of small molecules with NP.

Using purified, recombinant influenza virus (A/WSN/33) NP, which was fused to monomeric red fluorescent protein (mRFP), we succeeded in detecting 72 compounds as positive. Next, plaque assay was used to investigate whether the 72 compounds inhibited multiplication of the influenza virus (A/WSN/33). Among them, 9 compounds showed inhibitory activity against influenza virus multiplication (Table 2). Furthermore, to obtain the compound which shows high inhibition activity, we searched for the derivatives of compounds from RIKEN NPDepo and found three derivatives of compound 1, which is

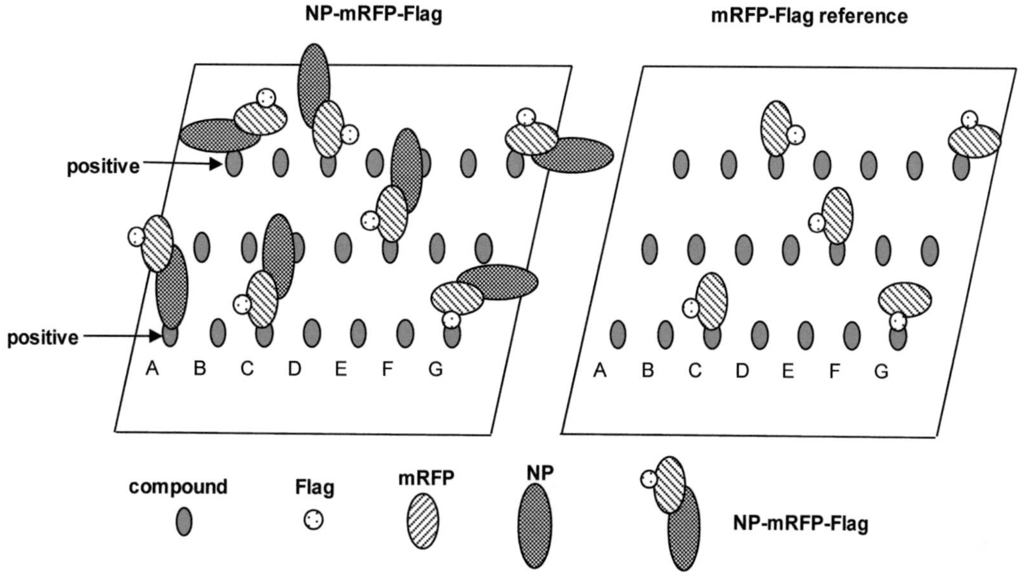

Approximately 2,000 compounds are spotted, with duplicates, on a glass plate using a photo-cross linker.

Fig. 6. Summary of compound screening using chemical array.

Methods	Targeting	Positive	Negative
Photo-crosslinked chemical array assay	Binding to NP	72	6,800
Plaque assay	Inhibition of viral replication	9	63
Plaque assay using derivatives	Inhibition of viral replication	1	8 (not determined)
Surface plasmon resonance	Binding of four derivatives to NP	4	0

Table 2. Screening for NP inhibitors from the NPDepo RIKEN Natural Products Depository.

artificial analog of mycalamide. Among them, two derivatives showed lower inhibitory effect compared with compound 1, whereas compound 4 (Fig. 7, Table 2) showed strong activity reaching inhibition level up to 97% (Hagiwara et al., 2010).

Furthermore, surface plasmon resonance imaging experiments demonstrated that the binding activity of each compound to NP correlated with its antiviral activity. Finally, it was shown that these compounds bound NP within the N-terminal 110-amino acid region but their binding abilities were dramatically reduced when the N-terminal 13-amino acid tail was deleted, suggesting that the compounds might bind to this region, which mediates the nuclear transport of NP and its binding to viral RNA. These data suggest that compound binding to the N-terminal 13-amino acid tail region corresponding to an unconventional NLS may inhibit viral replication by inhibiting the nuclear transport of NP.

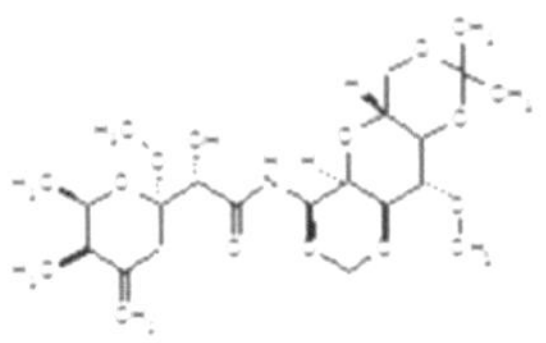

compound 1

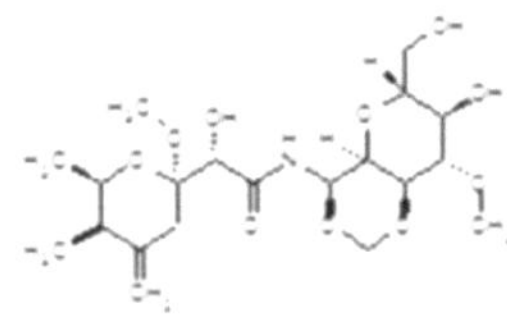

compound 2

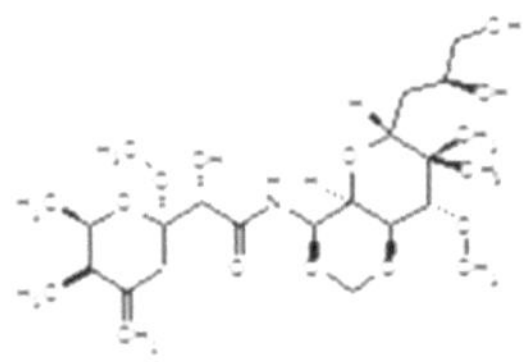

compound 3

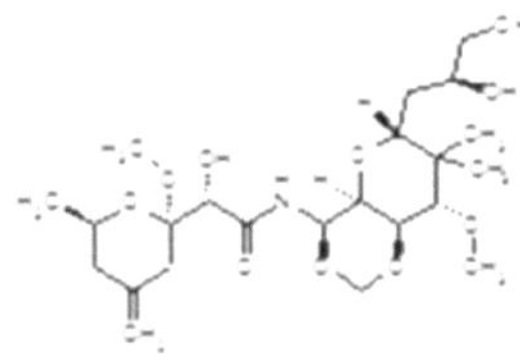

compound 4

Compound 1, which is artificial analog of mycalamide was finally selected as the anti-influenza virus agent. Compound 4 was the derivative of compound 1 that showed the strongest activity in inhibiting influenza virus multiplication.

Fig. 7. Chemical structure of three derivatives of compound 1.

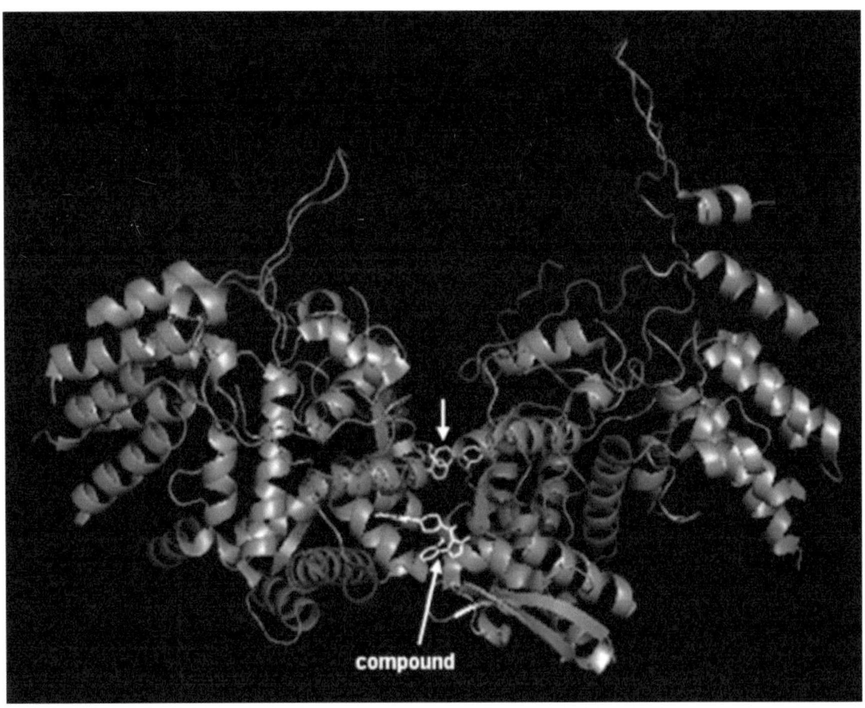

The positions of the compounds are highlighted in white and indicated by arrows.
The compounds induce the aggregation of NP. This structure is based on the available structural information for NP (PDB code: 3RO5).

Fig. 8. Structure of influenza virus NP bound to compounds.

7. Alternative anti-influenza virus compounds targeting NP

As described earlier, we first experimentally identified NP as a valuable drug target for inhibiting the influenza virus (Hagiwara et al., 2010). Interestingly, two other compounds that inhibit the function of NP have been reported. One compound, called nucleozin, was randomly screened from a commercial chemical library. Nucleozin inhibits nuclear localization of NP by inducing aggregation of NP (Kao et al., 2010). Furthermore, some nucleozin derivatives have been developed (Gerritz et al., 2011; Su et al., 2010) and the co-crystal structures of NP and these nucleozin derivatives were also reported (Gerritz et al., 2011). The crystal structures indicated that two derivatives bound to the NP dimer (Fig. 8) and might induce the aggregation of NP, thereby inhibiting nuclear transport of NP and thereby influenza virus multiplication.

Another compound was screened *in silico* and found to inhibit construction of the NP trimer. The compound interacts with E339-R416 salt bridge in the tail-loop binding pocket and thereby inhibits functional oligomerization of NP, which would in turn inhibit the multiplication of the influenza virus (Shen et al., 2011).

Using three different methods (direct binding, random screening, and *in silico* screening), compounds that inhibit the function of NP have been obtained. The results strongly suggest that NP is a good target for the development of an anti-influenza virus drug.

8. Conclusions

Influenza A viruses are responsible for seasonal epidemics and high mortality pandemics. Influenza A virus has a segmented genome of eight negative-strand RNA segments, which are packaged into virions as RNPs. In addition to RNA, RNP contains the viral NP and the three subunits of the RNA-dependent RNA polymerase, PB1, PB2, and PA. The NP is expressed in the early stage of infection and plays important roles in numerous steps of viral replication. NP also is relatively well conserved compared with viral surface spike proteins. Using three different methods, direct binding, random screening, and *in silico* screening, several small molecules that interact with NP and inhibit virus multiplication were discovered. Since there are currently only two types of drugs available for the treatment of influenza virus infection, M2 inhibitors and NA inhibitors, the discovery of a novel mechanism of inhibition of influenza virus replication may supply the field of drug development with an effective new strategy.

9. Acknowledgments

This study was supported in part by a Japan Advanced Molecular Imaging Program (J-AMP), by a RIKEN Program for Drug Discovery and Medical Technology Platforms, and by the Chemical Biology Research Project (RIKEN).

10. References

Air, G.M. & Laver, W.G. (1989). The neuraminidase of influenza virus. *Proteins*, Vol.6, No.4, pp. 341-356, ISSN 0887-3585

Akkina, R.K.; Chambers, T.M.; Londo, D.R. & Nayak, D.P. (1987). Intracellular localization of the viral polymerase proteins in cells infected with influenza virus and cells expressing PB1 protein from cloned cDNA. *Journal of Virology*, Vol.61, No.7, pp. 2217-2224, ISSN 0022-538X

Albo, C.; Valencia, A. & Portela, A. (1995). Identification of an RNA binding region within the N-terminal third of the influenza A virus nucleoprotein. *Journal of Virology*, Vol.69, No.6, pp. 3799-3806, ISSN 0022-538X

Barman, S.; Adhikary, L.; Chakrabarti, A.K.; Bernas, C.; Kawaoka, Y. & Nayak, D.P. (2004). Role of transmembrane domain and cytoplasmic tail amino acid sequences of influenza a virus neuraminidase in raft association and virus budding. *Journal of Virology*, Vol.78, No.10, pp. 5258-5269, ISSN 0022-538X

Besselaar, T.G.; Naidoo, D.; Buys, A.; Gregory, V.; McAnerney, J.; Manamela, J.M.; Blumberg, L. & Schoub, B.D. (2008). Widespread oseltamivir resistance in influenza A viruses (H1N1), South Africa. *Emerging infectious diseases*, Vol.14, No.11, pp. 1809-1810, ISSN 1080-6040

Biswas, S.K.; Boutz, P.L. & Nayak, D.P. (1998). Influenza virus nucleoprotein interacts with influenza virus polymerase proteins. *Journal of Virology*, Vol.72, No.7, pp. 5493-5501, ISSN 0022-538X

Bouloy, M.; Plotch, S.J. & Krug, R.M. (1978). Globin mRNAs are primers for the transcription of influenza viral RNA in vitro. *Proceedings of the National Academy of Sciences of the United States of America*, Vol.75, No.10, pp. 4886-4890, ISSN 0027-8424

Bright, R.A.; Medina, M.J.; Xu, X.Y.; Perez-Oronoz, G.; Wallis, T.R.; Davis, X.H.M.; Povinelli, L.; Cox, N.J. & Klimov, A.I. (2005). Incidence of adamantane resistance among influenza A (H3N2) viruses isolated worldwide from 1994 to 2005: a cause for concern. *Lancet*, Vol.366, No.9492, pp. 1175-1181, ISSN 0140-6736

Bright, R.A.; Shay, D.K.; Shu, B.; Cox, N.J. & Klimov, A.I. (2006). Adamantane resistance among influenza A viruses isolated early during the 2005-2006 influenza season in the United States. *The Journal of the American Medical Association*, Vol.295, No.8, pp. 891-894, ISSN 0098-7484

Bryson, Y.J.; Monahan, C.; Pollack, M. & Shields, W.D. (1980). A prospective double-blind study of side effects associated with the administration of amantadine for influenza A virus prophylaxis. *The Journal of infectious diseases*, Vol.141, No.5, pp.543-547, ISSN 0022-1899

Bui, M.; Whittaker, G. & Helenius, A. (1996). Effect of M1 protein and low pH on nuclear transport of influenza virus ribonucleoproteins. *Journal of Virology*, Vol.70, No.12, pp. 8391-8401, ISSN 0022-538X

Compans, R.W.; Content, J. & Duesberg, P.H. (1972) Structure of the ribonucleoprotein of influenza virus. *Journal of Virology*, Vol.10, No.4, pp. 795-800, ISSN 0022-538X

Cooper, N.J.; Sutton, A.J.; Abrams, K.R.; Wailoo, A.; Turner, D. & Nicholson, K.G. (2003). Effectiveness of neuraminidase inhibitors in treatment and prevention of influenza A and B: systematic review and meta-analyses of randomised controlled trials. *British medical journal*, Vol.326, No.7401, pp. 1235, ISSN 0959-535X

Cronshaw, J.M.; Krutchinsky, A.N.; Zhang, W.; Chait, B.T. & Matunis, M.J. (2002). Proteomic analysis of the mammalian nuclear pore complex. *The Journal of cell biology*, Vol.158, No.5, pp. 915-927, ISSN 0021-9525

Cros, J.F. & Palese, P. (2003). Trafficking of viral genomic RNA into and out of the nucleus: influenza, Thogoto and Borna disease viruses. *Virus research*, Vol.95, No.1-2, pp. 3-12, ISSN 0168-1702

Cros, J.F.; García-Sastre, A. & Palese, P. (2005). An unconventional NLS is critical for the nuclear import of the influenza A virus nucleoprotein and ribonucleoprotein. *Traffic*, Vol.6, No.3, pp. 205-213, ISSN 1398-9219

Davey, J.; Dimmock, N.J. & Colman, A. (1985). Identification of the sequence responsible for the nuclear accumulation of the influenza virus nucleoprotein in Xenopus oocytes. *Cell*, Vol.40, No.3, pp. 667-675, ISSN 0092-8674

Davies, W.L.; Grunert, R.R.; Haff R.F.; Mcgahen J.W.; Neumayer E.M.; Paulshock M.; Watts J.C.; Wood, T.R.; Hermann E.C. & Hoffmann, C.E. (1964). Antiviral activity of 1-adamantanamine (amantadine). *Science*, Vol.144, No.362, pp. 862-863, ISSN 0036-8075

de Wit, E.; Spronken, M.I.; Rimmelzwaan, G.F.; Osterhaus, A.D. & Fouchier, R.A. (2006). Evidence for specific packaging of the influenza A virus genome from conditionally defective virus particles lacking a polymerase gene. *Vaccine*, Vol.24, No.44-46, pp. 6647-6650, ISSN 0264-410X

Dharan, N.J.; Gubareva, L.V.; Meyer, J.J.; Okomo-Adhiambo, M.; McClinton, R.C.; Marshall, S.A.; St George, K.; Epperson, S.; Brammer, L.; Klimov, A.I.; Bresee, J.S.; Fry, A.M. & Oseltamivir-Resistance Working Group. (2009). Infections with oseltamivir-resistant influenza A(H1N1) virus in the United States. *The Journal of the American Medical Association*, Vol.301, No.10, pp. 1034-1041, ISSN 0098-7484

Digard, P.; Elton, D.; Bishop, K.; Medcalf, E.; Weeds, A. & Pope, B. (1999). Modulation of nuclear localization of the influenza virus nucleoprotein through interaction with actin filaments. *Journal of Virology*, Vol.73, No.3, pp. 2222-2231, ISSN 0022-538X

Dolin, R.; Reichman, R.C.; Madore, H.P.; Maynard, R.; Linton, P.N. & Webber-Jones, J. (1982). A controlled trial of amantadine and rimantadine in the prophylaxis of influenza A infection. *The New England journal of medicine*, Vol.307, No.10, pp. 580-584, ISSN 0028-4793

Dworetzky, S.I. & Feldherr, C.M. (1988). Translocation of RNA-coated gold particles through the nuclear pores of oocytes. *The Journal of cell biology*, Vol.106, No.3, pp. 575-584, ISSN 0021-9525

Elton, D.; Medcalf, E.; Bishop, K. & Digard, P. (1999). Oligomerization of the influenza virus nucleoprotein: identification of positive and negative sequence elements. *Virology*, Vol.260, No.1, pp. 190-200, ISSN 0042-6822

Fahrenkrog, B. & Aebi, U. (2003). The nuclear pore complex: nucleocytoplasmic transport and beyond. *Nature reviews. Molecular cell biology*, Vol.4, No.10, pp. 757-766, ISSN 1471-0072

Fouchier, R.A.M.; Munster, V.; Wallensten, A.; Bestebroer, T.M.; Herfst, S.; Smith, D.; Rimmelzwaan, G.F.; Olsen, B. & Osterhaus, A.D.M.E. (2005). Characterization of a novel influenza a virus hemagglutinin subtype (H16) obtained from black-headed gulls. *Journal of Virology*, Vol.79, No.5, pp. 2814-2822, ISSN 0022-538X

Fujii, Y.; Goto, H.; Watanabe, T.; Yoshida, T. & Kawaoka, Y. (2003). Selective incorporation of influenza virus RNA segments into virions. *Proceedings of the National Academy of Sciences of the United States of America*, Vol.100, No.4, pp. 2002-2007, ISSN 0027-8424

Furuta, Y.; Takahashi, K.; Kuno-Maekawa, M.; Sangawa, H.; Uehara, S.; Kozaki, K.; Nomura, N.; Egawa, H. & Shiraki, K. (2005). Mechanism of action of T-705 against influenza virus. *Antimicrobial agents and chemotherapy*, Vol.49, No.3, pp. 981-986, ISSN 0066-4804

Gabriel, G.; Klingel, K.; Otte, A.; Thiele, S.; Hudjetz, B.; Arman-Kalcek, G.; Sauter, M.; Shmidt, T.; Rother, F.; Baumgarte, S.; Keiner, B.; Hartmann, E.; Bader, M.; Brownlee, G.G.; Fodor, E. & Klenk, H.D. (2011). Differential use of importin-α isoforms governs cell tropism and host adaptation of influenza virus. *Nature communications*, Vol.2, pp. 156, ISSN 2041-1723

Gerritz, S.W.; Cianci, C.; Kim, S.; Pearce, B.C.; Deminie, C.; Discotto, L.; McAuliffe, B.; Minassian, B.F.; Shi, S.; Zhu, S.; Zhai, W.; Pendri, A.; Li, G.; Poss, M.A.; Edavettal, S.; McDonnell, P.A.; Lewis, H.A.; Maskos, K.; Mörtl, M.; Kiefersauer, R.; Steinbacher, S.; Baldwin, E.T.; Metzler, W.; Bryson, J.; Healy, M.D.; Philip, T.; Zoeckler, M.; Schartman, R.; Sinz, M.; Leyva-Grado, V.H.; Hoffmann, H.H.; Langley, D.R.; Meanwell, N.A. & Krystal, M. (2011). Inhibition of influenza virus replication via small molecules that induce the formation of higher-order nucleoprotein oligomers. *Proceedings of the National Academy of Sciences of the United States of America*, Vol.108, No.37, pp. 15366-15371, ISSN 0027-8424

Goldfarb, D.S.; Corbett, A.H.; Mason, D.A.; Harreman, M.T. & Adam, S.A. (2004). Importin alpha: a multipurpose nuclear-transport receptor. *Trends in cell biology*, Vol.14, No.9, pp. 505-514, ISSN 0962-8924

Gómez-Puertas, P.; Albo, C.; Pérez-Pastrana, E.; Vivo, A. & Portela, A. (2000). Influenza virus matrix protein is the major driving force in virus budding. *Journal of Virology*, Vol.74, No.24, pp. 11538-11547, ISSN 0022-538X

Gruenbaum, Y.; Margalit, A.; Goldman, R.D.; Shumaker, D.K. & Wilson, K.L. (2005). The nuclear lamina comes of age. *Nature reviews. Molecular cell biology*, Vol.6, No.1, pp. 21-31, ISSN 1471-0072

Hagiwara, K.; Kondoh, Y.; Ueda, A.; Yamada, K.; Goto, H.; Watanabe, T.; Nakata, T.; Osada, H. & Aida, Y. (2010). Discovery of novel antiviral agents directed against the influenza A virus nucleoprotein using photo-cross-linked chemical arrays. *Biochemical and biophysical research communications*, Vol.394, No.3, pp. 721-727, ISSN 0006-291X

Harel, A. & Forbes, D.J. (2004). Importin beta: conducting a much larger cellular symphony. *Molecular cell*, Vol.16, No.3, pp. 319-330, ISSN 1097-2765

Hauge, S.H.; Dudman, S.; Borgen, K.; Lackenby, A. & Hungnes, O. (2009). Oseltamivir-resistant influenza viruses A (H1N1), Norway, 2007-08. *Emerging infectious diseases*, Vol.15, No.2, pp. 155-162, ISSN 1080-6040

Hayden, F.G.; Osterhaus, A.D.; Treanor, J.J.; Fleming, D.M.; Aoki, F.Y.; Nicholson, K.G.; Bohnen, A.M.; Hirst, H.M.; Keene, O. & Wightman, K. (1997). Efficacy and safety of the neuraminidase inhibitor zanamivir in the treatment of influenza virus infections. GG167 Influenza Study Group. *The New England journal of medicine*, Vol.337, No.13, pp. 874-880, ISSN 0028-4793

Heiny, A.T.; Miotto, O.; Srinivasan, K.N.; Khan, A.M.; Zhang, G.L.; Brusic, V.; Tan, T.W. & August, J.T. (2007). Evolutionarily conserved protein sequences of influenza A viruses, avian and human, as vaccine targets. *PLoS one*, Vol.2, No.11, pp. e1190, ISSN 1932-6203

Herold, A.; Truant, R.; Wiegand, H. & Cullen, B.R. (1998). Determination of the functional domain organization of the importin alpha nuclear import factor. *The Journal of cell biology*, Vol.143, No.2, pp. 309-318, ISSN 0021-9525

Herz, C.; Stavnezer, E.; Krug R. & Gurney, T Jr. (1981). Influenza virus, an RNA virus, synthesizes its messenger RNA in the nucleus of infected cells. Cell, Vol.26, No.3, pp. 391-400, ISSN 0092-8674

Hinshaw, V.S.; Air, G.M.; Gibbs, A.J.; Graves, L.; Prescott, B. & Karunakaran, D. (1982). Antigenic and genetic-characterization of a novel hemagglutinin subtype of influenza-A viruses from gulls. *Journal of Virology*, Vol.42, No.3, pp. 865-872, ISSN 0022-538X

Hurt, A.C.; Ernest, J.; Deng, Y.M.; Iannello, P.; Besselaar, T.G.; Birch, C.; Buchy, P.; Chittaganpitch, M.; Chiu, S.C.; Dwyer, D.; Guigon, A.; Harrower, B.; Kei, I.P.; Kok, T.; Lin, C.; McPhie, K.; Mohd, A.; Olveda, R.; Panayotou, T.; Rawlinson, W.; Scott, L.; Smith, D.; D'Souza, H.; Komadina, N.; Shaw, R.; Kelso, A. & Barr, I.G. (2009). Emergence and spread of oseltamivir-resistant A(H1N1) influenza viruses in Oceania, South East Asia and South Africa. *Antiviral research*, Vol.83, No.1, pp. 90-93, ISSN 0166-3542

Jones, I.M.; Reay, P.A. & Philpott, K.L. (1986). Nuclear location of all three influenza polymerase proteins and a nuclear signal in polymerase PB2. *The EMBO journal*, Vol.5, No.9, pp. 2371-2376, ISSN 0261-4189

Kanoh, N.; Asami, A.; Kawatani, M.; Honda, K.; Kumashiro, S.; Takayama, H.;Simizu, S.; Amemiya, T.; Kondoh, Y.; Hatakeyama, S.; Tsuganezawa, K.; Utata, R.; Tanaka, A.; Yokoyama, S.; Tashiro, H. & Osada, H. (2006). Photo-cross-linked small-molecule microarrays as chemical genomic tools for dissecting protein–ligand interactions. *Chemistry, an Asian journal*, Vol.1, No.6, pp. 789-797, ISSN 1861-4728

Kao, R.Y.; Yang, D.; Lau, L.S.; Tsui, W.H.; Hu, L.; Dai, J.; Chan, M.P.; Chan, C.M.; Wang, P.; Zheng, B.J.; Sun, J.; Huang, J.D.; Madar, J.; Chen, G.; Chen, H.; Guan, Y. & Yuen, KY. (2010). Identification of influenza A nucleoprotein as an antiviral target. *Nature biotechnology*, Vol.28, No.6, pp. 600-605, ISSN 1087-0156

Kawaoka, Y.; Yamnikova, S.; Chambers, T.M.; Lvov, D.K. & Webster, R.G. (1990). Molecular characterization of a new hemagglutinin, subtype H14, of influenza A virus. *Virology*, Vol.179, No.2, pp. 759-767, ISSN 0042-6822

Ketha, K.M. & Atreya, C.D. (2008). Application of bioinformatics-coupled experimental analysis reveals a new transport-competent nuclear localization signal in the nucleoprotein of influenza A virus strain. *BMC cell biology*, Vol.9, pp. 22, ISSN 1471-2121

Keyser, L.A.; Karl, M.; Nafziger, A.N. & Bertino, J.S. (2000). Comparison of central nervous system adverse effects of amantadine and rimantadine used as sequential prophylaxis of influenza A in elderly nursing home patients. *Archives of internal medicine*, Vol.160, No.10, pp. 1485-1488, ISSN 0003-9926

Kim, C.U.; Lew, W.; Williams, M.A.; Liu, H.T.; Zhang, L.J.; Swaminathan, S.; Bischofberger, N.; Chen, M.S.; Mendel, D.B.; Tai, C.Y.; Laver, W.G. & Stevens, R.C. (1997). Influenza neuraminidase inhibitors possessing a novel hydrophobic interaction in the enzyme active site: design, synthesis, and structural analysis of carbocyclic sialic acid analogues with potent anti-influenza activity. *Journal of the American Chemical Society*, Vol.119, No.4, pp. 681-690, ISSN 0002-7863

Klumpp, K.; Ruigrok, R.W.H. & Baudin, F. (1997). Roles of the influenza virus polymerase and nucleoprotein in forming a functional RNP structure. *EMBO Journal*, Vol.16, No.6, pp.1248-1257, ISSN 0261-4189

Kobayashi, M.; Toyoda, T.; Adyshev, D.M.; Azuma, Y. & Ishihama, A. (1994). Molecular dissection of influenza virus nucleoprotein: deletion mapping of the RNA binding domain. *Journal of Virology*, Vol.68, No.12, pp. 8433-8436, ISSN 0022-538X

Kobe, B. (1999). Autoinhibition by an internal nuclear localization signal revealed by the crystal structure of mammalian importin alpha. *Nature structural biology*, Vol.6, No.4, pp. 388-397, ISSN 1072-8368

Koehler, A.N.; Shamji, A.F. & Schreiber, S.L. (2003). Discovery of an inhibitor of a transcription factor using small molecule microarrays and diversity-oriented synthesis. *American Chemical Society*, Vol.125, No.28, pp. 8420-8421, ISSN 0002-7863

Kubo, S.; Tomozawa, T.; Kakuta, M.; Tokumitsu, A. & Yamashita, M. (2010). Laninamivir prodrug CS-8958, a long-acting neuraminidase inhibitor, shows superior anti-influenza virus activity after a single administration. *Antimicrobial agents and chemotherapy*, Vol.54, No.3, pp. 1256-1264, ISSN 0066-4804

Kuruvilla, F.G.; Shamji, A.F.; Sternson, S.M.; Hergenrother, P.J. & Schreiber, S.L. (2002). Dissecting glucose signalling with diversity-oriented synthesis and small-molecule microarrays. *Nature*, Vol.416, No.6881, pp. 653-657, ISSN 0028-0836

Li, Z.; Watanabe, T.; Hatta, M.; Watanabe, S.; Nanbo, A.; Ozawa, M.; Kakugawa, S.; Shimojima, M.; Yamada, S.; Neumann, G. & Kawaoka, Y. (2009). Mutational analysis of conserved amino acids in the influenza A virus nucleoprotein. *Journal of Virology*, Vol.83, No.9, pp. 4153-4162, ISSN 0022-538X

Liang, Y.; Huang, T.; Ly, H.; Parslow, T.G. & Liang, Y. (2008). Mutational analyses of packaging signals in influenza virus PA, PB1, and PB2 genomic RNA segments. *Journal of Virology*, Vol.82, No.1, pp. 229-236, ISSN 0022-538X

Martin, K. & Helenius, A. (1991). Transport of incoming influenza virus nucleocapsids into the nucleus. *Journal of Virology*, Vol.65, No.1, pp. 232-244, ISSN 0022-538X

Martín-Benito, J.; Area, E.; Ortega, J.; Llorca, O.; Valpuesta, J.M.; Carrascosa, J.L. & Ortín, J. (2001). Three-dimensional reconstruction of a recombinant influenza virus ribonucleoprotein particle. *EMBO reports*, Vol.2, No.4, pp. 313-317, ISSN 1469-221X

Matlin, K.S.; Reggio, H.; Helenius, A. & Simons, K. (1981). Infectious entry pathway of influenza virus in a canine kidney cell line. *The Journal of cell biology*, Vol.91, No.3, pp. 601-613, ISSN 0021-9525

Miyazaki, I.; Simizu, S.; Ichimiya, H.; Kawatani, M. & Osada, H. (2008). Robust and systematic drug screening method using chemical arrays and the protein library: identification of novel inhibitors of carbonic anhydrase II. *Bioscience, biotechnology, and biochemistry*, Vol.72, No.10, pp. 2739-2749, ISSN 0916-8451

Momose, F.; Basler, C.F.; O'Neill, R.E.; Iwamatsu, A.; Palese, P. & Nagata, K. (2001). Cellular splicing factor RAF-2p48/NPI-5/BAT1/UAP56 interacts with the influenza virus nucleoprotein and enhances viral RNA synthesis. *Journal of Virology*, Vol.75, No.4, pp. 1899-1908, ISSN 0022-538X

Monto, A.S.; Fleming, D.M.; Henry, D.; de Groot, R.; Makela, M.; Klein, T.; Elliott, M.; Keene, O.N. & Man, C.Y. (1999). Efficacy and safety of the neuraminidase inhibitor zanamivirin the treatment of influenza A and B virus infections. *The Journal of infectious diseases*, Vol.180, No.2, pp. 254-261, ISSN 0022-1899

Muramoto, Y.; Takada, A.; Fujii, K.; Noda, T.; Iwatsuki-Horimoto, K.; Watanabe, S.; Horimoto, T.; Kida, H. & Kawaoka, Y. (2006). Hierarchy among viral RNA (vRNA) segments in their role in vRNA incorporation into influenza A virions. *Journal of Virology*, Vol.80, No.5, pp. 2318-2325, ISSN 0022-538X

Nagata, K.; Kawaguchi, A. & Naito, T. (2008). Host factors for replication and transcription of the influenza virus genome. *Reviews in medical virology*, Vol.18, No.4, pp. 247-260, ISSN 1052-9276

Neumann, G.; Castrucci, M.R. & Kawaoka, Y. (1997). Nuclear import and export of influenza virus nucleoprotein. *Journal of Virology*, Vol.71, No.12, pp. 9690-9700, ISSN 0022-538X

Neumann, G.; Brownlee, G.G.; Fodor, E. & Kawaoka, Y. (2004). Orthomyxovirus replication, transcription, and polyadenylation. *Current topics in microbiology and immunology*, Vol.283, pp. 121-143, ISSN 0070-217X

Ng, A.K.; Zhang, H.; Tan, K.; Li, Z.; Liu, J.H.; Chan, P.K.; Li, S.M.; Chan, W.Y.; Au, S.W.; Joachimiak, A.; Walz, T.; Wang, J.H. & Shaw, P.C. (2008). Structure of the influenza virus A H5N1 nucleoprotein: implications for RNA binding, oligomerization, and vaccine design. *The FASEB journal*, Vol.22, No.10, pp. 3638-3647, ISSN 0892-6638

Ng, A.K.; Wang, J.H. & Shaw, P.C. (2009). Structure and sequence analysis of influenza A virus nucleoprotein. *Science in China. Series C, Life sciences*, Vol.52, No.5, pp. 439-449, ISSN 1006-9305

Nguyen, H.T.; Sheu, T.G.; Mishin, V.P.; Klimov, A.I. & Gubareva, L.V. (2010). Assessment of pandemic and seasonal influenza A (H1N1) virus susceptibility to neuraminidase inhibitors in three enzyme activity inhibition assays. *Antimicrobial agents and chemotherapy*, Vol.54, No.9, pp. 3671-3677, ISSN 0066-4804

Nicholson, K.G.; Aoki, F.Y.; Osterhaus, A.D.; Trottier, S.; Carewicz, O.; Mercier, C.H.; Rode, A.; Kinnersley, N. & Ward, P. (2000). Efficacy and safety of oseltamivir in treatment of acute influenza: a randomised controlled trial. Neuraminidase Inhibitor Flu Treatment Investigator Group. *Lancet*, Vol.355, No.9218, pp. 1845-1850, ISSN 0140-6736

Nieto A, de la Luna S, Bárcena J, Portela A, Ortín J. (1994). Complex structure of the nuclear translocation signal of influenza virus polymerase PA subunit. *The Journal of general virology*, Vol.75, pp. 29-36, ISSN 0022-1317

Noda, T.; Sagara, H.; Yen, A.; Takada, A.; Kida, H.; Cheng, R.H. & Kawaoka, Y. (2006). Architecture of ribonucleoprotein complexes in influenza A virus particles. *Nature*, Vol.439, No.7075, pp. 490-492, ISSN 0028-0836

Noton, S.L.; Simpson-Holley, M.; Medcalf, E.; Wise, H.M.; Hutchinson, E.C.; McCauley, J.W. & Digard, P. (2009). Studies of an influenza A virus temperature-sensitive mutant identify a late role for NP in the formation of infectious virions. *Journal of Virology*, Vol.83, No.2, pp. 562-571, ISSN 0022-538X

O'Neill, R.E.; Jaskunas, R.; Blobel, G.; Palese, P. & Moroianu, J. (1995). Nuclear import of influenza virus RNA can be mediated by viral nucleoprotein and transport factors required for protein import. *The Journal of biological chemistry*, Vol.270, No.39, pp. 22701-22704, ISSN 0021-9258

Ortega, J.; Martin-Benito, J.; Zurcher, T.; Valpuesta, J.M.; Carrascosa, J.L. & Ortin, J. (2000). Ultrastructural and functional analyses of recombinant influenza virus ribonucleoproteins suggest dimerization of nucleoprotein during virus amplification. *Journal of Virology*, Vol.74, No.1, pp. 156-163, ISSN 0022-538X

Ozawa, M.; Fujii, K.; Muramoto, Y.; Yamada, S.; Yamayoshi, S.; Takada, A.; Goto, H.; Horimoto, T. & Kawaoka, Y. (2007). Contributions of two nuclear localization signals of influenza A virus nucleoprotein to viral replication. *Journal of Virology*, Vol.81, No.1, pp. 30-41, ISSN 0022-538X

Palese, P. (1977). The genes of influenza virus. *Cell*, Vol.10, No.1, pp. 1-10, ISSN 0092-8674

Pinto, L.H.; Holsinger, L.J. & Lamb R.A. (1992). Influenza virus M2 protein has ion channel activity. *Cell*, Vol.69, No.3, pp. 517-528, ISSN 0092-8674

Plotch, S.J.; Bouloy, M. & Krug, R.M. (1979). Transfer of 5'-terminal cap of globin mRNA to influenza viral complementary RNA during transcription in vitro. *Proceedings of the National Academy of Sciences of the United States of America*, Vol.76, No.4, pp. 1618-1622, ISSN 0027-8424

Quimby, B.B. & Dasso, M. (2003). The small GTPase Ran: interpreting the signs. *Current opinion in cell biology*, Vol.15, No.3, pp. 338-344, ISSN 0955-0674

Robertson, J.S.; Schubert, M. & Lazzarini, R.A. (1981). Polyadenylation sites for influenza virus mRNA. *Journal of Virology*, Vol.38, No.1, pp. 157-163, ISSN 0022-538X

Rohm, C.; Zhou, N.A.; Suss, J.C.; Mackenzie, J. & Webster, R.G. (1996). Characterization of a novel influenza hemagglutinin, H15: Criteria for determination of influenza a subtypes. *Virology*, Vol.217, No.2, pp. 508-516, ISSN 0042-6822

Rossman, J.S.; Jing, X.; Leser, G.P. & Lamb, R.A. (2010a). Influenza virus M2 protein mediates ESCRT-independent membrane scission. *Cell*, Vol.142, No.6, pp. 902-913, ISSN 0092-8674

Rossman, J.S.; Jing, X.; Leser, G.P.; Balannik, V.; Pinto, L.H. & Lamb, R.A. (2010b). Influenza virus M2 ion channel protein is necessary for filamentous virion formation. *Journal of Virology*, Vol.84, No.10, pp. 5078-5088, ISSN 0022-538X

Rout, M.P.; Aitchison, J.D.; Suprapto, A.; Hjertaas, K.; Zhao, Y. & Chait, B.T. (2000). The yeast nuclear pore complex: composition, architecture, and transport mechanism. *The Journal of cell biology*, Vol.148, No.4, pp. 635-651, ISSN 0021-9525

Ruigrok, R.; Baudin, F.; Petit, I. & Weissenhorn, W. (2001). Role of influenza virus M1 protein in the viral budding process. *International Congress Series*, Vol.1219, pp. 397-404, ISSN0960-1643

Shen, Y.F.; Chen, Y.H.; Chu, S.Y.; Lin, M.I.; Hsu, H.T.; Wu, P.Y.; Wu, C.J.; Liu, H.W.; Lin, F.Y.; Lin, G.; Hsu, P.H.; Yang, A.S.; Cheng, Y.S.; Wu, Y.T.; Wong, C.H. & Tsai, M.D. (2011). E339...R416 salt bridge of nucleoprotein as a feasible target for influenza virus inhibitors. *Proceedings of the National Academy of Sciences of the United States of America*, Vol.108, No.40, pp. 16515-16520, ISSN 0027-8424

Shu, L.L.; Bean, W.J. & Webster, R.G. (1993). Analysis of the evolution and variation of the human influenza A virus nucleoprotein gene from 1933 to 1990. *Journal of Virology*, Vol.67, No.5, pp. 2723-2729, ISSN 0022-538X

Stegmann, T.; Morselt, H.W.; Scholma, J. & Wilschut J. (1987). Fusion of influenza virus in an intracellular acidic compartment measured by fluorescence dequenching. *Biochimica et Biophysica Acta*, Vol.904, No.1, pp. 165-170, ISSN 0006-3002

Steinhauer, D.A. & Holland, J.J. (1987). Rapid evolution of RNA viruses. *Annual review of microbiology*, Vol.41, pp. 409-433, ISSN 0066-4227

Stewart, M. (2000). Insights into the molecular mechanism of nuclear trafficking using nuclear transport factor 2 (NTF2). *Cell structure and function*, Vol.25, No.4, pp. 217-225, ISSN 0386-7196

Stiver, H.G. (2004). The threat and prospects for control of an influenza pandemic. *Expert review of vaccines*, Vol.3, No.1, pp. 35-42, ISSN 1476-0584

Su, C.Y.; Cheng, T.J.; Lin, M.I.; Wang, S.Y.; Huang, W.I.; Lin-Chu, S.Y.; Chen, Y.H.; Wu, C.Y.; Lai, M.M.; Cheng, W.C.; Wu, Y.T.; Tsai, M.D.; Cheng, Y.S. & Wong, C.H. (2010). High-throughput identification of compounds targeting influenza RNA-dependent RNA polymerase activity. *Proceedings of the National Academy of Sciences of the United States of America*, Vol.107,No.45, pp. 19151-19156, ISSN 0027-8424

Terry, L.J.; Shows, E.B. & Wente, S.R. (2007). Crossing the nuclear envelope: hierarchical regulation of nucleocytoplasmic transport. *Science*, Vol.318, No.5855, pp. 1412-1416, ISSN 0036-8075

Tran, T.H.; Nguyen, T.L.; Nguyen, T.D.; Luong, T.S.; Pham, P.M.; Nguyen, V.C.; Pham, T.S.; Vo, C.D.; Le, T.Q.; Ngo, T.T.; Dao, B.K.; Le, P.P.; Nguyen, T.T.; Hoang, T.L.; Cao, V.T.; Le, T.G.; Nguyen, D.T.; Le, H.N.; Nguyen, K.T.; Le, H.S.; Le, V.T.; Christiane, D.; Tran, T.T.; Menno de, J.; Schultsz, C.; Cheng, P.; Lim, W.; Horby, P.; Farrar, J. & World Health Organization International Avian Influenza Investigative Team. (2004). Avian influenza A (H5N1) in 10 patients in Vietnam. *The New England journal of medicine*, Vol.350, No.12, pp. 1179-1188, ISSN 0028-4793

Ungchusak, K.; Auewarakul, P.; Dowell, S.F.; Kitphati, R.; Auwanit, W.; Puthavathana, P.; Uiprasertkul, M.; Boonnak, K.; Pittayawonganon, C.; Cox, N.J.; Zaki, S.R.; Thawatsupha, P.; Chittaganpitch, M.; Khontong, R.; Simmerman, J.M. & Chunsutthiwat, S. (2005). Probable person-to-person transmission of avian influenza A (H5N1). *The New England journal of medicine*, Vol.352, No.4, pp. 333-340, ISSN 0028-4793

Vanvoris, L.P.; Betts, R.F.; Hayden, F.G.; Christmas, W.A. & Douglas, R.G. (1981). Successful treatment of naturally occurring influenza A/USSR/77 H1N1. *The Journal of the American Medical Association*, Vol.245, No.11, pp. 1128-1131, ISSN 0098-7484

Varghese, J.N.; McKimm-Breschkin, J.L.; Caldwell, J.B.; Kortt, A.A. & Colman, P.M. (1992). The structure of the complex between influenza virus neuraminidase and sialic acid, the viral receptor. *Proteins*, Vol.14, No.3, pp. 327-332, ISSN 0887-3585

Varghese, J.N.; Epa, V.C. & Colman, P.M. (1995). Three-dimensional structure of the complex of 4-guanidino-Neu5Ac2en and influenza virus neuraminidase. *Protein science*, Vol.4, No.6, pp. 1081-1087, ISSN 0961-8368

von Itzstein, M.; Wu, W.Y.; Kok, G.B.; Pegg, M.S.; Dyason, J.C.; Jin, B.; Phan, T.V.; Smythe, M.L.; White, H.F.; Oliver, S.W.; Colman, P.M.; Varghese, J.N.; Ryan, D.M.; Woods, J.M.; Bethell, R.C.; Hotham, V.J.; Cameron, J.M. & Penn, C.R. (1993). Rational design of potent sialidase-based inhibitors of influenza virus replication. *Nature*, Vol.363, No.6428, pp. 418-423, ISSN 0028-0836

Wang, C.; Takeuchi, K.; Pinto, L.H. & Lamb, R.A. (1993). Ion channel activity of influenza A virus M2 protein: characterization of the amantadine block. *Journal of Virology*, Vol.67, No.9, pp. 5585-5594, ISSN 0022-538X

Wang, P.; Palese, P. & O'Neill, R.E. (1997). The NPI-1/NPI-3 (karyopherin alpha) binding site on the influenza a virus nucleoprotein NP is a nonconventional nuclear localization signal. *Journal of Virology*, Vol.71, No.3, pp. 1850-1856, ISSN 0022-538X

Wang, H.; Feng, Z.; Shu, Y.; Yu, H.; Zhou, L.; Zu, R.; Huai, Y.; Dong, J.; Bao, C.; Wen, L.; Wang, H.; Yang, P.; Zhao, W.; Dong, L.; Zhou, M.; Liao, Q.; Yang, H.; Wang, M.; Lu, X.; Shi, Z.; Wang, W.; Gu, L.; Zhu, F.; Li, Q.; Yin, W.; Yang, W.; Li, D.; Uyeki, T.M. & Wang, Y. (2008). Probable limited person-to-person transmission of highly pathogenic avian influenza A (H5N1) virus in China. *Lancet*, Vol.371, No.9622, pp. 1427-1434, ISSN 0140-6736

Weber, F.; Kochs, G.; Gruber, S. & Haller, O. (1998). A classical bipartite nuclear localization signal on Thogoto and influenza A virus nucleoproteins. *Virology*, Vol.250, No.1, pp. 9-18, ISSN 0042-6822

Webster, R.G.; Bean, W.J.; Gorman, O.T.; Chambers, T.M. & Kawaoka, Y. (1992). Evolution and ecology of influenza A viruses. *Microbiological reviews*, Vol.56, No.1, pp. 152-179, ISSN 0146-0749

White, J, Kartenbeck, J. & Helenius, A. (1982). Membrane fusion activity of influenza virus. *The EMBO journal*, Vol.1, No.2, pp. 217-222, ISSN 0021-9525

Wingfiel, W.L.; Pollack, D. & Grunert, R.R. (1969). Therapeutic efficacy of amantadine HCl and rimantadine HCl in naturally occurring influenza A2 respiratory illness in man. *The New England journal of medicine*, Vol.281, No.11, pp. 579-584, ISSN 0028-4793

Wise, H.M.; Foeglein, A.; Sun, J.; Dalton, R.M.; Patel, S.; Howard, W.; Anderson, E.C.; Barclay, W.S. & Digard, P. (2009). A complicated message: Identification of a novel PB1-related protein translated from influenza A virus segment 2 mRNA. *Journal of Virology*, Vol.83, No.16, pp. 8021-8031, ISSN 0022-538X

World Health Organization. (1980). A revision of the system of nomenclature for influenza viruses: a WHO memorandum. *Bulletin of the World Health Organization*, Vol.58, No.4, pp. 585-591

Yamashita, M. (2011). Laninamivir and its prodrug, CS-8958: long-acting neuraminidase inhibitors for the treatment of influenza. *Antiviral chemistry & chemotherapy*, Vol.21, No.2, pp. 71-84, ISSN 0956-3202

Ye, Q.; Krug, R.M. & Tao, Y.J. (2006). The mechanism by which influenza A virus nucleoprotein forms oligomers and binds RNA. *Nature*, Vol.444, No.7122, pp. 1078-1082, ISSN 0028-0836

7

Targeting Norovirus: Strategies for the Discovery of New Antiviral Drugs

Joana Rocha-Pereira and Maria São José Nascimento
Laboratório de Microbiologia, Departamento de Ciências Biológicas, Faculdade de Farmácia, Universidade do Porto, Porto, Portugal

1. Introduction

Gastroenteritis is globally responsible for great morbidity and mortality among all ages. In the developing countries, it still represents one of the top causes of death for children <5 years of age, resulting in 1,8 million fatalities every year (Boschi-Pinto et al., 2008; Bryce et al., 2005). Viruses are responsible for the majority of cases of gastroenteritis with rotaviruses and noroviruses being the major pathogens.

Noroviruses are today recognized as the leading cause of foodborne outbreaks and sporadic cases of gastroenteritis worldwide (Glass et al., 2009; Patel et al., 2009). Nowadays, they are even considered the second most important agent of severe childhood diarrhea after rotavirus (Koopmans, 2008; Patel et al., 2008; Ramani & Kang, 2009) but the importance of norovirus in this age group is expected to increase in the upcoming years, as a consequence of the implementation of routine rotavirus vaccination (Koo et al., 2010).

The recognition of the clinical importance of norovirus only began in the late 1990s when sensitive routine diagnostic methods became available. In fact, the first norovirus (the *Norwalk* virus) was discovered in 1972 (Kapikian et al., 1972) but more than twenty years were necessary to disclose the important role of these viruses as human pathogens. Noroviruses are now on the upswing and a fundamental question is being raised: are norovirus really emerging? (Widdowson et al., 2005)

Despite the increasing attention given to norovirus today and the significant morbidity and mortality associated with norovirus gastroenteritis, no specific antiviral drugs or vaccines are yet available for treatment or prevention of norovirus illness. Only recently, a recombinant intranasal vaccine has entered a phase I clinical trial (El-Kamary et al., 2010; Vinje, 2010)

This chapter will highlight the importance of finding specific antiviral therapy for norovirus infection and explore biological features of norovirus, pointing out directions to stop or control this important human pathogen.

1.1 Clinical disease, transmission and epidemiology

Norovirus gastroenteritis is generally acute and self-limited, but in infants, elderly, and immunocompromised individuals it may be more severe and prolonged since they are more susceptible to complications due to dehydration (Green, 2007; Patel et al., 2008). After an incubation period of 24–48 h, there is an acute onset of symptoms of nausea, vomiting, abdominal cramps, myalgias, and intense non-bloody diarrhea which usually resolves in 2–3 days (Green, 2007). The median duration of illness can be longer, lasting up to six weeks in infants and young children (Kirkwood & Streitberg, 2008; Murata et al., 2007; Patel et al., 2009). Prolonged shedding is also documented in transplant patients and other immunosuppressed individuals, with symptoms lasting over two years (Hutson et al., 2004; Widdowson et al., 2005). Deaths have been reported in elderly during outbreaks in nursing homes, hospitals and cruise ships (Gotz et al., 2002; Lopman et al., 2004; Patel et al., 2008). Repeated associations of norovirus infections with clinical outcomes other than gastroenteritis have been reported (CDC, 2002; Chen et al., 2009; Kawano et al., 2007; Marshall et al., 2007; Turcios-Ruiz et al., 2008). Moreover, norovirus RNA has been detected in the blood of children with norovirus gastroenteritis and in the cerebrospinal fluid of a child with encephalopathy (Ito et al., 2006; Takanashi et al., 2009). This data suggests that norovirus infection is probably not limited to the intestine and could disseminate to systemic sites.

Noroviruses are transmitted by the fecal-oral route either directly from person-to-person or indirectly through consumption of contaminated food (fresh fruit, vegetables, shellfish and bakery products), water (drinking, ice or swimming) or following exposure to contaminated environmental surfaces and to airborne vomitus droplets (Green, 2007). Concerns about a potential zoonotic transmission have been raised given the close genetic relatedness between norovirus found in humans and animals and the presence of antibodies to animal strains in humans (Bank-Wolf et al., 2010).

Norovirus outbreaks are notably extensive and often occur in semi-closed environments (nursing homes, hospitals, day-care centers, schools, cruise ships and restaurants) that favor person-to-person transmission (Glass et al., 2009; Patel et al., 2009). Moreover, modern lifestyles make people more vulnerable to norovirus. More elderly people and infants live in communal settings, people eat more food outside the household (handled by potentially infected workers), consume more imported fresh fruit and vegetables from countries where crops are still irrigated with sewage-contaminated water and also more people are travelling and being exposed to norovirus in hotels, airplanes and cruise ships (Widdowson et al., 2005).

The very low infectious dose of norovirus (≈ 17 virus particles), their long persistence in the environment, withstanding sanitary measures effective against other microorganisms (freezing, heating and chlorination) combined with prolonged asymptomatic viral shedding make norovirus extremely infectious and explain the extensiveness of outbreaks (Duizer et al., 2004a; Siebenga et al., 2008; Teunis et al., 2008; Widdowson et al., 2005). Additionally, repeated infections can occur throughout life with re-exposure, likely due to the lack of lasting immunity and the lack of complete cross-protection against the diverse norovirus strains. (Donaldson et al., 2010; Patel et al., 2009).

Over the past years, a global increase in the number of norovirus outbreaks was noticed, with the GII.4 variants being accountable for the vast majority of cases. These GII.4 variants have become globally predominant and were responsible for four pandemics in the last two decades (Lindesmith et al., 2008; Siebenga et al., 2008). This emergence of dominants strains of norovirus causing worldwide epidemics suggests a pattern of epochal evolution resembling that of influenza (Glass et al., 2009).

1.2 Host susceptibility and virus-host interaction

Susceptibility to norovirus infection involves both acquired immunity and genetic resistance (Parrino et al., 1977). Volunteer studies found that some individuals were repeatedly susceptible to norovirus infection whereas others were repeatedly resistant (Parrino et al., 1977). Although it was initially unclear why some subjects did not develop illness, current research suggests that host genotype is a prominent factor in the development of norovirus infection since it depends on the presence of specific human histo-blood group antigen (HBGA) receptors in the gut of susceptible hosts (Lindesmith et al., 2003). Infection by norovirus relies on the recognition of HBGAs in the initial viral attachment and this key event most likely controls host susceptibility and resistance to norovirus (Hutson et al., 2004; Marionneau et al., 2002; Tan & Jiang, 2005, 2011).

HBGAs are complex carbohydrates linked to proteins or lipids on the surface of red blood cells and mucosal epithelia of the respiratory, genitourinary and digestive tracts, or present as free oligosaccharide in biological fluids such as milk and saliva. These antigens provide diversity within the human population and their biosynthesis is controlled by the enzyme products of alleles at the ABH, fucosyltransferase (FUT) 2, and FUT 3 loci (Hutson et al., 2004).

A number of distinct binding patterns of noroviruses to HBGAs have been described according to the ABO, Lewis and secretor types of the human HBGAs (Huang et al., 2003; Huang et al., 2005). This explains the correlation between secretor status and susceptibility to Norwalk virus infection, where secretor individuals with a wild-type *FUT2* gene (~80% of the population), who express HBGAs on gut epithelial cells and in body fluids, are susceptible to Norwalk virus infection, while nonsecretors, with a null *FUT2* allele, are completely resistant (Lindesmith et al., 2003).

The binding patterns of noroviruses to HBGAs are currently sorted into three major groups, the H, the A/B, and the Lewis binding groups (Tan & Jiang, 2011). While norovirus strains display distinct HBGA binding properties, collectively they can infect nearly all individuals due to their high genetic variability (Le Pendu et al., 2006). This highlights the highly adaptive nature of noroviruses and the likelihood of a long co-evolution of human noroviruses with their human host.

1.3 Classification and genome organization

Noroviruses are a genetically diverse group of viruses belonging to the genus *Norovirus* of the family *Caliciviridae* (Green, 2007). The Norwalk virus was the first norovirus to be discovered and associated to a gastroenteritis outbreak in an elementary school in Norwalk, Ohio, USA in 1968 and is today considered the prototype of the genus *Norovirus* (Kapikian et al., 1972).

The family *Caliciviridae* comprises, besides *Norovirus*, four accepted (*Sapovirus, Lagovirus, Vesivirus, Nebovirus)* and two tentative genera (*Recovirus, Valovirus*), that include human and non-human pathogenic viruses (Farkas et al., 2008; Green, 2007; Green et al., 2000; L'Homme et al., 2009). The two genera *Norovirus* (NoV) and *Sapovirus* (SaV) are the only that comprise human pathogenic agents, both causing acute gastroenteritis. The other genera include important veterinary pathogens such as the rabbit hemorrhagic disease virus (RHDV) which causes an often fatal hemorrhagic disease in rabbits in the genera *Lagovirus*, the feline calicivirus (FCV) which causes a respiratory disease in domestic and wild cat species in the genera *Vesivirus*, and the Newbury-1 virus which infect bovines in the genera *Nebovirus*. The tentative genera *Recovirus*, comprises the Tulane virus (TV) isolated from stool samples of rhesus macaques whose pathogenicity remains to be elucidated (Farkas et al., 2008). The other tentative genera *Valovirus* comprises the St-Valérien-like viruses isolated from pig feces (L'Homme et al., 2009).

Noroviruses are today classified into five genogroups (GI-V) divided into at least 31 genetic clusters or genotypes based on sequence diversity in the complete capsid protein VP 1 (Zheng et al., 2006). Genogroups share > 60% amino acid identity in the VP 1 and each genetic cluster or genotype shares > 80% identity in amino acid sequence of VP 1 (Green et al., 2000; Zheng et al., 2006). Human noroviruses have been associated with GI, GII and GIV and bovine and murine noroviruses belong to GIII and GV, respectively (Wobus et al., 2004; Zheng et al., 2006). GII also contains swine strains and GIV comprises the feline (lion) and canine strains (Martella et al., 2007; Martella et al., 2008; Mesquita et al., 2010).

Noroviruses are small icosahedric non-enveloped viruses of 27-32 nm with a positive-sense single stranded (ss) RNA genome of 7.4–7.7 kb, organized into three open reading frames (ORF1-3) (Fig 1). The 5′ proximal region of the norovirus genome encodes a polyprotein of six/seven nonstructural protein products in a single ORF (ORF1). ORF2 encodes the major structural capsid protein VP1 and ORF3 the minor structural protein VP2. Norovirus genome is covalently linked, at the 5′ end, to a viral protein called VPg (virion protein, genome-linked) and is polyadenlyated at the 3′ end (Green, 2007).

The ORF1 of norovirus encodes the six/seven nonstructural proteins in the following order: the p48/ N-terminal protein (or NS1-2), the NTPase (NS3), the p22 (NS4), the VPg (NS5), the viral protease (Pro, NS6), and the viral RNA-dependent RNA polymerase (RdRp, NS7). Some of these proteins have defined activities such as NS3, an NTPase (nucleoside triphosphatase) (Pfister & Wimmer, 2001), NS6, a protease (Liu et al., 1996), and NS7, an RNA-dependent RNA polymerase (RdRp) (Fukushi et al., 2004; Rohayem et al., 2006a). Also, NS5 known as VPg, is a protein that is covalently attached to the 5′ ends of viral genomes in place of a typical 5′ cap and that can function as a primer in viral RNA replication (Burroughs & Brown, 1978; Rohayem et al., 2006b). The role of the remaining nonstructural proteins (NS1-2 and NS4) in norovirus replication is not yet well defined (Green, 2007). Available data suggests that NS1-2 and NS4, also known as N-term/p48 and p22, respectively, both contribute to norovirus replication complex formation on intracellular membranes, including that of the Golgi apparatus, and disrupt intracellular host protein trafficking (Ettayebi & Hardy, 2003; Fernandez-Vega et al., 2004; Hyde et al., 2009).

The major structural protein of norovirus, the VP1, is encoded by ORF2. Virions contain 180 copies or 90 dimers of VP1 that assemble into icosahedral particles (Prasad et al., 1999; Prasad et al., 1994). The VP1 protein is divided into a conserved internal shell domain (S) and a more variable protruding domain, the P domain, that forms the arch-like protrusions and is further subdivided into P1 and P2 domains (Fig. 1). The P2 subdomain is located at

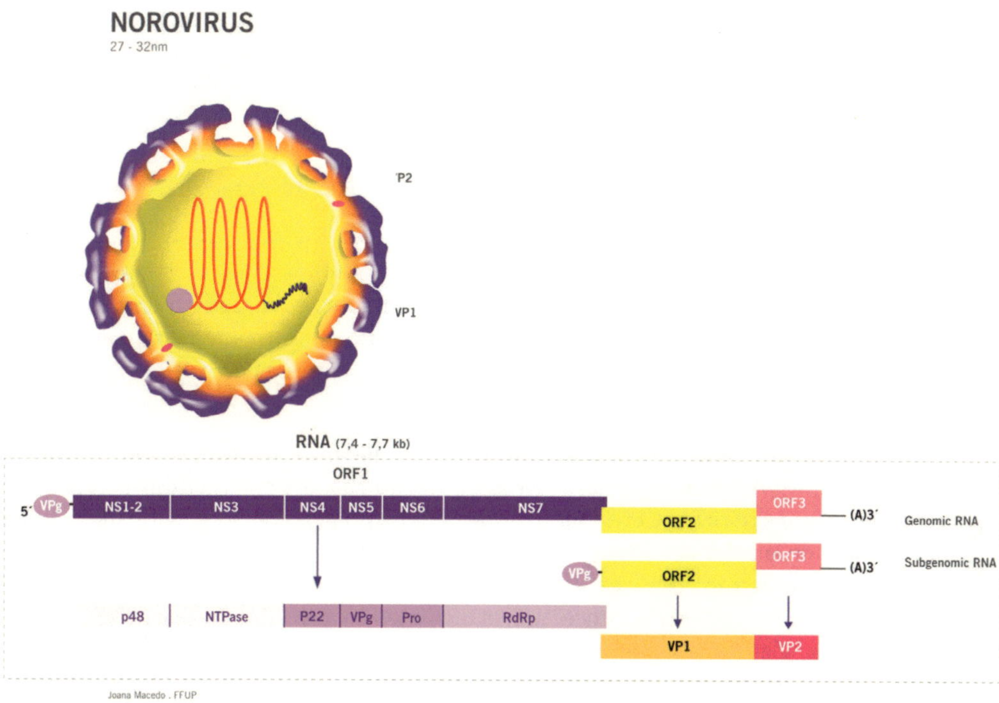

Fig. 1. Schematic representation of a viral particle and genome organization of norovirus. Genomic and subgenomic RNA of norovirus with the genome linked protein VPg at the 5′ end and the poly(A) tail at 3′ end is shown along with the nonstructural proteins (NS1-7) encoded by ORF1 as well as the structural proteins (VP1 and VP2), encoded by ORF2 and 3. See text for further details

the outmost surface of the viral capsid and comprises a hypervariable region, where resides the binding interface for HBGA association with norovirus (Bu et al., 2008; Cao et al., 2007; Choi et al., 2008; Tan et al., 2003). The VP2 is a small, basic structural protein encoded by the ORF3 which is present in one or two copies per virion (Glass et al., 2000; Hardy, 2005). Its function in viral replication is currently undefined but there is evidence that it increases the level of expression of VP1 and stabilizes virus-like particles (VLPs, generated through expression of the VP1) (Bertolotti-Ciarlet et al., 2003). The basic charge of VP2 suggests that it may function in encapsidation of the viral genome (Karst, 2010).

1.4 Replication of norovirus

The replication of norovirus has not been yet fully elucidated and most of the current knowledge is drawn by analogy with other (+)ssRNA viruses and studies with related animal caliciviruses. Norovirus is one of the positive-sense ssRNA viruses whose genome functions directly as the mRNA, beginning the infectious cycle with the synthesis of a precursor that only gives rise to the nonstructural proteins, including the RdRp enzyme that transcribes then one subgenomic mRNA encoding the structural proteins (VP1 and VP2) (Green, 2007). Like the other (+)ssRNA viruses , the replication of norovirus occurs in the cytoplasm. In Fig 2 is represented a scheme of the replication of norovirus.

In the first step, the viral attachment of the virion to the cell receptor, the P2 subdomain of the VP1 binds to a sugar residue, mostly to the HBGA carbohydrates in the case of human noroviruses but also to sialic acid or heparan sulfate (Hutson et al., 2002; Marionneau et al., 2002; Rydell et al., 2009; Stuart & Brown, 2007; Tamura et al., 2004; Taube et al., 2009). This interaction between VP1 and HBGA seems not to be enough for the entry of norovirus in host cells and the involvement of a membrane protein as a receptor or co-receptor for subsequent penetration/entry is suspected (Tan & Jiang, 2010).

Norovirus enters the cell using a non-clathrin-, non-caveolin-mediated endocytic pathway but dependent on dynamin II and cholesterol (Gerondopoulos et al., 2010; Perry & Wobus, 2010). Moreover, this entry step is pH-independent and no conformational changes in the capsid required for viral uncoating are observed with acidic intracellular pH (Perry et al., 2009).

After the internalization in the cell and uncoating of viral genome, the translation of ORF1 of the viral genomic RNA produces a large protein, the so called nonstructural polyprotein. The initiation of translation is dependent on the interaction of the VPg with the cellular translation initiation machinery (Daughenbaugh et al., 2003; Daughenbaugh et al., 2006). A co-translational processing releases the nonstructural proteins and their precursors (Sosnovtsev, 2010). The proteolytic processing is mediated by the viral protease (NS6) which is autocatalytically released from the polyprotein precursor (Putics et al., 2010).

The replication of norovirus is believed to occur in a replication complex (RC) formed by intracellular membranous structures which contain all the viral nonstructural proteins along with host proteins that will help viral replication as well as the viral RNA intermediate, ssRNA and double stranded RNA (dsRNA) (Hyde & Mackenzie, 2010; Hyde et al., 2009). The recruitment of host membranes (RE, Golgi, endossomes) necessary for the formation of the RC, is induced by the viral non structural proteins p48 (NS1-2) and p22 (NS4), through a modulation of the host cell secretory pathway (Denison, 2008; Hyde & Mackenzie, 2010; Sharp et al., 2010).

Once the RC is assembled, the RdRp (NS7) starts the synthesis of the antigenomic RNA (negative sense) from the genomic (positive sense) RNA template. The initiation of antigenomic RNA synthesis by the RdRp is dependent upon uridylylation of VPg that serves as a primer in the presence of the polyadenylated genomic RNA (Rohayem et al., 2006a; Rohayem et al., 2006b). This antigenomic RNA is then used as a template for synthesis of the new genomic RNA and of the subgenomic RNA.

The newly synthesized genomic RNA is either translated as a polyprotein precursor or used for packaging in the assembled viral protein core. The subgenomic RNA (positive sense) is translated as structural proteins, VP1 and VP2. Finally, the structural proteins are assembled and the genomic RNA packaged, followed by release of the mature virion from the cell. This late stages of replication are, however, poorly understood.

1.5 Surrogate models for the study of human norovirus

Human noroviruses are not cultivable in routine laboratory cell culture or primary tissue cultures (Duizer et al., 2004b). There has been a single report using a 3-D cell culture system demonstrated for the first time successful passage of both GI and GII norovirus *in vitro*

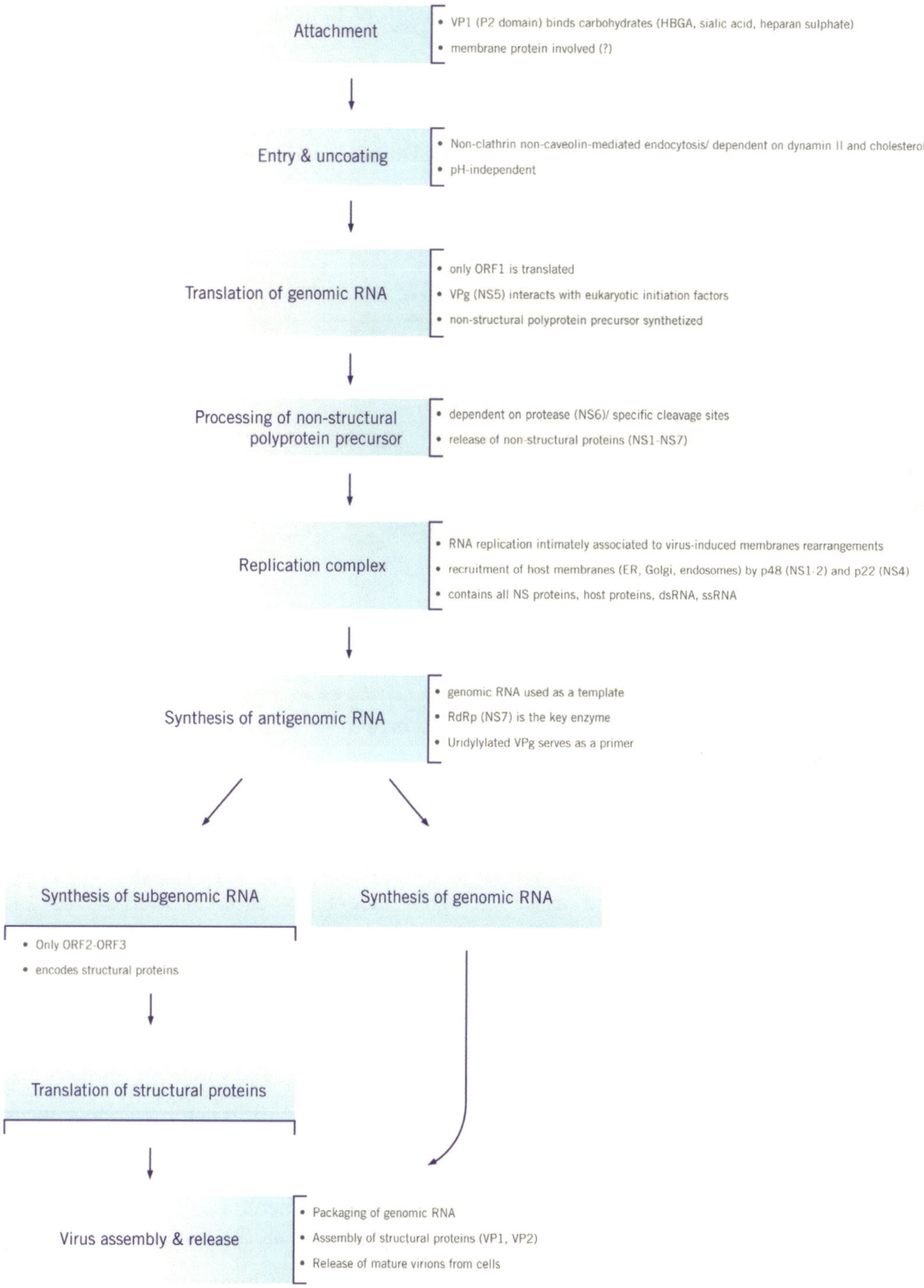

Fig. 2. Replication scheme of norovirus and key events.

(Straub et al., 2007) but several independent laboratories failed to reproduce such results (Papafragkou et al., 2009). For this reason, the study of human norovirus has been made using surrogate viruses.

Initially, surrogate models for norovirus infectivity included viruses from other genera within the family *Caliciviridae,* namely porcine enteric calicivirus, a *Sapovirus*, and the feline calicivirus (FCV), a *Vesivirus* (Doultree et al., 1999; Duizer et al., 2004a) (Fig.3).

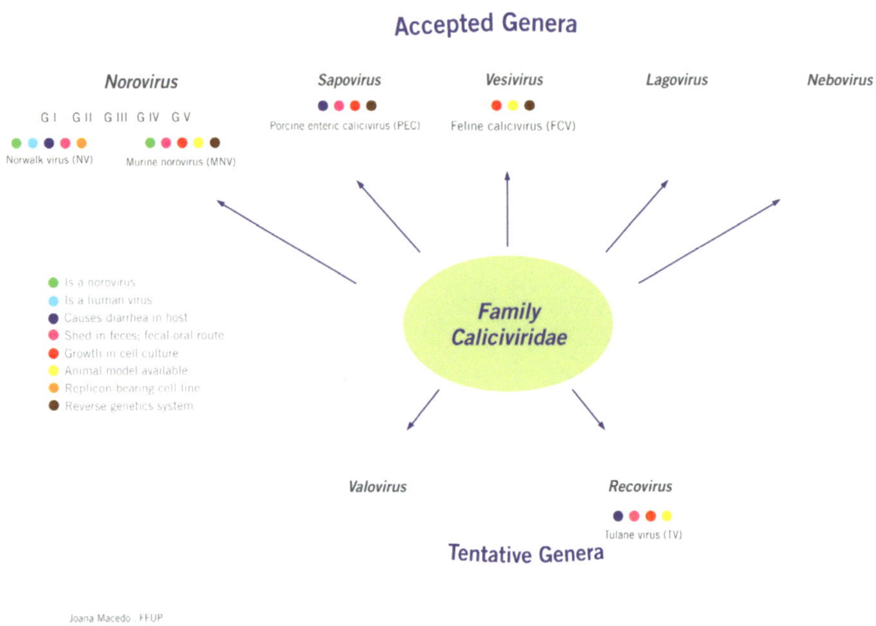

Fig. 3. Characteristics of the different surrogates models for human norovirus within the genera of the family *Caliciviridae*

FCV was then frequently used as a surrogate model for survival, persistence and inactivation studies of human noroviruses until the more recent discovery of murine norovirus (MNV) (Bae & Schwab, 2008; Cannon et al., 2006; Wobus et al., 2004; Wobus et al., 2006). MNV is a genogroup V norovirus and is to date the only *Norovirus* able to replicate both in cell culture and in a small animal model. Moreover, like human norovirus MNV is an enteric pathogen that spreads through the fecal-oral route and is shed at high levels in the feces (Karst et al., 2003; Wobus et al., 2004). On the other hand, the use of FCV was criticized because: (i) it does not belong to the genus *Norovirus*; (ii) it is a respiratory virus; (iii) it is not shed in feces and (iv) it cannot survive at low pH, a necessary characteristic of enteric viruses that must survive passage through the stomach (Bae & Schwab, 2008; Cannon et al., 2006; Duizer et al., 2004b; Wobus et al., 2006). Therefore, MNV is considered today the best surrogate model for human norovirus (Wobus et al., 2004; Wobus et al., 2006).

MNV has the size, shape, and buoyant density characteristic of human norovirus (Green, 2007; Karst et al., 2003). MNV genome has also the three ORFs characteristic of noroviruses (Wobus et al., 2006), but it has an additional ORF4 that overlaps ORF2 in a different reading frame (Thackray et al., 2007). ORF1 of MNV also encodes the nonstructural proteins and ORFs 2 and 3 encode the two proteins of the the viral capsid (Sosnovtsev et al., 2006). The conserved molecular features of MNV and human norovirus genomes suggest that many fundamental mechanisms of replication are conserved between murine and human noroviruses (Wobus et al., 2006). Although MNV infection seems to be asymptomatic in immunocompetent mice, it causes diarrhea and lethality in mice deficient in components of innate immunity (Karst et al., 2003; Mumphrey et al., 2007). Hence, the clinical presentation of MNV is different from the one of human norovirus, and for this reason MNV does not constitute yet the ideal model for studying human norovirus.

The recent discovery of the Tulane virus (TV), a novel calicivirus isolated from stool samples of rhesus macaques, together with the likelihood of this virus causing intestinal infection and the availability of a tissue culture system could make TV a valuable surrogate for human norovirus (Farkas et al., 2008).

An alternative approach to the study of norovirus RNA replication was established when a human norovirus replicon-bearing cell line was created by transfecting a plasmid containing most of the Norwalk virus genome into mammalian cell lines (Chang et al., 2006). These cell lines are capable of constitutively expressing the replicative enzymes and other nonstructural proteins, allowing the study of RNA replication and providing a platform for screening antiviral compounds.

Reverse genetics systems have been developed for some caliciviruses, namely for PEC, FCV, MNV and TV (Chang et al., 2005; Chaudhry et al., 2007; Sosnovtsev & Green, 1995; Ward et al., 2007; Wei et al., 2008; Wobus et al., 2004). These systems have helped to elucidate fundamental aspects of caliciviruses replication through the introduction of deliberate changes in certain genes and the analysis of the resultant effect in the virus phenotype. Reverse genetics systems represent also an important tool for the development of antivirals against norovirus (Putics et al., 2010).

Virus-like particles (VLPs) which result of the independent expression and self-assembly of the VP1 are also valuable tools that have been used in many research areas of norovirus (El-Kamary et al., 2010; Jiang et al., 1992). These VLPs are morphologically and antigenically indistinguishable from the native forms of viruses found in human stools, and retain the binding properties of native norovirus virions at least in terms of carbohydrate association (Jiang et al., 1992). VLPs have been used for the development of immunological assays, the study of virus-host interaction, structural studies of the norovirus capsid, investigation of antigenic relationships and as potential vaccine candidates (Green, 2007; Tan & Jiang, 2005).

2. Strategies to inhibit the replication of norovirus

The antiviral research of norovirus is still in its infancy and there are only few reports of antivirals for norovirus. Recently, a new chemical scaffold, the 2-styrylchromones, has shown anti-norovirus activity in the MNV surrogate model, opening the door to the search of anti-norovirus drugs among a wider range of novel compounds from different chemical families (Rocha-Pereira et al., 2010). Additionally, nitoxanide, a prodrug used to treat protozoal gastroenteritis has been reported to reduce the duration of norovirus gastroenteritis in a clinical trial although the mechanism of action remains unclear (Rossignol & El-Gohary, 2006).

In the following section, potential targets and strategies to inhibit norovirus life cycle are presented, based on the information available today on norovirus genome organization, functions of structural and nonstructural proteins, replication and virus-host interaction (Fig. 4). The predictable advantages and/or disadvantages of these strategies are discussed and some antiviral drugs previously identified as active against similar molecular targets in other plus stranded RNA viruses are suggested as a starting point.

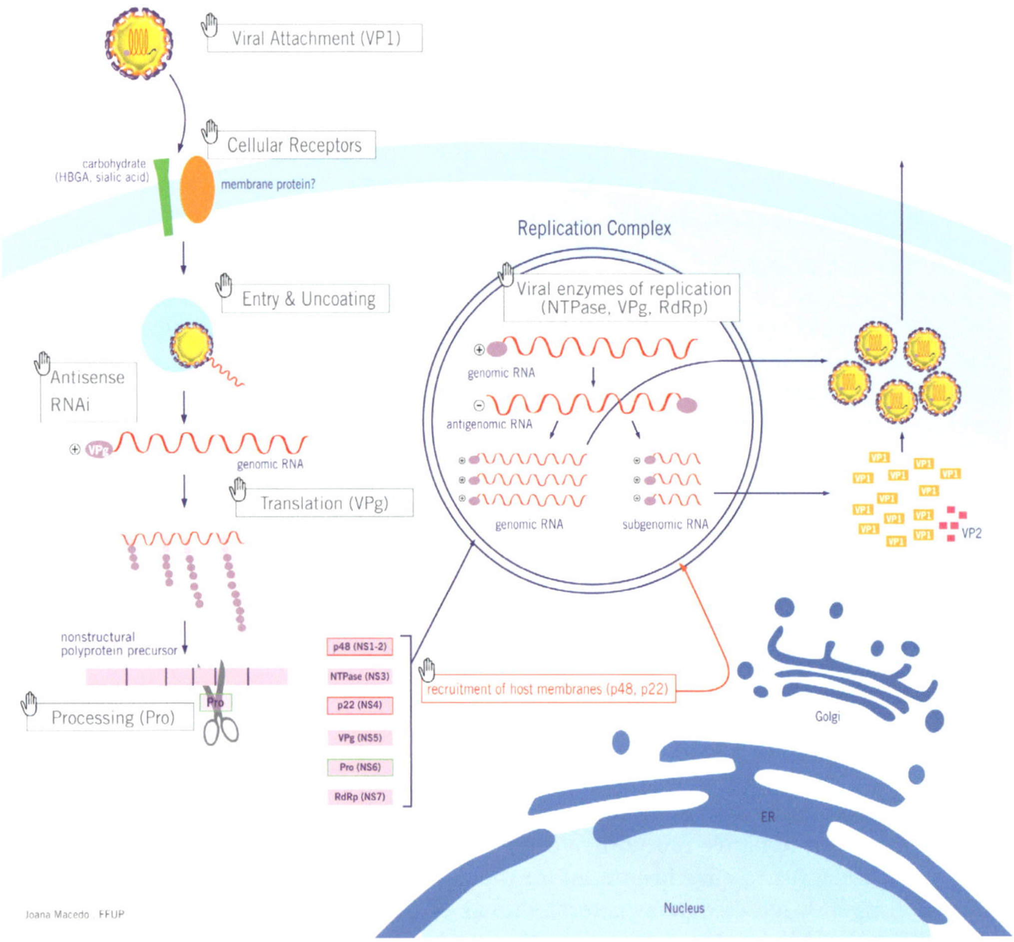

Fig. 4. Targeting the various steps of the replication of norovirus

2.1 Targeting cellular receptors of norovirus

Human noroviruses recognize HBGA carbohydrates present on cell surface, which are key players in the initial viral attachment, acting most likely as cellular receptors or co-receptors of norovirus (Hutson et al., 2002; Marionneau et al., 2002; Tan & Jiang, 2005, 2011)

Noroviruses present diverse binding patterns to HBGAs, being currently sorted into three major binding groups, the H, the A/B, and the Lewis binding group (Tan & Jiang, 2011). The interaction between noroviruses and HBGA is highly strain-specific rather than genogroup- or genotype-specific (Tan & Jiang, 2010). Hence, strains of the H, A/B and

Lewis binding groups can be found in both two major genogroups of human noroviruses (GI and GII).

The existence of only three HBGA-binding interfaces makes possible the design of antivirals against these targets in noroviruses. Any compound that targets a given HBGA binding interface may be capable of blocking infection of all strains that bind that same type of HBGA. Thus, only three different HBGA-binding interfaces would need to be targeted by compounds to block nearly all noroviruses in the GI and GII genogroups (Tan et al., 2009).

The strategy of targeting this first step of virus-receptor interaction could be of great interest to use as prophylactic therapy since it would be effective in preventing infections of individuals in high risk settings or that were in contact with an index case during an outbreak (Tan & Jiang, 2008). Furthermore, it would be expected that such compounds would be able to reduce the severity of symptoms in already infected individuals and likely reduce virus excretion, limiting its propagation to higher numbers of individuals (Tan & Jiang, 2008). Citrate, and other glycomimetics, showed to have the potential to block human noroviruses from binding to HBGAs (Hansman et al., 2011) providing a starting point for norovirus inhibitors.

However, there are predictable difficulties to this strategy, one of which being the fact that the early steps of norovirus life cycle are not yet fully disclosed. Recent findings of FCV and MNV binding to sialic acid (Rydell et al., 2009; Stuart & Brown, 2007; Taube et al., 2009) or heparan sulfate (Tamura et al., 2004) broadens the spectrum of sugar residues that interact with these viruses. Moreover, the identification of a membrane protein, the junctional adhesion molecule A (JAM-A), as a receptor for FCV (Makino et al., 2006) raises the hypothesis of this protein or other members of the Ig superfamily being also cellular receptors for caliciviruses, like they are for reoviruses and picornaviruses (Tan & Jiang, 2010). According to the proposed model for reoviruses, the virus interact firstly with a sugar residue like sialic acid, as a determinant of tropism that is responsible for initial virus attachment, and later use a membrane protein (JAM-1) to enter the host cell (Barton et al., 2001). The role of these two molecules in viral attachment and entry is likely to occur also in FCV, and one could even speculate that it could be extended to noroviruses since it is usual that viruses within the same family use similar cellular receptors (Tan & Jiang, 2010).

Much remains to be unraveled in this field, therefore there are still doubts about the selection of the best target for chemical compounds to block or interfere with virus attachment.

2.2 Targeting entry and uncoating of norovirus

In order to enter host cells, viruses take advantage of cellular processes entering by an endocytic pathway, most commonly a clathrin-mediated endocytosis. Viral entry can also occur via caveolin-mediated endocytosis, clathrin/caveolin-independent endocytosis, macropinocytosis, or phagocytosis (Marsh & Helenius, 2006). After entrance in the host cell, the uncoating of virus must occur in order to deliver the viral genome into the host cytoplasm. This event is often triggered by the acidic environment of endosomes but it can also occur after the binding of virus to cellular receptors (Tsai, 2007).

Studies with FCV showed this virus enters cells by clathrin-mediated endocytosis in a pH-dependent manner (Stuart & Brown, 2007). However, it was demonstrated that the entry of MNV is clathrin/caveolin-independent but mediated by dynamin II and cholesterol (Gerondopoulos et al., 2010; Perry & Wobus, 2010). In addition, studies with MNV show this virus is pH-independent and that a low intracellular pH does not trigger conformational changes in the capsid required for MNV uncoating (Perry et al., 2009). This difference in sensitivity to low pH between FCV and MNV was suggested to be related with the different routes of infection of these viruses (Perry et al., 2009). While MNV is an enteric virus that infects its host by the small intestine and retains infectivity for hours at a pH of 2 (similarly to the human Norwalk virus), FCV is a respiratory virus that significantly decreases infectivity at low pH (Cannon et al., 2006; Dolin et al., 1972).

Further understanding of the cellular mechanisms of norovirus entry and uncoating would bring out new antiviral targets.

2.3 Targeting structural proteins of norovirus

The VP1 is the major structural protein of norovirus and its P2 subdomain, which is located at the outmost surface of the viral capsid, comprises the binding surface for HBGA (Bu et al., 2008; Cao et al., 2007; Choi et al., 2008; Tan et al., 2003). The function of VP2 is currently undefined and there is not sufficient information to address this minor protein as an antiviral target.

The search of compounds targeting VP1 of norovirus was explored through a saliva-based enzyme immunoassay (EIA) that measures their capacity to block the binding of norovirus VLPs to HBGAs present in such biological fluid (Feng & Jiang, 2007). Different chemical compounds were found to be strong inhibitors of this binding being potential candidates for further development as antivirals for norovirus (Feng & Jiang, 2007), but one should be aware that a saliva-based EIA was used instead of a cellular system or animal model and this could be regarded as an handicap.

Antiviral drugs that target viral surface proteins of other RNA virus have been described, such as pleconaril, a picornavirus capsid-binding compound, but resulted in a not entirely successfully strategy (Field & Vere Hodge, 2008). The problem with this kind of drugs relies on their low genetic barrier since the viral surface proteins can undergo variations without compromising viral fitness, easily allowing resistant strains to emerge (Field & Vere Hodge, 2008). The same problem would most likely take place with norovirus given its well known antigenic variation. A strategy could be the use of combination therapy of this class of compounds together with drugs against well conserved nonstructural proteins with critical functions. This would avoid or at least delay the development of resistance.

2.4 Targeting nonstructural proteins

The six/seven nonstructural proteins of norovirus are the p48/ N-terminal protein (NS1-2), the NTPase (NS3), the p22 (NS4), the VPg (NS5), the viral protease (Pro, NS6), and the viral RNA-dependent RNA polymerase (RdRp, NS7). Since noroviruses share some similarities with picornaviruses, the nomenclature and functions of these ORF1-encoded proteins of norovirus was initially predicted through comparative sequence analysis of their picornavirus counterparts. Hence, the norovirus RdRp was called 3D-like, the protease was called 3C-like, the p22 was called 3A-like, the NTPase was named 2C-like and the p48/N-term was related to the 2B protein (Green, 2007). This resemblance could be important for the search of antivirals against norovirus since the known strategies and targets for inhibiting the replication of picornavirus might be also effective for norovirus.

Although a detailed knowledge of the role of nonstructural proteins is still not available, some important clues have raised from studies with MNV which showed that all these proteins play a role in norovirus replication and are associated with the replication complex (RC) and the viral RNA intermediate dsRNA (Hyde et al., 2009). There is also evidence that the replication complex of MNV is associated with host membranes, namely of the endoplasmic reticulum (ER), the Golgi apparatus and endossomes which suffer virus-induced rearrangements (Hyde et al., 2009; Wobus et al., 2004). These and other features of each nonstructural protein are described below, as well as how these could be used for the discovery of antiviral drugs against norovirus.

2.4.1 p48

The role of p48 or NS1-2 is not yet well defined but it is thought to be comparable to that of the analogous picornavirus 2B protein, which participates in intracellular membrane changes that occur during virus replication (Sosnovtsev, 2010). Studies with Norwalk virus indicated that the p48 may interfere with disassembly of the Golgi complex and cellular protein trafficking (Ettayebi & Hardy, 2003; Fernandez-Vega et al., 2004) while studies with MNV and FCV point out that p48 is associated with the recruitment of ER membranes to the RC (Bailey et al., 2009; Hyde & Mackenzie, 2010). This recruitment of membranes is vital to the synthesis of new viral proteins by the actively replicating noroviruses (Hyde et al., 2009; Wobus et al., 2004). Hence, the impairment of the mechanisms controlled by p48 in the membrane rearrangements could be a good strategy to stop the norovirus life cycle.

2.4.2 NTPase

The NTPase or NS3 shares sequence motifs with other viral NTPases, namely the picornaviruses 2C protein and the flaviviruses NS3 helicase/NTPase. It has also been classified in the superfamily 3 of RNA helicases (Hardy, 2005; Pfister & Wimmer, 2001). The role of these enzymes consists in catalyzing the hydrolysis reaction of nucleoside triphosphates and using the released energy to unwind the viral nucleic acids (Kwong et al., 2005). However, until now there is only experimental data confirming the NTPase but not the helicase activity of this nonstructural protein of norovirus (Hardy, 2005).

In recent years, substantial efforts have been made to identify inhibitors of such proteins, since they are well conserved and essential for viral replication. The thiazolobenzimidazoles were identified as potent inhibitors of picornaviruses, showing one of these compounds, TBZE-029 [1-(2,6-difluorophenyl)-6-trifluoromethyl-1*H*,3*H*-thiazolo[3,4-a]benzimidazole] to target the protein 2C of coxsackievirus B3 (De Palma et al., 2008a; De Palma et al., 2008c). These and other picornavirus 2C-targeting compounds, such as MRL-1237 [1-(4-fluorophenyl)-2-(4-imino-1,4-dihydropyridin-1-yl) methylbenzimidazole hydrochloride] and HBB [2-(α-hydroxybenzyl)-benzimidazole] (De Palma et al., 2008a; De Palma et al., 2008c; Norder et al., 2011) could as well be inhibitors of the NTPase of norovirus. The multiple mechanisms through which compounds could inhibit the helicase/NTPase have been extensively described elsewhere (Rohayem et al., 2010). The search of norovirus NTPase inhibitors could result in the development of an innovative antiviral strategy and at the same time reveal functional details of this enzyme of norovirus.

2.4.3 p22

The function of p22 or NS4 in norovirus life cycle is also not yet fully understood. This protein occupies in norovirus genome a position similar to that of the 3A protein in picornavirus genomes but they share only limited sequence similarity (Green, 2007; Hardy, 2005). The 3A protein is known to inhibit the protein trafficking from the ER to Golgi apparatus, a function central to the cellular homeostasis (Wessels et al., 2006). A similar function has been recently described for Norwalk virus p22 (Sharp et al., 2010). It was reported that this protein contains a well-conserved motif that mimics the normal ER export signal, leading to the inhibition of protein trafficking to Golgi, inducing its disassembly and ultimately inhibiting cellular protein secretion (Sharp et al., 2010). Since this motif is highly conserved in human noroviruses, it may constitute a new target for the design of anti-norovirus drugs (Sharp et al., 2010).

Besides, based on what has been described for picornavirus 3A protein, one of the consequences of the inhibition of cellular protein secretion by p22 could be a more severe infection due to the decrease of surface MHC class I proteins and normal cytokine release that leads to a reduction of clearance in infected cells (Sharp et al., 2010; Wessels et al., 2006).

Additionally, there is evidence suggesting that p22 is part of the norovirus RC participating in the recruitment of membranes from the late secretory pathway (Golgi and endossomes) to the RC, being the main viral protein known to be responsible for the recruitment of endossome membranes (Hyde & Mackenzie, 2010).

Two compounds, enviroxime and TTP-8307, have shown to inhibit the *in vitro* replication of enteroviruses and rhinoviruses by targeting the nonstructural protein 3A (De Palma et al., 2009; Heinz & Vance, 1995). Therefore, these compounds are good candidates to be evaluated for their ability to inhibit p22 and the norovirus replication.

2.4.4 VPg

The VPg or NS5 is covalently linked to the 5′-end of the norovirus RNA genome and plays an important role in the replication of norovirus. Initiation of RNA synthesis by viral RdRp is dependent upon uridylylation of VPg that serves as a primer in the presence of the polyadenylated genomic RNA (Rohayem et al., 2006a; Rohayem et al., 2006b). This "protein-primed" initiation occurs after the annealing of the elongated VPg-poly(U) to the poly(A) tail of the viral genome (Rohayem et al., 2006a; Rohayem et al., 2006b).

The inhibition of this uridylylation step or prevention of annealing to the poly(A) tail through a disruption of interaction between VPg and the viral genome or the RdRp could be an effective manner to stop the norovirus life cycle and therefore a good antiviral strategy (Rohayem et al., 2010).

It is known that the initiation of translation of norovirus proteins is dependent on the interaction of the VPg with eIF4F complex (eukaryotic initiation factor 4F), a key component of the cellular translation initiation machinery (Daughenbaugh et al., 2003; Daughenbaugh et al., 2006). The interaction of the VPg with individual eIF4F components has been described. A direct interaction with eIF4E (cap binding protein) was firstly demonstrated with the VPg of Norwalk virus (Goodfellow et al., 2005). A similar interaction with this component was also seen with FCV and MNV but, in these viruses, the key requirement for

RNA translation was shown to be the interaction with another component of the complex, the eIF4A (a RNA helicase) (Chaudhry et al., 2006). This was demonstrated by the inhibitor of eIF4A hippuristanol which blocked the translation of both FCV and MNV viral proteins *in vitro* (Chaudhry et al., 2006). However, the potential use of hippuristanol in therapy is limited by the fact that this compound is also an inhibitor of cellular protein synthesis, therefore expected to be cytotoxic. Panteamine is another compound that has the potential of interfering with VPg/ eIF4F complex, since it stimulates the helicase/NTPase activity of eIF4A, dysregulating its function within the eIF4F complex (Bordeleau et al., 2006). Therefore, these classes of compounds could potentially be explored as antivirals for norovirus but with less cytotoxic derivatives.

2.4.5 Protease

The norovirus protease or NS6 is a cysteine protease that is responsible for processing the nonstructural polyprotein precursor into the six/seven nonstructural proteins (Green, 2007). The atomic structure of the norovirus protease has been resolved (Nakamura et al., 2005). A two-domain structure was identified as being similar to other viral cysteine proteases, like those of picornavirus 3C proteases that show a chymotrypsin-like fold with a cysteine as the active-site nucleophile (Nakamura et al., 2005; Zeitler et al., 2006).

Similarly to what happens with the picornavirus 3C protease, the scissile bonds of the calicivirus proteases are restricted to a few number of dipeptides, revealing a very high specificity of substrate recognition in the cleavage sites of these enzymes which have also shown to be highly conserved among all caliciviruses (Sosnovtsev, 2010). Hence, the development of substrate-like peptides that block the protease active site constitutes an interesting strategy to inhibit the protease of norovirus. The inhibitors of the 3C protease of picornavirus, such as ruprintrivir, may potentially inhibit the norovirus protease given the overall similarity between the proteases of these viruses. (Binford et al., 2005; De Palma et al., 2008c; Leyssen et al., 2008).

The detailed structural information available for norovirus protease constitutes a good basis for the rational design of protease inhibitors and a valuable tool for the *in silico* screening of large compound libraries (Tan & Jiang, 2008). The recent development of functional assays for the detection of protease activity of calicivirus, using fluorogenic substrate peptides (Zeitler et al., 2006) or bioluminescence technologies (Oka et al., 2011) can constitute useful tools for the screening of protease inhibitors.

However, the role of norovirus protease appears to be more extensive. An association of the protease of MNV with mitochondria was suggested since they were found to co-localize within the cell (Hyde & Mackenzie, 2010). In this case, the protease could be implicated in an up-regulation of apoptosis of norovirus, which is known to occur via a mitochondrial-mediated apoptotic pathway involving caspase-9 (Bok et al., 2009). The involvement of viral protease with apoptotic pathways has been described for their picornavirus counterparts (Drahos & Racaniello, 2009). An association of proteases with mitochondria was linked, in hepatitis A and C viruses, to a cleavage of the mitochondrial antiviral signaling protein (MAVS) (Yang et al., 2007). Since MAVS induces antiviral responses of interferon and NF-kB, one may implicate viral proteases in prevention of immune signaling (Hyde & Mackenzie, 2010).

Whether the protease of MNV plays a role in prevention of immune signaling through the cleavage of MAVS is currently under investigation (Hyde & Mackenzie, 2010). It is known so far that the innate immune response against MNV starts with the recognition of viral RNA by MDA-5 (McCartney et al., 2008), the cytosolic receptor which initiates the antiviral signaling cascade by interacting with MAVS, its downstream partner.

In conclusion, targeting protease may be one of the most promising approaches to inhibit norovirus replication given the important function of this protein.

2.4.6 RNA-dependent RNA polymerase

The RdRp or NS7 is the central enzyme of replication, being responsible for the synthesis of the genomic, subgenomic and antigenomic RNA of norovirus. Given its critical role in norovirus replication, the RdRp constitutes one of the most important antiviral targets.

The crystal structure of the norovirus RdRp in an enzymatically active form has been resolved and overall showed catalytic and structural elements characteristic of RdRp of other positive stranded RNA viruses (Ferrer-Orta et al., 2006; Nakamura et al., 2005; Ng et al., 2004). However, its carboxyl terminus folds into the active site cleft of the enzyme which constitutes a distinctive aspect of the norovirus RdRp deserving special attention when designing an RdRp inhibitor (Hardy, 2005; Ng et al., 2004). It would be expected that a compound that could interrupt the interaction between the carboxyl-terminus and the active site cleft of the RdRp would hamper norovirus replication (Tan & Jiang, 2008).

A more accurate picture of how the RdRp of Norwalk virus functions was provided recently when the crystal structure of the Norwalk virus polymerase was resolved bound to the RNA primer template and to its natural substrate, a nucleoside triphosphate (NTP) (Zamyatkin et al., 2008). This ternary RdRp·RNA·NTP complex revealed details underlying the nucleotidyl transfer reaction, which is thought to be highly conserved among viral polymerases. This complex was also resolved bound to a potent inhibitor of picornavirus polymerases, the 5-nitrocytidine triphosphate (NCT), revealing differences between NCT and NTP complexes, which indicate a novel mechanism of inhibition of the RdRp that should be explored in the design of anti-norovirus compounds mimicking natural nucleosides and nucleotides (Zamyatkin et al., 2008).

A functional assay was developed for the detection of norovirus RdRp activity (Rohayem et al., 2006a; Rohayem et al., 2006b) and the inhibitory activity of some nucleoside analogs such as 2'-arauridine-5'-triphosphate and 3'-deoxyuridine-5'-triphosphate has been reported (Rohayem et al., 2010). Nucleoside analogs display similar mechanisms of inhibition of RdRps and some, like 2'-C-methylcytidine, 2'-C-methyladenosine and 4'-azidocytidine have shown a broad spectrum of activity against plus stranded RNA viruses, such as picornavirus and HCV (De Palma et al., 2008b; Goris et al., 2007; Klumpp et al., 2006). Hence, this class of compounds has great potential to be inhibitors of the norovirus RdRp and ought to be studied as antiviral drugs.

Ribavirin is a guanosine analogue with broad-spectrum activity against RNA virus. Although it was discovered over 30 years ago, its mechanism of action still remains controversial. Ribavirin was formally approved to treat chronic HCV infections in combination with pegylated interferon and in aerosol form to treat pediatric respiratory syncytial virus (RSV) infections (Graci & Cameron, 2006). It has also been used against a number of other viruses such as Lassa fever virus, Crimean Congo hemorrhagic fever, hantaviruses and severe acute respiratory syndrome coronavirus (SARS-CoV) (Haagmans & Osterhaus, 2006; Leyssen et al., 2008). Ribavirin has shown to be active against norovirus in the Norwalk replicon model and the MNV model (Chang & George, 2007). The main mechanism of action in the Norwalk replicon model was associated with the depletion of GTP in the cells since the addition of guanosine moderately reversed the antiviral effect of ribavirin (Chang & George, 2007). This depletion of intracellular GTP could be due to the inhibition of the cellular inosine monophosphate dehydrogenase (IMPDH) by ribavirin (Graci & Cameron, 2006; Leyssen et al., 2005). Mycophenolic acid (MPA), a potent noncompetitive inhibitor of IMPDH, also showed to inhibit Norwalk virus replication (Chang & George, 2007).

Another of the proposed mechanisms of ribavirin is an increased mutation frequency via incorporation of ribavirin into newly synthesized genomes leading to error catastrophe (Graci & Cameron, 2006). However, ribavirin seemed not to induce catastrophic mutations in norovirus since there was no increase in the mutation rates in the ribavirin-treated Norwalk replicon-bearing cells (Chang & George, 2007).

Overall, this data indicates that ribavirin or its analogs, such as EICAR (5-ethynyl-1-β-D-ribofuranosylimidazole-4-carboxamide) and viramidine, could constitute a promising starting point in the development of inhibitors of norovirus replication.

2.5 Targeting the norovirus genome

The norovirus RNA genome or viral transcripts also constitute an important target to inhibit the replication of norovirus. Antisense oligonucleotides and siRNAs (small interfering RNA) can be designed to target conserved regions of the norovirus genome with the aim of disrupting viral replication. For that, these oligonucleotides need to fulfill some requisites, namely the target sequence has to be involved in viral replication, accessible for oligonucleotide hybridization and conserved among different viral strains (Spurgers et al., 2008).

The existence of conserved secondary structures among calicivirus genomes opens the possibility of designing an oligonucleotide that would present a broad spectrum activity among noroviruses or troughout the family *Caliciviridae*. These conserved structures include 5′ terminal stem-loops, 3′ terminal hairpins, a stem-loop just upstream of the ORF1/2 junction in the antigenomic strand and a stem-loop at the 5′ end of the polymerase coding region with a motif characteristic of picornavirus *cis*-acting replication elements (*cre* elements) that dictate VPg uridylylation (Simmonds et al., 2008; Victoria et al., 2009). Some of these structures were found to be critical for the replication of MNV and for its infectivity (Simmonds et al., 2008). By using MNV reverse genetics system it was demonstrated that the disruption of the 5′-stem loops or the 3′-hairpins strongly impaired MNV replication *in vitro* (Simmonds et al., 2008). Moreover, a polypyrimidine tract located at the 3′-end of the genome has been incriminated in regulating viral fitness and virulence of MNV *in vivo* (Bailey et al., 2010). The important roles played by these conserved RNA structures in norovirus replication and virulence makes them potentially good antiviral targets.

The 5'-UTR (untranslated region) sequence of the norovirus genome has already been successfully targeted by an antisense strategy. A panel of peptide-conjugated phosphorodiamidiate morpholino oligomers (PPMOs) specific for the 5'-UTR of MNV proved to be effective in inhibiting its replication *in vitro* (Bok et al., 2008). Also, a consensus PPMO (designated *Noro 1.1*), designed to target the corresponding region of several diverse human norovirus genotypes, inhibited Norwalk virus protein expression in replicon-bearing cells (Bok et al., 2008). Moreover, PMOs targeting the 5'-UTR of the FCV genome were used successfully in three clinical trials during FCV outbreaks in kittens (Smith et al., 2008). Overall, these studies suggests that PPMOs directed against the relatively conserved 5'-end of the norovirus genome may show broad antiviral activity against this genetically diverse group of viruses and might translate into a successful clinical application but only further studies in animal models will say.

An alternative nucleic acid-based strategy is the use of RNA interference (RNAi) for silencing the viral genome. A wide range of viruses have been inhibited with RNAi (Leonard & Schaffer, 2006) and concerning calicivirus the first preliminary results have been published (Bergmann & Rohayem, 2010; Rohayem et al., 2010). In this study, siRNAs targeting the 5'-UTR and the subgenomic region of the FCV genome were successful in inhibiting FCV replication *in vitro*, namely by reducing infectivity, reducing the levels of viral genomic RNA and inhibiting viral translation.

2.6 Other strategies to stop norovirus replication

The enhancement of the host cell's antiviral mechanisms may constitute a valuable strategy to inhibit norovirus replication. Interferons (IFNs) are critical components of the innate immune response which establish an antiviral state of cells through interactions with IFN receptors expressed in nearly all nucleated cells. The binding of IFNs to their receptors triggers activation of STATs (signal transducer and activator of transcription) and cascade events which results in the induction of various antiviral proteins, such as RNA-dependent protein kinase (PKR) and RNase L (Samuel, 2001). However, many viruses are armed with anti-IFN mechanisms, such as those counteracting the STATs and inhibiting IFN synthesis (Samuel, 2001).

Interferons, both type I (IFN-α) and type II (IFN-γ), showed to inhibit the replication of norovirus in the Norwalk replicon model (Chang & George, 2007; Chang et al., 2006). Norwalk virus did not present a strong anti-IFN mechanism in the replicon-bearing cells, and this may be a reason for its high sensitivity to IFNs (Chang & George, 2007; Chang et al., 2006). It was also demonstrated that IFN responses were critical to control MNV infection *in vivo* and inhibited viral replication *in vitro* (Karst et al., 2003; Wobus et al., 2004). Both type I and type II IFNs block the translation of viral proteins of MNV but while type II IFN-mediated inhibition is dependent on the well-characterized interferon-induced antiviral molecule PKR, type I IFN-mediated inhibition occur through a PKR-independent process (Changotra et al., 2009). This data suggests that IFN may be a good therapeutic option for norovirus gastroenteritis.

The cellular pathway of cholesterol biosynthesis has been shown to be upregulated during the replication of several viruses, including HIV and HCV (Giguere & Tremblay, 2004; Ye, 2007). A study using Norwalk replicon system demonstrated that cholesterol pathways were also important in the replication of norovirus (Chang, 2009). Statins, such as simvastatin and lovastatin, are well known drugs that interfere with cholesterol pathways by inhibiting *de novo* synthesis of cholesterol through inhibition of HMG-CoA (3-hydroxy-3-methyl glutaryl-coenzyme A), reducing plasma cholesterol levels by upregulating low density lipoprotein receptor (LDLR) and promoting the uptake of LDL bound cholesterol to cells. It has been demonstrated that the use of statins resulted in a reduction of HCV replication through blockage of protein geranylgeranylation and the proper formation of viral replicase complexes (Ye, 2007; Ye et al., 2003). On the contrary, the inhibition of cholesterol biosynthesis using statins significantly enhanced the replication of Norwalk virus which was correlated with an increased expression of LDLR (Chang, 2009). It was postulated that LDLR could play an important direct role in virus replication such as participating in viral replication complexes as an essential cofactor (Chang, 2009).

The activity of acyl-CoA:cholesterol acyltransferase (ACAT) is also an important factor for cholesterol biosynthesis. Unlike statins, treatment with ACAT inhibitors such as Cl-976, Sandoz 58-035, YIC-C8-434 and pyripyropene resulted in reduced levels of Norwalk replication and interestingly, in reduced levels of LDLR (Chang, 2009). This data indicate that ACAT may be a novel target for inhibiting norovirus replication and its inhibitors could be further developed as anti-norovirus drugs.

3. Final remarks

Antiviral therapy is still not available today for norovirus and certainly a long road still lies ahead. A significant progress has been made in the elucidation of the replication strategy of norovirus, for which the use of surrogate viruses, the generation of a Norwalk replicon model, the available crystal structures of norovirus proteins were landmark developments that helped this giant pursuit.

In this chapter, we review and speculate about potential targets and antiviral strategies. Many were the targets suggested, however we believe that priority should be given to viral enzymes of replication, such as the RdRp and protease. Besides being key enzymes in norovirus life cycle, they are conserved across this genetically diverse group of viruses and divergent enough from cellular enzymes for their inhibitors to have good selectivity and minimal toxicity. Moreover, viral enzymes of replication are in general less prone to variation than structural proteins, minimizing the emergence of drug resistance.

As the understanding of norovirus replication deepens, one could look forward to new opportunities for the development of innovative antiviral strategies targeting this important human pathogen in a near future.

4. Acknowledgments

We thank Joana Macedo (Faculdade de Farmácia, Universidade do Porto) for designing the figures of this chapter. Thanks are due to FCT – Fundação para a Ciência e a Tecnologia for the PhD grant of J. Rocha-Pereira (SFRH/BD/48156/2008).

5. References

Bae, J. & Schwab, K.J. (2008). Evaluation of murine norovirus, feline calicivirus, poliovirus, and MS2 as surrogates for human norovirus in a model of viral persistence in surface water and groundwater. *Appl Environ Microbiol* Vol.No. 2 pp. (477-484).

Bailey, D., Kaiser, W.J., Hollinshead, M., Moffat, K., Chaudhry, Y., Wileman, T., Sosnovtsev, S.V. & Goodfellow, I.G. (2009). Feline calicivirus p32, p39 and p30 proteins localize to the endoplasmic reticulum to initiate replication complex formation. *J Gen Virol* Vol.No. Pt 3 pp. (739-749).

Bailey, D., Karakasiliotis, I., Vashist, S., Chung, L.M., Reese, J., McFadden, N., Benson, A., Yarovinsky, F., Simmonds, P. & Goodfellow, I. (2010). Functional analysis of RNA structures present at the 3' extremity of the murine norovirus genome: the variable polypyrimidine tract plays a role in viral virulence. *J Virol* Vol.No. 6 pp. (2859-2870).

Bank-Wolf, B.R., Konig, M. & Thiel, H.J. (2010). Zoonotic aspects of infections with noroviruses and sapoviruses. *Vet Microbiol* Vol.No. 3-4 pp. (204-212).

Barton, E.S., Forrest, J.C., Connolly, J.L., Chappell, J.D., Liu, Y., Schnell, F.J., Nusrat, A., Parkos, C.A. & Dermody, T.S. (2001). Junction adhesion molecule is a receptor for reovirus. *Cell* Vol.No. 3 pp. (441-451).

Bergmann, M. & Rohayem, J. (2010). Inhibition of Calicivirus Replication in Mammalian Cells by RNAi. *Antiviral Research* Vol.No. 1 pp. (A53).

Bertolotti-Ciarlet, A., Crawford, S.E., Hutson, A.M. & Estes, M.K. (2003). The 3' end of Norwalk virus mRNA contains determinants that regulate the expression and stability of the viral capsid protein VP1: a novel function for the VP2 protein. *J Virol* Vol.No. 21 pp. (11603-11615).

Binford, S.L., Maldonado, F., Brothers, M.A., Weady, P.T., Zalman, L.S., Meador, J.W., 3rd, Matthews, D.A. & Patick, A.K. (2005). Conservation of amino acids in human rhinovirus 3C protease correlates with broad-spectrum antiviral activity of rupintrivir, a novel human rhinovirus 3C protease inhibitor. *Antimicrob Agents Chemother* Vol.No. 2 pp. (619-626).

Bok, K., Cavanaugh, V.J., Matson, D.O., Gonzalez-Molleda, L., Chang, K.O., Zintz, C., Smith, A.W., Iversen, P., Green, K.Y. & Campbell, A.E. (2008). Inhibition of norovirus replication by morpholino oligomers targeting the 5'-end of the genome. *Virology* Vol.No. 2 pp. (328-337).

Bok, K., Prikhodko, V.G., Green, K.Y. & Sosnovtsev, S.V. (2009). Apoptosis in murine norovirus-infected RAW264.7 cells is associated with downregulation of survivin. *J Virol* Vol.No. 8 pp. (3647-3656).

Bordeleau, M.E., Cencic, R., Lindqvist, L., Oberer, M., Northcote, P., Wagner, G. & Pelletier, J. (2006). RNA-mediated sequestration of the RNA helicase eIF4A by Pateamine A inhibits translation initiation. *Chem Biol* Vol.No. 12 pp. (1287-1295).

Boschi-Pinto, C., Velebit, L. & Shibuya, K. (2008). Estimating child mortality due to diarrhoea in developing countries. *Bull World Health Organ* Vol.No. 9 pp. (710-717).

Bryce, J., Boschi-Pinto, C., Shibuya, K. & Black, R.E. (2005). WHO estimates of the causes of death in children. *Lancet* Vol.No. 9465 pp. (1147-1152).

Bu, W., Mamedova, A., Tan, M., Xia, M., Jiang, X. & Hegde, R.S. (2008). Structural basis for the receptor binding specificity of Norwalk virus. *J Virol* Vol.No. 11 pp. (5340-5347).

Burroughs, J.N. & Brown, F. (1978). Presence of a covalently linked protein on calicivirus RNA. *J Gen Virol* Vol.No. 2 pp. (443-446).

Cannon, J.L., Papafragkou, E., Park, G.W., Osborne, J., Jaykus, L.A. & Vinje, J. (2006). Surrogates for the study of norovirus stability and inactivation in the environment: A comparison of murine norovirus and feline calicivirus. *J Food Prot* Vol.No. 11 pp. (2761-2765).

Cao, S., Lou, Z., Tan, M., Chen, Y., Liu, Y., Zhang, Z., Zhang, X.C., Jiang, X., Li, X. & Rao, Z. (2007). Structural basis for the recognition of blood group trisaccharides by norovirus. *J Virol* Vol.No. 11 pp. (5949-5957).

CDC (2002). Outbreak of acute gastroenteritis associated with Norwalk-like viruses among British military personnel--Afghanistan, May 2002. *MMWR Morb Mortal Wkly Rep* Vol.No. 22 pp. (477-479).

Chang, K.O. (2009). Role of cholesterol pathways in norovirus replication. *J Virol* Vol.No. 17 pp. (8587-8595).

Chang, K.O. & George, D.W. (2007). Interferons and ribavirin effectively inhibit Norwalk virus replication in replicon-bearing cells. *J Virol* Vol.No. 22 pp. (12111-12118).

Chang, K.O., Sosnovtsev, S.S., Belliot, G., Wang, Q., Saif, L.J. & Green, K.Y. (2005). Reverse genetics system for porcine enteric calicivirus, a prototype sapovirus in the Caliciviridae. *J Virol* Vol.No. 3 pp. (1409-1416).

Chang, K.O., Sosnovtsev, S.V., Belliot, G., King, A.D. & Green, K.Y. (2006). Stable expression of a Norwalk virus RNA replicon in a human hepatoma cell line. *Virology* Vol.No. 2 pp. (463-473).

Changotra, H., Jia, Y., Moore, T.N., Liu, G., Kahan, S.M., Sosnovtsev, S.V. & Karst, S.M. (2009). Type I and type II interferons inhibit the translation of murine norovirus proteins. *J Virol* Vol.No. 11 pp. (5683-5692).

Chaudhry, Y., Nayak, A., Bordeleau, M.E., Tanaka, J., Pelletier, J., Belsham, G.J., Roberts, L.O. & Goodfellow, I.G. (2006). Caliciviruses differ in their functional requirements for eIF4F components. *J Biol Chem* Vol.No. 35 pp. (25315-25325).

Chaudhry, Y., Skinner, M.A. & Goodfellow, I.G. (2007). Recovery of genetically defined murine norovirus in tissue culture by using a fowlpox virus expressing T7 RNA polymerase. *J Gen Virol* Vol.No. Pt 8 pp. (2091-2100).

Chen, S.Y., Tsai, C.N., Lai, M.W., Chen, C.Y., Lin, K.L., Lin, T.Y. & Chiu, C.H. (2009). Norovirus infection as a cause of diarrhea-associated benign infantile seizures. *Clin Infect Dis* Vol.No. 7 pp. (849-855).

Choi, J.M., Hutson, A.M., Estes, M.K. & Prasad, B.V. (2008). Atomic resolution structural characterization of recognition of histo-blood group antigens by Norwalk virus. *Proc Natl Acad Sci U S A* Vol.No. 27 pp. (9175-9180).

Daughenbaugh, K.F., Fraser, C.S., Hershey, J.W. & Hardy, M.E. (2003). The genome-linked protein VPg of the Norwalk virus binds eIF3, suggesting its role in translation initiation complex recruitment. *EMBO J* Vol.No. 11 pp. (2852-2859).

Daughenbaugh, K.F., Wobus, C.E. & Hardy, M.E. (2006). VPg of murine norovirus binds translation initiation factors in infected cells. *Virol J* Vol.No. pp. (33).

De Palma, A.M., Heggermont, W., Lanke, K., Coutard, B., Bergmann, M., Monforte, A.M., Canard, B., De Clercq, E., Chimirri, A., Purstinger, G., Rohayem, J., van Kuppeveld, F. & Neyts, J. (2008a). The thiazolobenzimidazole TBZE-029 inhibits enterovirus replication by targeting a short region immediately downstream from motif C in the nonstructural protein 2C. *J Virol* Vol.No. 10 pp. (4720-4730).

De Palma, A.M., Purstinger, G., Wimmer, E., Patick, A.K., Andries, K., Rombaut, B., De Clercq, E. & Neyts, J. (2008b). Potential use of antiviral agents in polio eradication. *Emerg Infect Dis* Vol.No. 4 pp. (545-551).

De Palma, A.M., Thibaut, H.J., van der Linden, L., Lanke, K., Heggermont, W., Ireland, S., Andrews, R., Arimilli, M., Al-Tel, T.H., De Clercq, E., van Kuppeveld, F. & Neyts, J. (2009). Mutations in the nonstructural protein 3A confer resistance to the novel enterovirus replication inhibitor TTP-8307. *Antimicrob Agents Chemother* Vol.No. 5 pp. (1850-1857).

De Palma, A.M., Vliegen, I., De Clercq, E. & Neyts, J. (2008c). Selective inhibitors of picornavirus replication. *Med Res Rev* Vol.No. 6 pp. (823-884).

Denison, M.R. (2008). Seeking membranes: positive-strand RNA virus replication complexes. *PLoS Biol* Vol.No. 10 pp. (e270).

Dolin, R., Blacklow, N.R., DuPont, H., Buscho, R.F., Wyatt, R.G., Kasel, J.A., Hornick, R. & Chanock, R.M. (1972). Biological properties of Norwalk agent of acute infectious nonbacterial gastroenteritis. *Proc Soc Exp Biol Med* Vol.No. 2 pp. (578-583).

Donaldson, E.F., Lindesmith, L.C., Lobue, A.D. & Baric, R.S. (2010). Viral shape-shifting: norovirus evasion of the human immune system. *Nat Rev Microbiol* Vol.No. 3 pp. (231-241).

Doultree, J.C., Druce, J.D., Birch, C.J., Bowden, D.S. & Marshall, J.A. (1999). Inactivation of feline calicivirus, a Norwalk virus surrogate. *J Hosp Infect* Vol.No. 1 pp. (51-57).

Drahos, J. & Racaniello, V.R. (2009). Cleavage of IPS-1 in cells infected with human rhinovirus. *J Virol* Vol.No. 22 pp. (11581-11587).

Duizer, E., Bijkerk, P., Rockx, B., De Groot, A., Twisk, F. & Koopmans, M. (2004a). Inactivation of caliciviruses. *Appl Environ Microbiol* Vol.No. 8 pp. (4538-4543).

Duizer, E., Schwab, K.J., Neill, F.H., Atmar, R.L., Koopmans, M.P. & Estes, M.K. (2004b). Laboratory efforts to cultivate noroviruses. *J Gen Virol* Vol.No. Pt 1 pp. (79-87).

El-Kamary, S.S., Pasetti, M.F., Mendelman, P.M., Frey, S.E., Bernstein, D.I., Treanor, J.J., Ferreira, J., Chen, W.H., Sublett, R., Richardson, C., Bargatze, R.F., Sztein, M.B. & Tacket, C.O. (2010). Adjuvanted intranasal Norwalk virus-like particle vaccine elicits antibodies and antibody-secreting cells that express homing receptors for mucosal and peripheral lymphoid tissues. *J Infect Dis* Vol.No. 11 pp. (1649-1658).

Ettayebi, K. & Hardy, M.E. (2003). Norwalk virus nonstructural protein p48 forms a complex with the SNARE regulator VAP-A and prevents cell surface expression of vesicular stomatitis virus G protein. *J Virol* Vol.No. 21 pp. (11790-11797).

Farkas, T., Sestak, K., Wei, C. & Jiang, X. (2008). Characterization of a rhesus monkey calicivirus representing a new genus of Caliciviridae. *J Virol* Vol.No. 11 pp. (5408-5416).

Feng, X. & Jiang, X. (2007). Library screen for inhibitors targeting norovirus binding to histo-blood group antigen receptors. *Antimicrob Agents Chemother* Vol.No. 1 pp. (324-331).

Fernandez-Vega, V., Sosnovtsev, S.V., Belliot, G., King, A.D., Mitra, T., Gorbalenya, A. & Green, K.Y. (2004). Norwalk virus N-terminal nonstructural protein is associated with disassembly of the Golgi complex in transfected cells. *J Virol* Vol.No. 9 pp. (4827-4837).

Ferrer-Orta, C., Arias, A., Escarmis, C. & Verdaguer, N. (2006). A comparison of viral RNA-dependent RNA polymerases. *Curr Opin Struct Biol* Vol.No. 1 pp. (27-34).

Field, H.J. & Vere Hodge, R.A. (2008). Antiviral Agents. In: *Desk Encyclopedia of General Virology*, B.W.J. Mahy & M.H.V. Van Regenmortel, pp. 292-304, Elsevier Ltd.

Fukushi, S., Kojima, S., Takai, R., Hoshino, F.B., Oka, T., Takeda, N., Katayama, K. & Kageyama, T. (2004). Poly(A)- and primer-independent RNA polymerase of Norovirus. *J Virol* Vol.No. 8 pp. (3889-3896).

Gerondopoulos, A., Jackson, T., Monaghan, P., Doyle, N. & Roberts, L.O. (2010). Murine norovirus-1 cell entry is mediated through a non-clathrin-, non-caveolae-, dynamin- and cholesterol-dependent pathway. *J Gen Virol* Vol.No. Pt 6 pp. (1428-1438).

Giguere, J.F. & Tremblay, M.J. (2004). Statin compounds reduce human immunodeficiency virus type 1 replication by preventing the interaction between virion-associated host intercellular adhesion molecule 1 and its natural cell surface ligand LFA-1. *J Virol* Vol.No. 21 pp. (12062-12065).

Glass, P.J., White, L.J., Ball, J.M., Leparc-Goffart, I., Hardy, M.E. & Estes, M.K. (2000). Norwalk virus open reading frame 3 encodes a minor structural protein. *J Virol* Vol.No. 14 pp. (6581-6591).

Glass, R.I., Parashar, U.D. & Estes, M.K. (2009). Norovirus gastroenteritis. *N Engl J Med* Vol.No. 18 pp. (1776-1785).

Goodfellow, I., Chaudhry, Y., Gioldasi, I., Gerondopoulos, A., Natoni, A., Labrie, L., Laliberte, J.F. & Roberts, L. (2005). Calicivirus translation initiation requires an interaction between VPg and eIF4E. *Embo Reports* Vol.No. 10 pp. (968-972).

Goris, N., De Palma, A., Toussaint, J.F., Musch, I., Neyts, J. & De Clercq, K. (2007). 2'-C-methylcytidine as a potent and selective inhibitor of the replication of foot-and-mouth disease virus. *Antiviral Res* Vol.No. 3 pp. (161-168).

Gotz, H., de, J.B., Lindback, J., Parment, P.A., Hedlund, K.O., Torven, M. & Ekdahl, K. (2002). Epidemiological investigation of a food-borne gastroenteritis outbreak caused by Norwalk-like virus in 30 day-care centres. *Scand J Infect Dis* Vol.No. 2 pp. (115-121).

Graci, J.D. & Cameron, C.E. (2006). Mechanisms of action of ribavirin against distinct viruses. *Rev Med Virol* Vol.No. 1 pp. (37-48).

Green, K.Y. (2007). Caliciviridae: The Noroviruses. In: *Fields Virology*, D.M. Knipe & P.M. Howley, pp. 949-979, Lippincott Williams & Wilkins

Green, K.Y., Ando, T., Balayan, M.S., Berke, T., Clarke, I.N., Estes, M.K., Matson, D.O., Nakata, S., Neill, J.D., Studdert, M.J. & Thiel, H.J. (2000). Taxonomy of the caliciviruses. *J Infect Dis* Vol.No. pp. (S322-330).

Haagmans, B.L. & Osterhaus, A.D. (2006). Coronaviruses and their therapy. *Antiviral Res* Vol.No. 2-3 pp. (397-403).

Hansman, G.S., Shahzad-ul-Hussan, S., McLellan, J.S., Chuang G.-Y., Georgiev, I., Shimoike T., Katayama, K., Bewley, C. A. & Kwong. P. D. (2011) Structural basis for norovirus inhibition and fucose mimicry by citrate, *J Virol* (Epub ahead of print 26 Oct 2011)

Hardy, M.E. (2005). Norovirus protein structure and function. *FEMS Microbiol Lett* Vol.No. 1 39 pp. (1-8).

Heinz, B.A. & Vance, L.M. (1995). The antiviral compound enviroxime targets the 3A coding region of rhinovirus and poliovirus. *J Virol* Vol.No. 7 pp. (4189-4197).

Huang, P., Farkas, T., Marionneau, S., Zhong, W., Ruvoen-Clouet, N., Morrow, A.L., Altaye, M., Pickering, L.K., Newburg, D.S., LePendu, J. & Jiang, X. (2003). Noroviruses bind to human ABO, Lewis, and secretor histo-blood group antigens: identification of 4 distinct strain-specific patterns. *J Infect Dis* Vol.No. 1 pp. (19-31).

Huang, P., Farkas, T., Zhong, W., Tan, M., Thornton, S., Morrow, A.L. & Jiang, X. (2005). Norovirus and histo-blood group antigens: demonstration of a wide spectrum of strain specificities and classification of two major binding groups among multiple binding patterns. *J Virol* Vol.No. 11 pp. (6714-6722).

Hutson, A.M., Atmar, R.L. & Estes, M.K. (2004). Norovirus disease: changing epidemiology and host susceptibility factors. *Trends Microbiol* Vol.No. 6 pp. (279-287).

Hutson, A.M., Atmar, R.L., Graham, D.Y. & Estes, M.K. (2002). Norwalk virus infection and disease is associated with ABO histo-blood group type. *J Infect Dis* Vol.No. 9 pp. (1335-1337).

Hyde, J.L. & Mackenzie, J.M. (2010). Subcellular localization of the MNV-1 ORF1 proteins and their potential roles in the formation of the MNV-1 replication complex. *Virology* Vol.No. 1 pp. (138-148).

Hyde, J.L., Sosnovtsev, S.V., Green, K.Y., Wobus, C., Virgin, H.W. & Mackenzie, J.M. (2009). Mouse norovirus replication is associated with virus-induced vesicle clusters originating from membranes derived from the secretory pathway. *J Virol* Vol.No. 19 pp. (9709-9719).

Ito, S., Takeshita, S., Nezu, A., Aihara, Y., Usuku, S., Noguchi, Y. & Yokota, S. (2006). Norovirus-associated encephalopathy. *Pediatr Infect Dis J* Vol.No. 7 pp. (651-652).

Jiang, X., Wang, M., Graham, D.Y. & Estes, M.K. (1992). Expression, self-assembly, and antigenicity of the Norwalk virus capsid protein. *J Virol* Vol.No. 11 pp. (6527-6532).

Kapikian, A.Z., Wyatt, R.G., Dolin, R., Thornhill, T.S., Kalica, A.R. & Chanock, R.M. (1972). Visualization by immune electron microscopy of a 27-nm particle associated with acute infectious nonbacterial gastroenteritis. *J Virol* Vol.No. 5 pp. (1075-1081).

Karst, S.M. (2010). Pathogenesis of Noroviruses, Emerging RNA Viruses. *Viruses* Vol.No. 3 pp. (748-781).

Karst, S.M., Wobus, C.E., Lay, M., Davidson, J. & Virgin, H.W.t. (2003). STAT1-dependent innate immunity to a Norwalk-like virus. *Science* Vol.No. 5612 pp. (1575-1578).

Kawano, G., Oshige, K., Syutou, S., Koteda, Y., Yokoyama, T., Kim, B.G., Mizuochi, T., Nagai, K., Matsuda, K., Ohbu, K. & Matsuishi, T. (2007). Benign infantile convulsions associated with mild gastroenteritis: a retrospective study of 39 cases including virological tests and efficacy of anticonvulsants. *Brain Dev* Vol.No. 10 pp. (617-622).

Kirkwood, C.D. & Streitberg, R. (2008). Calicivirus shedding in children after recovery from diarrhoeal disease. *J Clin Virol* Vol.No. 3 pp. (346-348).

Klumpp, K., Leveque, V., Le Pogam, S., Ma, H., Jiang, W.R., Kang, H., Granycome, C., Singer, M., Laxton, C., Hang, J.Q., Sarma, K., Smith, D.B., Heindl, D., Hobbs, C.J., Merrett, J.H., Symons, J., Cammack, N., Martin, J.A., Devos, R. & Najera, I. (2006). The novel nucleoside analog R1479 (4'-azidocytidine) is a potent inhibitor of NS5B-dependent RNA synthesis and hepatitis C virus replication in cell culture. *J Biol Chem* Vol.No. 7 pp. (3793-3799).

Koo, H.L., Ajami, N., Atmar, R.L. & DuPont, H.L. (2010). Noroviruses: The leading cause of gastroenteritis worldwide. *Discov Med* Vol.No. 50 pp. (61-70).

Koopmans, M. (2008). Progress in understanding norovirus epidemiology. *Curr Opin Infect Dis* Vol.No. 5 pp. (544-552).

Kwong, A.D., Rao, B.G. & Jeang, K.T. (2005). Viral and cellular RNA helicases as antiviral targets. *Nat Rev Drug Discov* Vol.No. 10 pp. (845-853).

L'Homme, Y., Sansregret, R., Plante-Fortier, E., Lamontagne, A.M., Ouardani, M., Lacroix, G. & Simard, C. (2009). Genomic characterization of swine caliciviruses representing a new genus of Caliciviridae. *Virus Genes* Vol.No. 1 pp. (66-75).

Le Pendu, J., Ruvoen-Clouet, N., Kindberg, E. & Svensson, L. (2006). Mendelian resistance to human norovirus infections. *Semin Immunol* Vol.No. 6 pp. (375-386).

Leonard, J.N. & Schaffer, D.V. (2006). Antiviral RNAi therapy: emerging approaches for hitting a moving target. *Gene Ther* Vol.No. 6 pp. (532-540).

Leyssen, P., Balzarini, J., De Clercq, E. & Neyts, J. (2005). The predominant mechanism by which ribavirin exerts its antiviral activity in vitro against flaviviruses and paramyxoviruses is mediated by inhibition of IMP dehydrogenase. *J Virol* Vol.No. 3 pp. (1943-1947).

Leyssen, P., De Clercq, E. & Neyts, J. (2008). Molecular strategies to inhibit the replication of RNA viruses. *Antiviral Res* Vol.No. 1 pp. (9-25).

Lindesmith, L., Moe, C., Marionneau, S., Ruvoen, N., Jiang, X., Lindblad, L., Stewart, P., LePendu, J. & Baric, R. (2003). Human susceptibility and resistance to Norwalk virus infection. *Nat Med* Vol.No. 5 pp. (548-553).

Lindesmith, L.C., Donaldson, E.F., Lobue, A.D., Cannon, J.L., Zheng, D.P., Vinje, J. & Baric, R.S. (2008). Mechanisms of GII.4 norovirus persistence in human populations. *PLoS Med* Vol.No. 2 pp. (e31).

Liu, B., Clarke, I.N. & Lambden, P.R. (1996). Polyprotein processing in Southampton virus: identification of 3C-like protease cleavage sites by in vitro mutagenesis. *J Virol* Vol.No. 4 pp. (2605-2610).

Lopman, B.A., Reacher, M.H., Vipond, I.B., Sarangi, J. & Brown, D.W. (2004). Clinical manifestation of norovirus gastroenteritis in health care settings. *Clin Infect Dis* Vol.No. 3 pp. (318-324).

Makino, A., Shimojima, M., Miyazawa, T., Kato, K., Tohya, Y. & Akashi, H. (2006). Junctional adhesion molecule 1 is a functional receptor for feline calicivirus. *J Virol* Vol.No. 9 pp. (4482-4490).

Marionneau, S., Ruvoen, N., Le Moullac-Vaidye, B., Clement, M., Cailleau-Thomas, A., Ruiz-Palacois, G., Huang, P., Jiang, X. & Le Pendu, J. (2002). Norwalk virus binds to histo-blood group antigens present on gastroduodenal epithelial cells of secretor individuals. *Gastroenterology* Vol.No. 7 pp. (1967-1977).

Marsh, M. & Helenius, A. (2006). Virus entry: open sesame. *Cell* Vol.No. 4 pp. (729-740).

Marshall, J.K., Thabane, M., Borgaonkar, M.R. & James, C. (2007). Postinfectious irritable bowel syndrome after a food-borne outbreak of acute gastroenteritis attributed to a viral pathogen. *Clin Gastroenterol Hepatol* Vol.No. 4 pp. (457-460).

Martella, V., Campolo, M., Lorusso, E., Cavicchio, P., Camero, M., Bellacicco, A.L., Decaro, N., Elia, G., Greco, G., Corrente, M., Desario, C., Arista, S., Banyai, K., Koopmans, M. & Buonavoglia, C. (2007). Norovirus in captive lion cub (Panthera leo). *Emerg Infect Dis* Vol.No. 7 pp. (1071-1073).

Martella, V., Lorusso, E., Decaro, N., Elia, G., Radogna, A., D'Abramo, M., Desario, C., Cavalli, A., Corrente, M., Camero, M., Germinario, C.A., Banyai, K., Di Martino, B.,

Marsilio, F., Carmichael, L.E. & Buonavoglia, C. (2008). Detection and molecular characterization of a canine norovirus. *Emerg Infect Dis* Vol.No. 8 pp. (1306-1308).
McCartney, S.A., Thackray, L.B., Gitlin, L., Gilfillan, S., Virgin, H.W. & Colonna, M. (2008). MDA-5 recognition of a murine norovirus. *PLoS Pathog* Vol.No. 7 pp. (e1000108).
Mesquita, J.R., Barclay, L., Jose Nascimento, M.S. & Vinje, J. (2010). Novel norovirus in dogs with diarrhea. *Emerg Infect Dis* Vol.No. 6 pp. (980-982).
Mumphrey, S.M., Changotra, H., Moore, T.N., Heimann-Nichols, E.R., Wobus, C.E., Reilly, M.J., Moghadamfalahi, M., Shukla, D. & Karst, S.M. (2007). Murine norovirus 1 infection is associated with histopathological changes in immunocompetent hosts, but clinical disease is prevented by STAT1-dependent interferon responses. *J Virol* Vol.No. 7 pp. (3251-3263).
Murata, T., Katsushima, N., Mizuta, K., Muraki, Y., Hongo, S. & Matsuzaki, Y. (2007). Prolonged norovirus shedding in infants <or=6 months of age with gastroenteritis. *Pediatr Infect Dis J* Vol.No. 1 pp. (46-49).
Nakamura, K., Someya, Y., Kumasaka, T., Ueno, G., Yamamoto, M., Sato, T., Takeda, N., Miyamura, T. & Tanaka, N. (2005). A norovirus protease structure provides insights into active and substrate binding site integrity. *J Virol* Vol.No. 21 pp. (13685-13693).
Ng, K.K., Pendas-Franco, N., Rojo, J., Boga, J.A., Machin, A., Alonso, J.M. & Parra, F. (2004). Crystal structure of norwalk virus polymerase reveals the carboxyl terminus in the active site cleft. *J Biol Chem* Vol.No. 16 pp. (16638-16645).
Norder, H., De Palma, A.M., Selisko, B., Costenaro, L., Papageorgiou, N., Arnan, C., Coutard, B., Lantez, V., De Lamballerie, X., Baronti, C., Sola, M., Tan, J., Neyts, J., Canard, B., Coll, M., Gorbalenya, A.E. & Hilgenfeld, R. (2011). Picornavirus non-structural proteins as targets for new anti-virals with broad activity. *Antiviral Res* Vol.No. 3 pp. (204-218).
Oka, T., Takagi, H., Tohya, Y., Murakami, K., Takeda, N., Wakita, T. & Katayama, K. (2011). Bioluminescence technologies to detect calicivirus protease activity in cell-free system and in infected cells. *Antiviral Res* Vol.No. 1 pp. (9-16).
Papafragkou, E., Hewitt, J., Park, G., Straub, T., Greening, G. & Vinje, J. (2009). Challenges of Culturing Human Norovirus in a 3-D Organoid Cell Culture Model. In Proceedings of *ASM.*109th General Meeting. Philadephia, PA, USA: 09-GM-A-2871-ASM.
Parrino, T.A., Schreiber, D.S., Trier, J.S., Kapikian, A.Z. & Blacklow, N.R. (1977). Clinical immunity in acute gastroenteritis caused by Norwalk agent. *N Engl J Med* Vol.No. 2 pp. (86-89).
Patel, M.M., Hall, A.J., Vinje, J. & Parashar, U.D. (2009). Noroviruses: a comprehensive review. *J Clin Virol* Vol.No. 1 pp. (1-8).
Patel, M.M., Widdowson, M.A., Glass, R.I., Akazawa, K., Vinje, J. & Parashar, U.D. (2008). Systematic literature review of role of noroviruses in sporadic gastroenteritis. *Emerg Infect Dis* Vol.No. 8 pp. (1224-1231).
Perry, J.W., Taube, S. & Wobus, C.E. (2009). Murine norovirus-1 entry into permissive macrophages and dendritic cells is pH-independent. *Virus Res* Vol.No. 1 pp. (125-129).
Perry, J.W. & Wobus, C.E. (2010). Endocytosis of murine norovirus 1 into murine macrophages is dependent on dynamin II and cholesterol. *J Virol* Vol.No. 12 pp. (6163-6176).

Pfister, T. & Wimmer, E. (2001). Polypeptide p41 of a Norwalk-like virus is a nucleic acid-independent nucleoside triphosphatase. *J Virol* Vol.No. 4 pp. (1611-1619).

Prasad, B.V., Hardy, M.E., Dokland, T., Bella, J., Rossmann, M.G. & Estes, M.K. (1999). X-ray crystallographic structure of the Norwalk virus capsid. *Science* Vol.No. 5438 pp. (287-290).

Prasad, B.V., Rothnagel, R., Jiang, X. & Estes, M.K. (1994). Three-dimensional structure of baculovirus-expressed Norwalk virus capsids. *J Virol* Vol.No. 8 pp. (5117-5125).

Putics, A., Vashist, S., Bailey, D. & Goodfellow, I. (2010). Murine norovirus translation, replication and reverse genetics In: *Caliciviruses: Molecular and Cellular Virology*, G.S. Hansman, X.J. Jiang & K.Y. Green, pp. 205-222, Caister Academic Press

Ramani, S. & Kang, G. (2009). Viruses causing childhood diarrhoea in the developing world. *Curr Opin Infect Dis* Vol.No. 5 pp. (477-482).

Rocha-Pereira, J., Cunha, R., Pinto, D.C.G.A., Silva, A.M.S. & Nascimento, M.S.J. (2010). (E)-2-Styrylchromones as potential anti-norovirus agents. *Bioorganic & Medicinal Chemistry* Vol.No. 12 pp. (4195-4201).

Rohayem, J., Bergmann, M., Gebhardt, J., Gould, E., Tucker, P., Mattevi, A., Unge, T., Hilgenfeld, R. & Neyts, J. (2010). Antiviral strategies to control calicivirus infections. *Antiviral Res* Vol.No. 2 pp. (162-178).

Rohayem, J., Jager, K., Robel, I., Scheffler, U., Temme, A. & Rudolph, W. (2006a). Characterization of norovirus 3Dpol RNA-dependent RNA polymerase activity and initiation of RNA synthesis. *J Gen Virol* Vol.No. Pt 9 pp. (2621-2630).

Rohayem, J., Robel, I., Jager, K., Scheffler, U. & Rudolph, W. (2006b). Protein-primed and de novo initiation of RNA synthesis by norovirus 3Dpol. *J Virol* Vol.No. 14 pp. (7060-7069).

Rossignol, J.F. & El-Gohary, Y.M. (2006). Nitazoxanide in the treatment of viral gastroenteritis: a randomized double-blind placebo-controlled clinical trial. *Aliment Pharmacol Ther* Vol.No. 10 pp. (1423-1430).

Rydell, G.E., Nilsson, J., Rodriguez-Diaz, J., Ruvoen-Clouet, N., Svensson, L., Le Pendu, J. & Larson, G. (2009). Human noroviruses recognize sialyl Lewis x neoglycoprotein. *Glycobiology* Vol.No. 3 pp. (309-320).

Samuel, C.E. (2001). Antiviral actions of interferons. *Clin Microbiol Rev* Vol.No. 4 pp. (778-809).

Sharp, T.M., Guix, S., Katayama, K., Crawford, S.E. & Estes, M.K. (2010). Inhibition of cellular protein secretion by norwalk virus nonstructural protein p22 requires a mimic of an endoplasmic reticulum export signal. *PLoS One* Vol.No. 10 pp. (e13130).

Siebenga, J.J., Beersma, M.F., Vennema, H., van Biezen, P., Hartwig, N.J. & Koopmans, M. (2008). High prevalence of prolonged norovirus shedding and illness among hospitalized patients: a model for in vivo molecular evolution. *J Infect Dis* Vol.No. 7 pp. (994-1001).

Simmonds, P., Karakasiliotis, I., Bailey, D., Chaudhry, Y., Evans, D.J. & Goodfellow, I.G. (2008). Bioinformatic and functional analysis of RNA secondary structure elements among different genera of human and animal caliciviruses. *Nucleic Acids Res* Vol.No. 8 pp. (2530-2546).

Smith, A.W., Iversen, P.L., O'Hanley, P.D., Skilling, D.E., Christensen, J.R., Weaver, S.S., Longley, K., Stone, M.A., Poet, S.E. & Matson, D.O. (2008). Virus-specific antiviral treatment for controlling severe and fatal outbreaks of feline calicivirus infection. *Am J Vet Res* Vol.No. 1 pp. (23-32).

Sosnovtsev, S. & Green, K.Y. (1995). RNA transcripts derived from a cloned full-length copy of the feline calicivirus genome do not require VpG for infectivity. *Virology* Vol.No. 2 pp. (383-390).

Sosnovtsev, S.V. (2010). Proteolytic cleavage and viral proteins In: *Caliciviruses: Molecular and Cellular Virology*, G.S. Hansman, X.J. Jiang & K.Y. Green, pp. 65-94, Caister Academic Press

Sosnovtsev, S.V., Belliot, G., Chang, K.O., Prikhodko, V.G., Thackray, L.B., Wobus, C.E., Karst, S.M., Virgin, H.W. & Green, K.Y. (2006). Cleavage map and proteolytic processing of the murine norovirus nonstructural polyprotein in infected cells. *J Virol* Vol.No. 16 pp. (7816-7831).

Spurgers, K.B., Sharkey, C.M., Warfield, K.L. & Bavari, S. (2008). Oligonucleotide antiviral therapeutics: antisense and RNA interference for highly pathogenic RNA viruses. *Antiviral Res* Vol.No. 1 pp. (26-36).

Straub, T.M., Honer zu Bentrup, K., Orosz-Coghlan, P., Dohnalkova, A., Mayer, B.K., Bartholomew, R.A., Valdez, C.O., Bruckner-Lea, C.J., Gerba, C.P., Abbaszadegan, M. & Nickerson, C.A. (2007). In vitro cell culture infectivity assay for human noroviruses. *Emerg Infect Dis* Vol.No. 3 pp. (396-403).

Stuart, A.D. & Brown, T.D. (2007). Alpha2,6-linked sialic acid acts as a receptor for Feline calicivirus. *J Gen Virol* Vol.No. Pt 1 pp. (177-186).

Takanashi, S., Hashira, S., Matsunaga, T., Yoshida, A., Shiota, T., Tung, P.G., Khamrin, P., Okitsu, S., Mizuguchi, M., Igarashi, T. & Ushijima, H. (2009). Detection, genetic characterization, and quantification of norovirus RNA from sera of children with gastroenteritis. *J Clin Virol* Vol.No. 2 pp. (161-163).

Tamura, M., Natori, K., Kobayashi, M., Miyamura, T. & Takeda, N. (2004). Genogroup II noroviruses efficiently bind to heparan sulfate proteoglycan associated with the cellular membrane. *J Virol* Vol.No. 8 pp. (3817-3826).

Tan, M., Huang, P., Meller, J., Zhong, W., Farkas, T. & Jiang, X. (2003). Mutations within the P2 domain of norovirus capsid affect binding to human histo-blood group antigens: evidence for a binding pocket. *J Virol* Vol.No. 23 pp. (12562-12571).

Tan, M. & Jiang, X. (2005). Norovirus and its histo-blood group antigen receptors: an answer to a historical puzzle. *Trends Microbiol* Vol.No. 6 pp. (285-293).

Tan, M. & Jiang, X. (2008). Norovirus gastroenteritis, increased understanding and future antiviral options. *Curr Opin Investig Drugs* Vol.No. 2 pp. (146-151).

Tan, M. & Jiang, X. (2010). Virus-Host Interaction and Cellular Receptors of Caliciviruses. In: *Caliciviruses: Molecular and Cellular Virology*, X.J.J.a.K.Y.G. Grant S. Hansman, pp. 111-130, Caister Academic Press

Tan, M. & Jiang, X. (2011). Norovirus-host interaction: Multi-selections by human histo-blood group antigens. *Trends Microbiol* Vol.No. 8 pp. (382-388).

Tan, M., Xia, M., Chen, Y., Bu, W., Hegde, R.S., Meller, J., Li, X. & Jiang, X. (2009). Conservation of carbohydrate binding interfaces: evidence of human HBGA selection in norovirus evolution. *PLoS One* Vol.No. 4 pp. (e5058).

Taube, S., Perry, J.W., Yetming, K., Patel, S.P., Auble, H., Shu, L., Nawar, H.F., Lee, C.H., Connell, T.D., Shayman, J.A. & Wobus, C.E. (2009). Ganglioside-linked terminal sialic acid moieties on murine macrophages function as attachment receptors for murine noroviruses. *J Virol* Vol.No. 9 pp. (4092-4101).

Teunis, P.F., Moe, C.L., Liu, P., Miller, S.E., Lindesmith, L., Baric, R.S., Le Pendu, J. & Calderon, R.L. (2008). Norwalk virus: how infectious is it? *J Med Virol* Vol.No. 8 pp. (1468-1476).

Thackray, L.B., Wobus, C.E., Chachu, K.A., Liu, B., Alegre, E.R., Henderson, K.S., Kelley, S.T. & Virgin, H.W.t. (2007). Murine noroviruses comprising a single genogroup exhibit biological diversity despite limited sequence divergence. *J Virol* Vol.No. 19 pp. (10460-10473).

Tsai, B. (2007). Penetration of nonenveloped viruses into the cytoplasm. *Annu Rev Cell Dev Biol* Vol.No. pp. (23-43).

Turcios-Ruiz, R.M., Axelrod, P., St John, K., Bullitt, E., Donahue, J., Robinson, N. & Friss, H.E. (2008). Outbreak of necrotizing enterocolitis caused by norovirus in a neonatal intensive care unit. *J Pediatr* Vol.No. 3 pp. (339-344).

Victoria, M., Colina, R., Miagostovich, M.P., Leite, J.P. & Cristina, J. (2009). Phylogenetic prediction of cis-acting elements: a cre-like sequence in Norovirus genome? *BMC Res Notes* Vol.No. pp. (176).

Vinje, J. (2010). A norovirus vaccine on the horizon? *J Infect Dis* Vol.No. 11 pp. (1623-1625).

Ward, V.K., McCormick, C.J., Clarke, I.N., Salim, O., Wobus, C.E., Thackray, L.B., Virgin, H.W.t. & Lambden, P.R. (2007). Recovery of infectious murine norovirus using pol II-driven expression of full-length cDNA. *Proc Natl Acad Sci U S A* Vol.No. 26 pp. (11050-11055).

Wei, C., Farkas, T., Sestak, K. & Jiang, X. (2008). Recovery of infectious virus by transfection of in vitro-generated RNA from tulane calicivirus cDNA. *J Virol* Vol.No. 22 pp. (11429-11436).

Wessels, E., Duijsings, D., Lanke, K.H., van Dooren, S.H., Jackson, C.L., Melchers, W.J. & van Kuppeveld, F.J. (2006). Effects of picornavirus 3A Proteins on Protein Transport and GBF1-dependent COP-I recruitment. *J Virol* Vol.No. 23 pp. (11852-11860).

Widdowson, M.A., Monroe, S.S. & Glass, R.I. (2005). Are noroviruses emerging? *Emerg Infect Dis* Vol.No. 5 pp. (735-737).

Wobus, C.E., Karst, S.M., Thackray, L.B., Chang, K.O., Sosnovtsev, S.V., Belliot, G., Krug, A., Mackenzie, J.M., Green, K.Y. & Virgin, H.W. (2004). Replication of Norovirus in cell culture reveals a tropism for dendritic cells and macrophages. *PLoS Biol* Vol.No. 12 pp. (e432).

Wobus, C.E., Thackray, L.B. & Virgin, H.W. (2006). Murine norovirus: a model system to study norovirus biology and pathogenesis. *J Virol* Vol.No. 11 pp. (5104-5112).

Yang, Y., Liang, Y.Q., Qu, L., Chen, Z.M., Yi, M.K., Li, K. & Lemon, S.M. (2007). Disruption of innate immunity due to mitochondrial targeting of a picornaviral protease precursor. *Proceedings of the National Academy of Sciences of the United States of America* Vol.No. 17 pp. (7253-7258).

Ye, J. (2007). Reliance of host cholesterol metabolic pathways for the life cycle of hepatitis C virus. *PLoS Pathog* Vol.No. 8 pp. (e108).

Ye, J., Wang, C., Sumpter, R., Jr., Brown, M.S., Goldstein, J.L. & Gale, M., Jr. (2003). Disruption of hepatitis C virus RNA replication through inhibition of host protein geranylgeranylation. *Proc Natl Acad Sci U S A* Vol.No. 26 pp. (15865-15870).

Zamyatkin, D.F., Parra, F., Alonso, J.M., Harki, D.A., Peterson, B.R., Grochulski, P. & Ng, K.K. (2008). Structural insights into mechanisms of catalysis and inhibition in Norwalk virus polymerase. *J Biol Chem* Vol.No. 12 pp. (7705-7712).

Zeitler, C.E., Estes, M.K. & Venkataram Prasad, B.V. (2006). X-ray crystallographic structure of the Norwalk virus protease at 1.5-A resolution. *J Virol* Vol.No. 10 pp. (5050-5058).

Zheng, D.P., Ando, T., Fankhauser, R.L., Beard, R.S., Glass, R.I. & Monroe, S.S. (2006). Norovirus classification and proposed strain nomenclature. *Virology* Vol.No. 2 pp. (312-323).

8

Single Domain Camelid Antibodies that Neutralize Negative Strand Viruses

Francisco Miguel Lopez Cardoso, Lorena Itatí Ibañez,
Bert Schepens and Xavier Saelens
*Department for Molecular Biomedical Research, Ghent,
Department of Biomedical Molecular Biology, Ghent University, Ghent,
Belgium*

1. Introduction

1.1 Conventional antibodies

Recombinant antibodies (Abs) are widely regarded as one of the main, if not the most promising tools against cancer and auto-immune, inflammatory, neurodegenerative and infectious diseases (Stiehm *et al.*, 2008). Conventional antibodies are complex molecules consisting of pairs of heavy and light chains, whose N-terminal domain is more variable than the rest of the protein sequence. The antibody heavy chain usually consists of three constant domains (CH1, CH2 and CH3) and a variable domain (VH). The light chain has only two domains, the constant light (CL) and the variable light (VL). Important Glycosylations on the CH2 domain are necessary for antibody effector functions, such as Antibody-Dependent Cellular Cytotoxicity (ADCC) and Complement–Dependent Cytolysis (CDC), and for regulating antibody half time in serum (Fig. 1, A). Antigen-binding is determined by the three hypervariable Complementary Determining Regions (CDR1, CDR2 and CDR3) present in both the VH and VL domains. These regions are located in juxtaposed loops, creating a continuous surface of ~ 1000 Å^2 that specifically binds to the epitope in an antigen. Although all CDRs can potentially make contact with the antigen, CDR3 contacts with the epitope are generally more extensive. The structural diversity of the antigen-binding sites of a conventional antibody depends on the size of the CDR3 in the VH and the conjunction with the VL at different angles and distances. These are grouped in three different classes, according to the size and type of antigen: cavities (fitting haptens), grooves (fitting peptides) and planar sites (fitting surface patches of proteins) (Johnson *et al.*, 2010).

1.2 The single variable domain of the heavy chain antibodies

In 1993 a surprising observation was made in members of the Artiodactyl Tylopoda family (camelids). Next to conventional IgG antibodies, camelids also naturally produce Heavy Chain antibodies (HCAbs) that lack the light chain (Hamers-Casterman *et al.*, 1993). Two years later, similar single chain antibodies were discovered in cartilaginous fish (sharks) (Greenberg *et al.*, 1995). Although the CH2 and CH3 of the HCAbs and the conventional Abs are highly homologous, there is no CH1 domain in the camelid HCAbs. The single variable domain, called VHH, is the only domain of HCAbs that makes contact with the antigen. Surprisingly, although the VHH have only three CDR regions, their affinity for antigens reaches the low nanomolar to even picomolar range, matching the best affinities of classical antibodies. When expressed as single domains (often referred to as nanobodies, Nb), the VHHs retain their strong epitope specificity and affinity, a feature that might be explained by the VHH architecture (Fig. 1, B). Just like the VHs of conventional antibodies, the amino acid (AA) sequence of VHHs is organised in three hypervariable regions (CDR1, CDR2 and CDR3) separated by four Framework regions (FR1-FR4) (Muyldermans *et al.*, 1994). As the

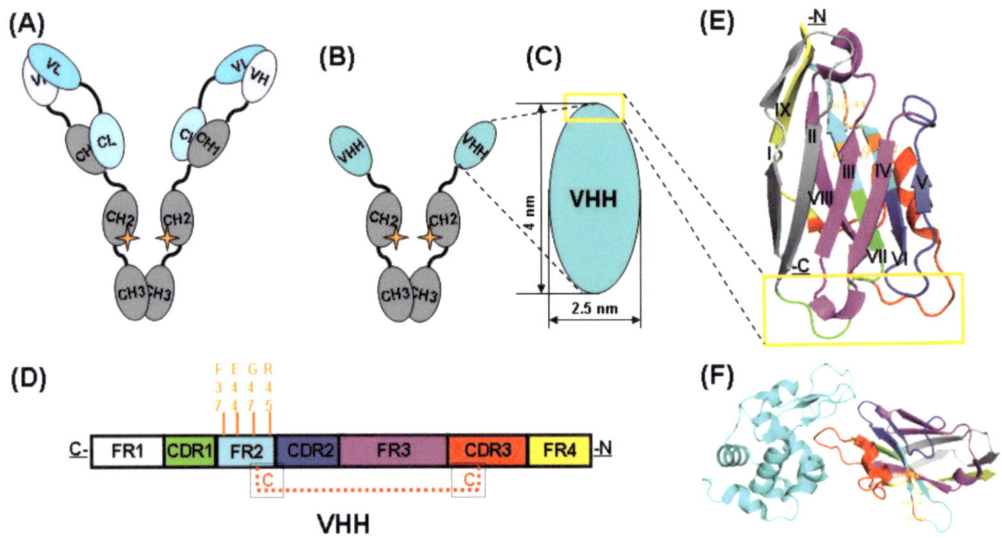

Fig. 1. Representative diagrams of a conventional antibody, an HCAb, and a VHH. (A) A conventional IgG antibody is a dimeric molecule, and each monomer comprises a heavy chain and a light chain. The heavy chain consists of the constant domains (CH1, CH2 and CH3) and the variable domain (VH). The light chain has only one conserved domain (CL) and a variable domain (VL). Important glycosylation sites (orange stars) are present in CH2, which are responsible for effector functions and the flexibility of the molecule. (B) The HCAb devoid of the light chain and CH1 contains the paratope (yellow box) present only in the single variable domain (VHH). (C) The VHH can be expressed as a prolate-shaped, soluble molecule of ~15 kDa. The yellow box shows the antigen binding site. (D) The VHH sequence is made of four Framework Regions (FR1, light gray; FR2, cyan; FR3, magenta and FR4, yellow), and three Complementary Determining Regions (CDR1, green; CDR2, blue and CDR3, red). Residues F37, E44, G47and R45 (orange) are located in the FR2 and mask a hydrophobic patch. C, C- terminal; N, N-terminal. The dotted red line represents a disulfide bond between the FR2 and the CDR3; this bond stabilizes the molecule and is present in dromedaries. (E) A three-dimensional structure of an anti lysozyme VHH, showing the Ig folding of β sheets, five strands in the front (roman numerals: I – V) and four strands in the back (VI – IX). The enlarged yellow box shows the antigen binding site, formed by juxtaposition of three CDRs. (F) The VHH shown in (F) is drawn in complex with lysozyme (light blue). A protruding paratope consisting mainly of CDR3 (red) recognizes and binds the catalytic cleft of lysozyme, inhibiting its activity.

AA sequence of the VHH FRs is highly similar to those of conventional VHs it was not surprising that the overall architecture of VHHs closely resembles that of VHs (Muyldermans *et al.*, 1994). Both VHH and VH domains fold into two β-sheets with the three CDRs that link these two sheets at one end of the barrel (or domain) (De Genst *et al.*, 2006; Desmyter *et al.*, 1996) (Fig. 1, C,E). However, there are striking structural differences between VHHs and conventional VH. Evidently, VHHs lack an interacting VL domain. Because of this, the hydrophobic amino acids present at the VH surface that is normally interacting with the VL, are substituted by hydrophilic AA (Fig.1, D). This enhances the solubility of VHH single domain proteins compared to engineered VH single domain proteins.

The absence of the additional CDRs in VHHs is likely compensated by structural features. First, the CDR3 regions of camelid VHHs are generally longer (13-17 amino acids) than the CDR3 regions of mouse and human VHs (9-12 and 9-17 AA respectively) (Wu *et al.*, 1993). In contrast to conventional Abs, in which the antigen binding surface is often a flat surface, a cavity or a groove, the long CDR3 loop may extend from the antigen binding surface (Desmyter *et al.*, 1996). This enlarges the paratope surface and hence the potential affinity and repertoire of camelid HCAbs. In addition, especially in dromedaries, the CDR1 and CDR3 regions contain a cysteine, which allows formation of a second disulfide bridge next to the single disulfide bridge in conventional VHs (Muyldermans *et al.*, 1994). This extra bridge likely stabilizes the CDR loops, thereby reducing their flexibility. This probably also contributes to the affinity (less entropy is lost upon antigen binding) and structural diversity of VHHs. Long extending CDR3 loops that are stabilized by an extra disulfide bridge can explain the tendency of VHHs to bind to clefts and concaves surfaces more readily than conventional antibodies do (Fig. 1, F) (De Genst *et al.*, 2006). Indeed comparison of multiple structures of hen egg white lysozyme interacting with either several conventional human antibodies or several camelid VHHs clearly illustrated that VHHs tends to bind to the concave substrate-binding pocket, whereas conventional antibodies favor epitopes on the "flat" surface of the antigen (Fig. 1, C). In addition, whereas each of the three CDRs of conventional VHs contributes considerably to the interaction with antigen, VHHs depended mainly on the CDR 3 loop for this interaction. Other antigens that are hard to target by conventional antibodies, but can be targeted by camelid VHHs are ion channels, GPCRs, haptens and enzymatic sites (Lauwereys *et al.*, 1998; Rasmussen *et al.*, 2011).

Next to an extended CDR3, the AA sequence of the H1 loop that precedes and comprises CDR1 appears to be particularly more variable in camelid VHHs than in conventional VHs. This might be interpreted as an extension of the VHH CDR1 (Vu *et al.*, 1997). Associated with this high variability in camelid VHHs, CH1 loops adopt conformations that deviate from the canonical H1 structures of conventional VHs (Barre *et al.*, 1994; Decanniere *et al.*, 1999; Decanniere *et al.*, 2000). Camelid VHH CH1 loops appear to fold into a more diverse repertoire of structures. The high variability in the AA sequence and conformations of the CH1 loop contribute to the VHH paratope size (850-1150 Å^2), which approaches that of conventional antibodies (VH + VL) (Desmyter *et al.*, 2002). Clearly, different biochemical and structural features of camelid VHHs compensate for the lack of a VL domain, thus allowing a broad repertoire of specific high affinity antigen interactions. In addition, due to their small size and typical extruding CDR3 regions, camelid VHH tend to bind in cavities that are not readily accessible for conventional antibodies. Next to these particular features,

VHH single domain protein is exceptionally stable and soluble, even under stringent conditions. As VHH are small and naturally monomeric, they can be easily formatted. In addition, the small size of VHHs allows them penetrate deeper into tissue (e.g. tumor tissue) and to occasionally cross the blood-brain barrier. On the down side, the small size of single domain VHH contributes to their rapid clearance from circulation.

Using display technologies, it is possible to select VHHs from large, synthetic or naive libraries (Verheesen *et al.*, 2006). The phage display generated from an immune VHH repertoire is the most widely and powerful technique used nowadays to rapidly select VHHs with the desired specificity (Arbabi Ghahroudi *et al.*, 1997). VHH are easily produced in bacterial or yeast systems in miligram quantities per liter of culture. Their stability, solubility, ease of production and small size make them excellent candidates for multivalent formatting. Tailor-made constructions using VHHs as building blocks enhance the avidity of the molecule even in a 3 log scale, and several constructions are being tested in clinical trials (Els Conrath *et al.*, 2001; Hmila *et al.*, 2010). Their high potential as therapeutics has prompted the creation in Belgium of the company Ablynx in 2001. Because of the publicity surrounding nanotechnology and the small size of the VHH, Ablynx named the VHH as "Nanobody (Nb)", and retains full intellectual property rights of the use of Nbs in therapeutics and diagnosis. The combined features of VHHs makes them ideal tools for many applications. In this chapter, we focus on the development and use of VHHs for anti-viral therapy. It is interesting to point out that only one monoclonal antibody is used today (Synagis) as a therapeutic against infectious disease (Groothuis & Simoes, 1993).

2. Influenza virus

The main prophylactic measure against influenza is vaccination. Therapeutic options for influenza are small molecule drugs targeting the viral proteins Neuraminidase (NA) or matrix protein 2 (M2). Influenza virus poses a great and continuous threat to humans and zoonotic infections also pose a dangerous challenge to human. In the last decade, two important viruses have emerged as pandemic or potentially pandemic outbreaks: the recent pandemic outbreak in the 2009 by the swine-derived H1N1 influenza virus (also called the Mexican Flu) and Highly Pathogenic Avian influenza (HPAV) viruses of the H5N1 subtype, mainly in Asiatic countries. The 2009 H1N1 pandemic presents an interesting case. It was a zoonotic infection that could be transmitted between humans, but had a low mortality rate. On the other hand, the HPAV H5N1 virus infections present a high replication efficiency, broader cell tropism and possible systemic spread in patients. Fulminant pneumonia, multi-organ failure caused by a high viral load and an intense inflammatory response (cytokine storm) are responsible of a mortality rate of 60 % (de Jong *et al.*, 2006). Vaccines to prevent HPAV infection are not available, but NA inhibitors (osetalmivir) are used as antiviral drugs. A combination of antiviral drugs and immunomodulators was used to control infection by HPAV H5N1 in patients, but its use was considered as a risk. On the other hand, passive immunization has been a successful alternative. Immunoglobulins in immune sera derived from animals or humans exposed to a homologous virus had been used to treat HPAV-infected humans (Luke & Subbarao, 2006; Zhou *et al.*, 2007). The genetic shift and drift of the influenza virus underline the need for new antiviral approaches. In addition, the emergence of drug resistant strains poses an extra concern. The Tamiflu Resistant strain (resulting mainly from the H274Y mutation, Wang *et al.*, 2002) is evidence of the urgent need for new anti-influenza drugs. It is also urgent to develop new and better antiviral tools against the zoonotic influenza virus, including HPAV. The characteristics of Nbs mentioned above makes them a potentially effective antiviral approach. Several attempts have been made to target conserved epitopes of proteins in the surface proteins of influenza viruses. The main antigenic target in influenza virus is the HA protein. However, the genetic shift of this viral protein, especially in its antigenic regions, complicates this approach. Even though this strategy has been successful in current seasonal vaccines, it is costly and far from optimal: it is not suitable for emerging pandemic viruses, as has been proven not suitable as an immediately available vaccine against the Mexican flu in 2009.

2.1 Targeting influenza HA: the Nb approach

The work of Hultberg and colleagues (Hultberg *et al.*, 2011) is the first report of the use of Nb technology as an antiviral tool against influenza. That study proved the binding of Nbs to an influenza protein and the neutralization of the binding of the virion to its cellular receptor in mammalian cells. These results are the proof of principle of the use of Nbs as antivirals. We discuss the most relevant results in scope of the potential further use of Nbs. To obtain Nbs directed against H5N1 viruses, llamas were immunized with recombinant H5N1 HA (H5, A/Vietnam/1203/04). The nanobody repertoire of the hyperimmune animals was cloned into a phage display library, and two promising HA-binding VHHs were isolated. The VHH of the HCab or Nb was cloned, produced as monovalent molecules, purified and screened for specific binding to the antigen, using as competitor the HA surrogate receptor fetuin. Two of the specific binders (B12 and C8) had high affinity to HA (K_D = 9.91 and 30.1 nM) as determined by surface plasmon resonance. In addition, in a MLV (H5) pseudotyped neutralization assay both Nbs neutralized the parental virus A/Vietnam/1203/04 and also another clade 1 virus (A/Vietnam/1194/04) with a minimal inhibition concentration (IC_{50}) of 75 nM. The possibility of cross reactivity among different H5N1 clades was also tested. The Nbs efficiency in neutralizing other clades of influenza virus decreased proportionally with the antigenic distance from the virus A/Vietnam/1203/04. Three viruses from clade 2.2 were inhibited by the monovalent Nbs in a similar range as clade 1 (IC_{50} = 50–150 nM). On the other hand, one virus of clade 2.3.4 and one virus from clade 2.5 showed little or no inhibition. As mentioned above, Nbs are potentially good building blocks for multivalent molecules due their small size, high affinity, and efficacy as a production platform. Bivalent and trivalent constructs were made, based on Nb C-8, using Gly4/Ser linkers (GS) of different lengths. The neutralization potential of the bivalent and trivalent constructs was greatly enhanced against the A/Vietnam/1194/04 virus ($IC_{50} \leq 1$ pM). Inhibition of this clade 1 virus was confirmed by a micronetralization assay in NIBRG-14 infected cells. NIBRG-14 is an engineered recombinant virus whose HA and NA are derived from the A/Vietnam/1194/04 virus. Surprisingly, in the bivalent and trivalent Nbs the IC_{50} neutralization activity (9 and 3 pM, respectively) decreased by more than 3 logs, compared to the monovalent Nb. These results show that the multimeric molecules outperformed a previously developed monoclonal antibody CR 261, against NIBRG-14 (Throsby *et al.*, 2008). These results were also confirmed in a hemagglutination inhibition assay, which showed an IC_{50} of 2 nM for the bivalent and trivalent construction, compared to 156 nm of the monovalent.

The multivalency format also resulted in the potential for neutralization of influenza virus of different clades. For three clade 2.2 viruses, two bivalent constructions of the Nb C-8 (9 GS and 15 GS) did not show any decrease in the IC_{50}. On the other hand, the 10 GS linker trivalent molecule showed a 10 to 40-fold increase in the neutralization potential, but the 20 GS linker trivalent showed only two-fold decrease in the IC_{50}, or none at all. Nevertheless, using the monovalent Nb the neutralization of virus from clades 2.3.4 or 2.5 was in the high nM range or absent, respectively. This result confirms the previous result showing that both bivalent and one trivalent (10GS) constructions decrease the IC_{50} to a low nM range. It is worth mentioning that the retroviral pseudovirus A/Vietnam/1194/04 and the influenza virus NIBRG-14 share the same HA, but different results were obtained using the MLV pseudotyped neutralization assay and the infected cells microneutralization. Using microneutralization, the reported IC_{50} of the monovalent, bivalent and trivalent molecules was reduced ten-fold as compared to the IC_{50} obtained by the pseudotyped neutralization. The difference in sensitivity of the assays emphasizes the need to confirm the neutralization results of the different influenza clades in infected cells based assays. The validation of the anti HA in an *in vivo* model was performed in a mouse model by our group (Ibañez *et al.*, 2011).

To confirm the *in vivo* efficacy of the Nbs, Ibañez and colleagues used an H5N1 NIBRG-14 mouse adapted virus strain (NIBRG-14 ma). It is important to point out that the Nbs were administered intranasally in all mouse experiments, in order to enhance penetration in the respiratory tract. Initially, to evaluate the antiviral potential using the bivalent Nb (C-8, 15 GS) *in vivo*, a dose of 5 mg/kg (100 μg) was used in mice. This dose completely prevented loss of body weight at 4, 24 and 48 h before a challenge with 1 LD_{50} of NIBRG-14 ma, compared to the controls after 4 days of monitoring. Using the same set up, on day 4 after challenge, no detectable lung virus titers were observed when mice had been treated at 4 and 24 hrs before challenge, and at 48 hrs the titer was 50-fold lower than in controls. These results suggested that the bivalent Nb provide strong protection against 1 LD_{50}, but it is important to consider the half life of the molecule. In previous *in vitro* results, the bivalent Nb neutralization activity was even 3 logs higher than that of the monovalent Nb, but *in vivo* there was also a significant improvement using the bivalent. The difference in virus neutralization capacity between the monovalent and bivalent Nbs and the minimal protective dose was assessed by administration of Nbs at different doses at 24 h before challenge with 1 LD_{50} NIBRG-14. The doses of Nbs ranged from 3 to 0.025 mg/kg, and complete neutralization was confirmed for the highest doses of both constructs. In addition, administration of the highest dose (60 μg, 3 mg/kg) of bivalent Nb 24 h before challenge with 4 LD_{50} also resulted in complete protection. The monovalent neutralization activity was dependent on the amount of Nb, but it was also statistically significant for doses of 6 or 1.2 μg of Nb per mouse. Remarkably, very low or no lung virus titer was detected in mice treated with the bivalent Nb, even for the lowest doses used (2.5–0.5 μg). These results strongly confirmed the neutralization efficacy of the bivalent Nb when used as prophylactic tool against a NIBRG-14 ma, a highly pathogenic influenza virus model.

The therapeutic efficacy of the bivalent Nb was also tested in the same model. The administration of 60 μg of bivalent Nb prevented the drop in body weight and showed a reduction in the lung viral titers when administered 4, 24 and 48 h after 1 LD_{50} challenge. On the other hand, 72 h after challenge, the drop in body weight was similar to that of the controls, but statistically significant reduction in lung viral titers was observed. The decrease in viral titers was also confirmed by measuring the amount of viral RNA by RT-PCR. In addition, 48 h after challenge of mice (treated with this dose of bivalent Nb) with 4 LD_{50} of NIBRG-14 ma, weight loss was observed and also a delay in mortality compared with the controls.

The antigenic site of the HA was mapped by selecting escape mutants in the presence of the monovalent or bivalent Nb. Three escape mutants were selected in the presence of monovalent Nb, K189E/N and N154D/S mutations were found, they are contiguous in the antigenic B site of the HA (Wiley *et al.*, 1981; Yamada *et al.*, 2006). It is noteworthy to mention that N154D/S removes an N-glycosylation site, a possible adaptation to mask an antigenic site (Fig. 2). The escape mutants selected in presence of the bivalent Nb presented not only the K189E/N mutation, but an additional D145N mutation located in the stalk of HA2, 40 residues upstream of the membrane anchor. The results of the hemaglutination assays and microneutralization experiments suggest that mutation K189N/E is necessary and sufficient to abolish binding to the Nb in a monovalent or bivalent conformation, indicating a close proximity between the antigenic B site and the receptor binding domain. Those results are the first one reported of the potential antiviral activity of a Nb against the influenza virus.

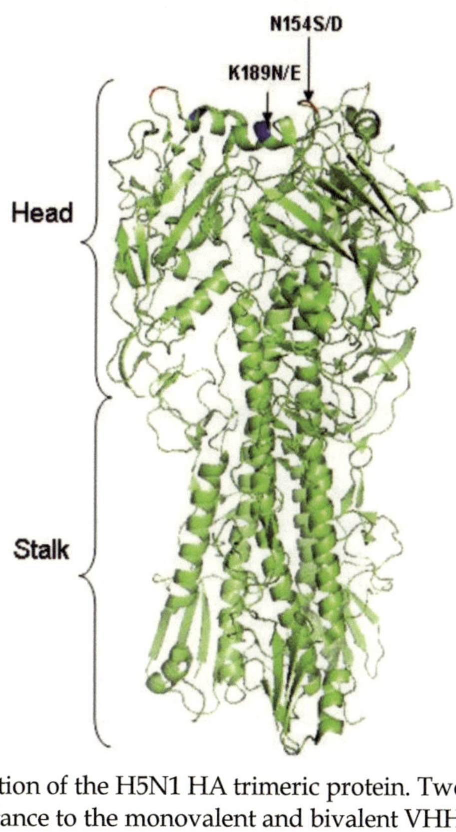

Fig. 2. Ribbon representation of the H5N1 HA trimeric protein. Two mutations in the head of the trimer confer resistance to the monovalent and bivalent VHH C-8. The mutation K189N/E was necessary and sufficient to prevent binding of both mono and bivalent VHHs. (PDB : 2IBX)

The Nb viral neutralization activity against a trimeric HA molecule (HA) was greatly enhanced when presented as bivalent and trimeric molecule, but the dynamics and details of the binding are not clear. It has been demonstrated that during intramolecular binding, a multivalent molecule has greater avidity than its monovalent counterpart. But a very interesting question is whether intermolecular binding occurs during Nb binding to the HA. In recent reports, the existence of intermolecular binding was proved to enhance an antiviral effect (Wang & Yang, 2010). Intermolecular binding could explain the increase in the neutralization activity: sterically, the hindrance of the HA for its cellular receptor is enhanced, and the flexibility of the HA is decreased.

3. RSV virus

Respiratory Syncytial Virus (RSV) infections are the leading cause of acute lower respiratory tract infections (ALRI) in children and associated hospitalizations world wide (Falsey *et al.*, 2005; Nair *et al.*, 2010). There is no specific antiviral therapy for RSV infection available. Each year 66, 000 – 199,000 children die worldwide due to RSV ALRI. Most pediatric cases of fatal RSV infections occur in developing countries. As RSV infections do not evoke protective immunity, infections occur throughout life, causing severe morbidity in young infants, the elderly, and immune-comprised adults (Boyce *et al.*, 2000; Falsey *et al.*, 2005).

Although high levels of RSV neutralizing antibodies correlate with lower frequencies of RSV-associated ALRI, no RSV vaccine is available (Glezen *et al.*, 1981). However, monthly administration of large amounts of a humanized RSV neutralizing antibody, palivizumab (Synagis), reduces RSV-associated hospitalization of high risk infants by about 78-39% (Groothuis & Simoes, 1993). Palivizumab is currently the sole monoclonal antibody that is approved for preventing viral infection. Palivizumab blocks fusion of the RSV membrane with the membrane of the target cell by binding to the RSV fusion protein (F) (Huang *et al.*, 2010). However, due to the high cost of palivizumab, there is an urgent need for new anti-virals that can prevent or treat RSV infections. RSV neutralizing Nbs have been developed as an alternative to existing antibodies (Hultberg *et al.*, 2011).

3.1 RSV binding VHHs antiviral effect: comparison with Synagis Mab.

To investigate if Nbs could be used for antiviral therapy, Nbs that bind to the palivizumab epitope were developed. For this purpose, two llamas were immunized with recombinant RSV A F protein (RSV F_{TM}-) lacking the transmembrane region (Hultberg *et al.*, 2011). This protein folds into trimers that resemble the native RSV F protein in its post-fusion conformation (Ruiz-Arguello *et al.*, 2004). Remarkably, RSV F_{TM}- proteins can be readily recognized by RSV F neutralizing antibodies that, just like palivizumab, bind to the antigenic site II (McLellan *et al.*, 2011; Swanson *et al.*, 2011). In this way, RSV F_{TM}- immunization can potentially induce RSV F antigenic site II specific camelid HCAbs. HCAbs that specifically bind to the RSV F antigenic region II were enriched by biopanning using RSV F_{TM}- protein and competitive elution in the presence of excess of palivizumab antibody. From these HCAbs, VHHs (or Nbs) were produced and tested for binding to the RSV F_{TM}- protein. Twelve VHHs that bound to the RSV F protein were tested for neutralization of RSV Long strain (RSV A subtype) virus in a micro-neutralization assay. Two VHHs (RSV-C4 and the RSV-D3) could neutralize RSV in the high nanomolar range (IC_{50}: 640 nM and 300 nM, respectively), which is similar to the neutralization activity as the Synagis Fab (IC_{50}: 549.2 nM) and about 100-fold less effective than the Synagis Mab (IC_{50}: 3.02 nM). However, in contrast to palivizumab, neither RSV-C4 nor RSV-D3 VHHs could neutralize RSV B subtype virus *in vitro*. On the contrary, another VHH (RSV-E4) could neutralize RSV B infection to some extent.

The epitopes of different VHHs were determined by antibody competition assays and diverse antibody escape RSV mutants. Whereas RSV-C4 and RSV-D3 VHHs readily competed with palivizumab for binding to recombinant RSV F_{TM}- or inactivated RSV virions, RSV-E4 competed with 101 Fab, which is known to bind to the antigenic region IV-VI (Wu *et al.*, 2007). These data are in line with the observation that AA substitutions within antigenic regions II and IV-VI, respectively, affected the binding of both RSV-D4 and RSV-C3 VHHs and RSV-E4 VHH. These data strongly suggest that both RSV-C3 and RSV-D4 bind to antigenic region II (palivizumab epitope) (Crowe *et al.*, 1998) whereas RSV-E4 VHH binds to antigenic regions IV-VI, explaining the observed differences in neutralization.

The affinity of the three VHHs, Synagis Mab and Synagis Fab was determined by Surface Plasmon Resonance using recombinant RSV F $_{TM-}$ as bait. The K_D of RSV-D3, RSV-E4 and RSV-E4 were in the low nanomolar range: 9.24 nM, 1.78 nM and 0.45 nM, respectively. Although RSV-D3 was more effective than RSV-C4 at neutralizing RSV A, it had a lower affinity for F_{TM}- than RSV-C4. However, the efficient binding of RSV-E4 VHH to a neutralizing epitope (antigenic region IV-VI) was not associated with neutralization of RSV A. This suggests that the affinity of VHHs for the recombinant RSV F_{TM}-, which likely represents the F protein in its post-fusion conformation, does not correlate directly with neutralization of living RSV (Table 1.)

	F-RSV-D3m	F-RSV-D3b	Synagys
In vitro neutralization (IC50, nM)	300	0.05 - 0.14 nM*	1.03 - 5.5 nM*
Prophylactic minimal protective dose (mg/kg)	ND	12 μg	ND
Prophylactic protective extension (mg/kg)	ND	48 hrs	ND
Therapeutisch protection extension	ND	24 hrs	ND

*Obtained from two different cell based assays, microneutralization and plaque assay

Table 1. Inhibition and protection of the RSV virus A binding by Nb RSV-D3. ND = not determined.

The avidity of a binding molecule can be increased by using a multivalent format (Rudge *et al.*, 2007; Wang & Yang, 2010). To increase the antiviral potential of RSV-D3 we formatted it into a bivalent molecule, by using a flexible linker, Gly_4/Ser (GS). Surprisingly, bivalent RSV-D3 VHHs with GC linkers of different sizes neutralized RSV A Long virus between 2421 and 4181 times more efficient than monovalent RSV-D3 VHHs, reaching picomolar range (IC_{50}: 190-110 pM). In contrast, Synagis Mab was only 200 times more efficient in neutralizing RSV A virus (IC_{50}: 6.5 nM) than its corresponding Fab fragment. In this way, bivalent RSV F specific VHHs outperform the Synagis antibody in RSV neutralization. Moreover, in contrast to its monovalent format, bivalent RSV-D3 could also neutralize RSV B1 strain virus. Also, neutralization was notably boosted against RSV A and B virus subtypes by linking two different VHHs (RSV-D3 and RSV-E4) which target different epitopes. The enhancement of the activity by linking two VHHs is likely due to the flexibility of the linker. Experiments aiming to characterize the binding dynamics of the RSV-D3 to the F protein are necessary for characterizing intra- or intermolecular binding.

The RSV F is responsible for fusion of the viral lipid membrane with the host membrane, but also participates in attachment of the RSV virions to target cells. In addition, it was recently demonstrated that RSV F protein can bind to nucleolin expressed at the surface of target cells, and that this interaction is crucial for RSV infection *in vitro* and *in vivo* (Tayyari *et al.*, 2011). After viral attachment, the RSV F protein mediates fusion of the viral membrane with the plasma membrane of the target cell, thereby releasing the viral genome into the cytoplasm of the host cell. This process involves a series of conformational changes in the F protein from a metastable pre-fusion to a stable post-fusion conformation. We recently demonstrated that bivalent RSV-D3 VHHs can prevent RSV infection both before and after viral attachment and can inhibit syncytia formation, but cannot hamper RSV attachment (Schepens *et al.*, 2011). Together, these observations constantly indicate that, by a similar mechanism as palivizumab, bivalent RSV-D3 VHHs prevent RSV infection by blocking fusion. Although the conformations of the RSV F antigenic regions II and IV-VI are maintained in the post-fusion form, it is more plausible that the RSV VHHs block viral fusion and syncytia formation by binding to the RSV F protein in either its pre-fusion or intermediate conformations (Fig. 3). Possibly, binding of the VHHs to the antigenic region II interferes with the conformational changes of the F protein that are required for fusion.

Immune compromised Balb/c mice (cyclophosphamide treatment) were used to test whether bivalent RSV-D3 VHHs can protect against RSV infection *in vivo* (Schepens *et al.*, 2011). As VHHs are known to remain active in the respiratory tract after nebulisation, bivalent RSV-D3 and control VHHs were administered intranasally (patent application WO 2009/147248). Prophylactic treatment of mice with 5 mg/kg of bivalent RSV-D3 VHH or palivizumab reduced RSV pulmonary titers below the detection limit of the RSV plaque assay. This strong reduction was confirmed by qPCR analysis. Remarkably, as low as 0.6 mg/kg bivalent RSV-D3 could prevent or strongly reduce (at least 100-fold) pulmonary RSV replication. In comparison, monovalent RSV-D3 VHH protected against pulmonary RSV replication about 25 times less efficiently than its bivalent counterpart. For prophylactic treatment to be valuable, even if is easy to administer, its effect should be long lasting. We demonstrate that intranasal administration of bivalent RSV-D3 VHHs can protect against RSV infection for at least 48 hours. Prophylactic treatment with palivizumab in high risk infants reduces RSV associated hospitalization, but no effective therapeutic is available. Therefore, RSV-D3 VHHs were also evaluated as therapeutic treatments. Intranasal administration of RSV-D3 VHHs 4 or 24 hours after infection strongly reduced pulmonary RSV replication (at least 100-fold). Plaque assays also indicated that administration of bivalent RSV-D3 VHHs 72 hours after RSV treatment can reduce pulmonary RSV replication. However, the lung homogenates used to quantify the pulmonary RSV titer in mice that were treated 72 hours after infection still contained neutralizing RSV VHHs. Therefore, it is not clear to which extent treatment at this time point reduced RSV replication *in vivo*. The potential of bivalent VHHs for preventing morbidity and pulmonary inflammation upon RSV infection was assessed in a non immunocompromised mouse model. Prophylactic administration of bivalent RSV-D3 VHHs (1 mg/kg) completely prevented body weight loss and pulmonary cell infiltration that was observed in mice treated with control VHHs. Therapeutic treatment with bivalent RSV-D3 VHHs 24 h after infection partially reduced body weight loss and pulmonary cell infiltration. These observations confirm the *in vivo* antiviral potential of neutralizing VHHs.

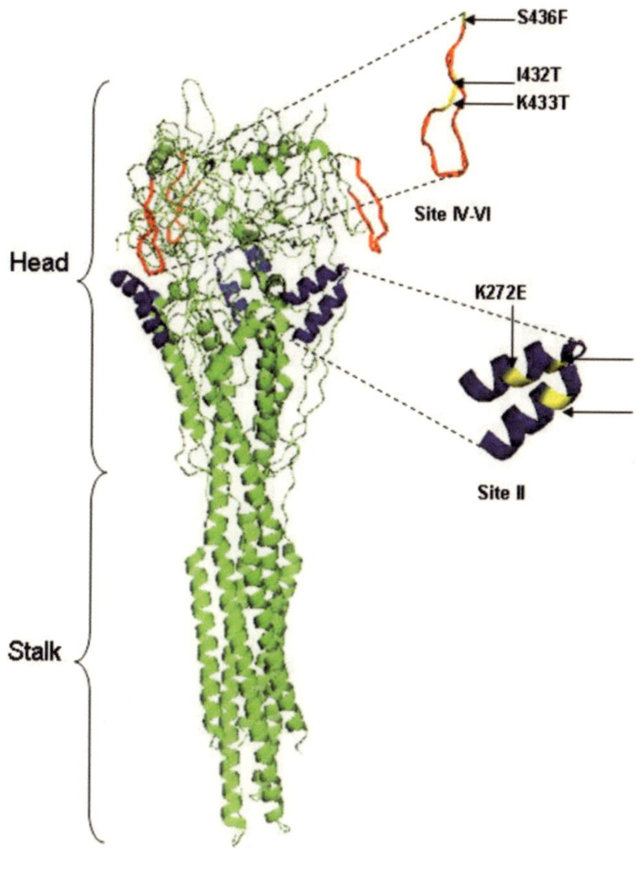

Fig. 3. Ribbon representation of the structure of the RSV F protein trimer in its post-fusion form. The head and stalk of this recombinant protein are depicted, lacking the fusion peptide, transmembrane region and cytoplasmic domain. The immunogenic epitopes recognized by Mab 101F (site II) and palimuzab (site IV-VI) are in red and blue, respectively, and the rest of the F protein is in green. The RSV-D3 and RSV-C4 resistant *in vitro* escape mutants are shown in yellow. Mutations I432T, K433T and S436F in site II disrupt the binding of the RSV-C4. The K262Y, N268I and K272E in the site IV-IV result in loss of binding of the RSV-D3 molecule. (PDB: 3RKI).

Currently Ablynx is preparing a phase I clinical trial to evaluate the safety of a trivalent RSV neutralizing VHH format consisting of three identical VHHs. Preclinical evaluation of this lead candidate can readily neutralize a broad spectrum of clinical RSV A and RSV B subtype viruses more efficiently than Synagis (abstract, 7th international RSV symposium, Rotterdam, 2010). *In vivo* studies demonstrated that both prophylactic and therapeutic treatment with this RSV neutralizing VHH can readily reduce RSV replication in the upper and lower respiratory tract of cotton rats (abstract, 7th international RSV symposium, Rotterdam, 2010).

In summary, neutralizing RSV VHHs are promising new candidates as anti-RSV therapeutics for different reasons. First, VHHs allow versatile formatting including the creation of multivalent formats by the use of flexible linkers. This feature enabled the creation of bivalent and trivalent VHH which can neutralize RSV at picomolar range, more than 1000-fold more efficient than their monovalent counterpart. Second, by linking two different VHHs which neutralize different virus strains (such as the RSV A versus the RSV B subtype strains) cross-reactive VHH constructs can be obtained. Moreover, as a result of avidity effects, cross linking VHH with different specificity can considerably improve the neutralizing activity. Third, the VHHs small size and protruding paratopes can contribute to its neutralization activity. As structural models and electron microscopic analysis indicate that the antigenic region II is located at the side of the RSV F protein trimer, at the dense surface of RSV virions, this region is likely more accessible for small and flexible VHH formats than for large and more rigid antibodies (McLellan *et al.*, 2011; Ruiz-Arguello *et al.*, 2004) (Fig. 3). Fourth, due to their high stability at stringent conditions, VHHs can be administered via nebulisation, which allows a rapid accumulation of high amounts of neutralizing VHH at the site of respiratory viral infections. In addition, due to the high stability of VHHs and the ease of intranasal or pulmonary administration, VHH therapy could potentially be applied more generally, even in developing countries.

4. Rabies virus

Rabies virus (RV) is a single stranded RNA virus of the *Rhabdoviridae* family, genus *Lyssavirus*. Infection with RV in humans causes acute encephalitis, with a mortality rate of almost 100%. It is transmitted to humans by bites from a carnivore or a quiroptera vector and most cases occur in Asia or Africa. The long incubation period following infection by RV presents a paradox, because of the absence or very weak antiviral immune response (Johnson *et al.*, 2010). The small amount of virus inoculated after infection and the neurotropism of RV are believed to contribute to the absence of effective antibodies in the patient. After the bite, wound cleaning can reduce the chances of a productive infection in humans. Passive immunization and vaccination promptly after exposure is the only effective therapeutic tool available now. Modern vaccines are inactivated virus produced from continuous cell cultures, like the vaccine by Aventis Pasteur (human diploid cells). Nevertheless, in underdeveloped countries, the established RV therapy (attenuated virus, Mab anti RV) is too expensive for most of the population. RV has a genome of 12 kDa coding for 5 proteins: nucleoprotein, phosphoprotein, matrix, RNA-dependent RNA polymerase and the Glycoprotein (RVG). In the virus particle, the RVG is the only viral protein exposed as a trimeric spike, and it is responsible for recognition of cellular receptors, virulence and antigenicity.

4.1 Nbs present a broad protection against Rabies virus

For more than 25 years, two well-defined antigenic sites in the RVG have been characterized by Mabs: antigenic sites II and III (Lafon *et al.*, 1990). Other epitopes have also been characterized, but their contribution to antigenicity is minor. Antigenic site III extends from 330 to 340 amino acids and is linear (Seif *et al.*, 1985). Mutations in this site affect virulence and the host range of the virus. On the contrary, antigenic site II is conformational and discontinuous and is determined by two regions, amino acids 34-42 and 198-200. Site II is responsible for about 70 % of the known Mabs against RVG (Benmansour *et al.*, 1991).

RGV is an interesting target for the VHH platform because alternative cost effective antirabies tools are needed. By using an approach similar to those previously discussed for influenza and RSV, a llama was immunized with recombinant RVG and five VHHs were obtained (Rab - E8, H7, F8, E6 and C12). The neutralizing activity of those VHHs was validated against 10 Rabies genotype 1 viruses: 3 laboratory strains (CVS-11 as prototype, ERA, CB-1) and 7 field isolates and one rabies genotype 5 virus (EBL-V1) was included to validate broad cross neutralization. A cell based assay was used, the Rapid Fluorescent Focus Inhibition Test (RFFIT) (Vene *et al.*, 1998). This assay has been internationally recognized as the *in vitro* standard for testing virus neutralizing antibodies. Mab 8-32, which recognizes antigenic site II of RVG was also included as positive control (Montano-Hirose *et al.*, 1993). VHHs F8, E6, H7 and C12 neutralized the genotype 1 strains: CB-1 and ERA with an IC_{50} in the low nanomolar range and the CVS-11 strain in the low to high nanomolar range. They could also neutralize several RV field isolates. On the other hand, E8 efficiently neutralized only CB-1 and CVS-11, in the low and high nanomolar range, respectively. C12 and E6 had better neutralization activity than Mab 8-2 against the ERA and CB-1 strains. Using a similar approach as described above for influeza and RSV, the authors also generated the bivalent against the Rabies genotype 1 CVS -11 and the genotype 5 EBLV-1. Bivalent monoparatopic VHHs were constructed using a Gly4/Ser linker, using the 12, H7, E8 and F8 VHHs. The neutralization IC_{50} of these constructions was reduced from two to 180-fold relative to the monovalent protein, indicating enhancement of the neutralization. Nevertheless, the best results were obtained when biparatopic molecules were used. The E6/H7 and the H7/F8 molecules increased the neutralization potency by a 2 log factor, while the E8/H7 increased 3 log-fold, compared with the monovalents. E8/H7 even outperformed Mab 8 -2 against the CVS-11. On the contrary, in the case of the genotype 5 strain EBLV-1, the monovalent molecules showed modest neutralization or none at all. The enhanced neutralization of biparatopic molecules was confirmed by E8/C12, which presented an increase in the neutralization potential of 147-fold (IC_{50} = 3.76 nM) relative to the monovalent moiety, but not as low as Mab 8 - 2 (IC_{50} = 0.12 nM). The results of competition assays of the 5 VHHs against the Mab 8- 2 showed that E6, E8, F8 and H7 compete for the same epitope. On the other hand, C12 did not compete which indicates that it recognizes a different epitope. The difference in epitope recognition could be one of the causes of the strong and broad effect of biparatopic molecules, especially for E8/C12. Experiments using VHHs against Rabies mutant virus, carrying substitutions in the known residues in the antigenic site II could localize the exact binding sites of these new antibodies. For example, it has been reported that substitution K198E of the glycoprotein abolish the binding of the Mab 8–2 (Montano-Hirose *et al.*, 1993). Unfortunately, the crystallographic structure of the RVG protein has not been reported. The use of vesicular stomatitis virus glycoprotein is accepted as a modeling reference and as a surrogate template for RVG structure (Cibulski *et al.*, 2009; Tomar *et al.*, 2010). We used the alignment of this protein with the RVG as reference to show the possible structure of antigenic site II (Fig. 4). The purpose of this estimate is to show the tendency of the VHHs to recognize conformational rather than linear epitopes. In line with the results of the neutralizing VHHs against influenza and RSV, the results of the broadness and the strong potency against both RV genotypes indicate the RV neutralizing VHHs as a promising. Nevertheless, in contrast with the previous cases of the influenza and RSV VHHs, there is not *in vivo* validation of the RV neutralizing VHHs available.

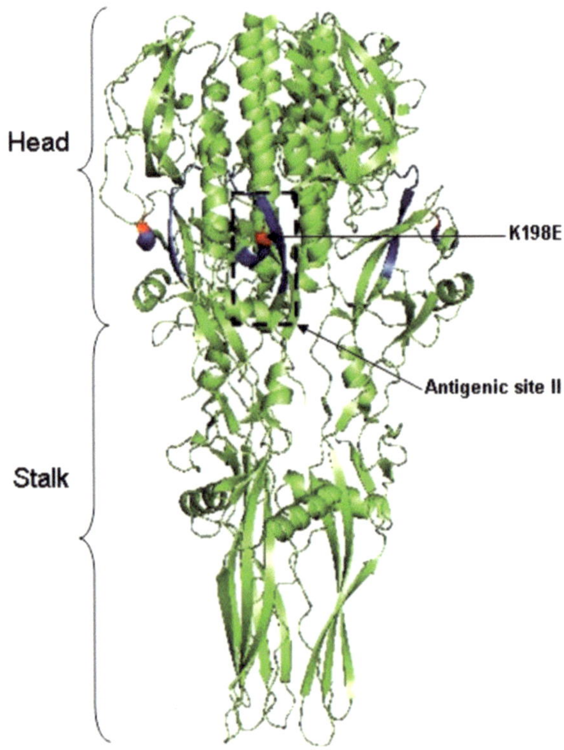

Fig. 4. Schematic representation of the vesicular stomatitis virus protein G trimer. This protein is taken as reference to depict the amino acids corresponding to the antigenic site II of the Rabies Virus glycoprotein (residues 34-42, and 198-200, in blue). The localization of the K198E mutation that prevents the binding of the Mab 8-2 is shown in red. The VHHs E8, F8, E6 and H7 compete with the Mab 8- 2 for the binding, which means that their epitopes might be within antigenic site II. (PDB: 2CMZ).

5. Conclusion

The Nb platform is a new and promising antiviral tool. The ease of producing Nbs in bacterial and lower eukaryotic cells, and the possibility of producing tailor-made constructions makes them an attractive and cost effective alternative to some established antiviral drugs. This approach may be useful for the treatment of infectious orphan diseases (including viral) and in developing countries, where the "standard" prophylaxis or therapy is prohibitively expensive or not available. In this work we have discussed findings on recently developed Nbs directed against three viruses affecting humans: the generation and *in vitro* validation of the Nbs or VHHs against influenza H5N1, RSV and RV (Hultberg *et al.*,

2011); as well as the *in vivo* validation of the influenza HA binding VHH (Ibañez *et al.*, 2011) and RSV (Schepens *et al.*, 2011). In the case of protection against influenza infection the bivalent format of the Nbs proved superior *in vitro* and *in vivo*. But, as indicated by the successful *in vivo* validation of one of the H5N1 strains, it is imperative to extend this validation to other influenza strains. Furthermore, it would be worthwhile to isolate and characterize Nbs that recognize conserved domains in HA, such as the stalk. In line with the influenza results, the activity of RSV and RVG neutralizing Nbs was significantly higher for the bivalent than the monovalent format: both the cross neutralization activity and potency were higher. Those results manifest the advantages of using a multimeric format against multimeric viral targets. The enhanced antiviral potential of the multimeric format could be due to increased avidity and/or the intra- or intermolecular binding could contribute in the enhancement. Experiments to assess the binding mechanism could lead to further improvements. The results overall confirm two important points: the high potential of the Nbs as prophylactic and therapeutic tools, and the possibility of using Nbs directed against other infectious diseases. There is limited function and sequence similarity among the three proteins used as antigens (HA, RSVF and RVG) other than their trimeric architecture and antigenicity. Nevertheless, the HA and the RVG are functionally similar and both are involved in the cellular receptor binding, whereas RSVF participates also in virion receptor binding, it s main function is in membrane fusion. In all three cases, showed capacity to neutralize the viral target by blocking binding or hampering necessary conformational changes, indicating the great versatility and efficiency of the antiviral discussed here. In competition assays, the recognition of non conventional epitopes by these antiviral was not observed, but could be the focus of research. Nbs recognized well known antigenic sites that are also targeted by Mabs. The HA, RSV F and RVG are not enzymes, and lack extensive antigenic clefts. This could be one reason why Nbs showed preference for recognition of "classical" epitopes in these viral proteins. If the presence of antigenic clefts could lead to recognition of non "classical" epitopes in the viral proteins, targeting viral enzymes could be an interesting approach. Enzymes such as the influenza Neuraminidase are potential targets. This viral sialidase presents a catalytic cleft, in which the framework and substrate contact residues are conserved in most of the influenza strains. The coming years will probably bring potent novel anti-viral Nbs directed against different viruses and it is likely that some of these Nbs will reach clinical trials.

6. Acknowledgement

We are grateful to Dr. Amin Bredan for editing the text. M.C. holds a VIB international PhD fellowship. L.I.I. was a beneficiary of the Belgian Federal Sciences Administration (Federale Wetenschapsbeleid, BELSPO) and was supported by Ghent University IOF grant Stepstone IOF08/STEP/001. B.S. is a postdoctoral fellow of FWO-Flanders.

7. References

Arbabi Ghahroudi, M., Desmyter, A., Wyns, L., Hamers, R. & Muyldermans, S. (1997). Selection and identification of single domain antibody fragments from camel heavy-chain antibodies. *FEBS letters* 414, 521-526.

Barre, S., Greenberg, A. S., Flajnik, M. F. & Chothia, C. (1994). Structural conservation of hypervariable regions in immunoglobulins evolution. In *Nat Struct Biol*, pp. 915-920.

Benmansour, A., Leblois, H., Coulon, P., Tuffereau, C., Gaudin, Y., Flamand, A. & Lafay, F. (1991). Antigenicity of rabies virus glycoprotein. In *J Virol*, pp. 4198-4203.

Boyce, T. G., Mellen, B. G., Mitchel, E. F., Wright, P. F. & Griffin, M. R. (2000). Rates of hospitalization for respiratory syncytial virus infection among children in medicaid. In *J Pediatr*, pp. 865-870.

Cibulski, S. P., Sinigaglia, M., Rigo, M. M., Antunes, D. A., Vieira, G. F., Fulber, C. C., Chies, J. A. B., Franco, A. C. & Roehe, P. M. (2009). Structure modelling of Rabies Virus Glycoprotein. In *5th International Conference of the Brazilian Association for Bioinformatics and Computational Biology*. Rio de Janeiro.

Crowe, J. E., Firestone, C. Y., Crim, R., Beeler, J. A., Coelingh, K. L., Barbas, C. F., Burton, D. R., Chanock, R. M. & Murphy, B. R. (1998). Monoclonal antibody-resistant mutants selected with a respiratory syncytial virus-neutralizing human antibody fab fragment (Fab 19) define a unique epitope on the fusion (F) glycoprotein. *Virology* 252, 373-375.

De Genst, E., Silence, K., Decanniere, K., Conrath, K., Loris, R., Kinne, J., Muyldermans, S. & Wyns, L. (2006). Molecular basis for the preferential cleft recognition by dromedary heavy-chain antibodies. In *Proc Natl Acad Sci*, pp. 4586-4591.

de Jong, M. D., Simmons, C. P., Thanh, T. T., Hien, V. M., Smith, G. J., Chau, T. N., Hoang, D. M., Chau, N. V., Khanh, T. H., Dong, V. C., Qui, P. T., Cam, B. V., Ha do, Q., Guan, Y., Peiris, J. S., Chinh, N. T., Hien, T. T. & Farrar, J. (2006). Fatal outcome of human influenza A (H5N1) is associated with high viral load and hypercytokinemia. In *Nature medicine*, pp. 1203-1207.

Decanniere, K., Desmyter, A., Lauwereys, M., Ghahroudi, M. A., Muyldermans, S. & Wyns, L. (1999). A single-domain antibody fragment in complex with RNase A: non-canonical loop structures and nanomolar affinity using two CDR loops. In *Structure*, pp. 361-370.

Decanniere, K., Muyldermans, S. & Wyns, L. (2000). Canonical antigen-binding loop structures in immunoglobulins: more structures, more canonical classes? In *J Mol Biol*, pp. 83-91.

Desmyter, A., Spinelli, S., Payan, F., Lauwereys, M., Wyns, L., Muyldermans, S. & Cambillau, C. (2002). Three camelid VHH domains in complex with porcine pancreatic alpha-amylase. Inhibition and versatility of binding topology. In *The Journal of biological chemistry*, pp. 23645-23650.

Desmyter, A., Transue, T. R., Ghahroudi, M. A., Thi, M. H., Poortmans, F., Hamers, R., Muyldermans, S. & Wyns, L. (1996). Crystal structure of a camel single-domain VH antibody fragment in complex with lysozyme. In *Nat Struct Biol*, pp. 803-811.

Els Conrath, K., Lauwereys, M., Wyns, L. & Muyldermans, S. (2001). Camel single-domain antibodies as modular building units in bispecific and bivalent antibody constructs. *The Journal of biological chemistry* 276, 7346-7350.

Falsey, A. R., Hennessey, P. A., Formica, M. A., Cox, C. & Walsh, E. E. (2005). Respiratory syncytial virus infection in elderly and high-risk adults. In *The New England journal of medicine*, pp. 1749-1759.

Glezen, W. P., Paredes, A., Allison, J. E., Taber, L. H. & Frank, A. L. (1981). Risk of respiratory syncytial virus infection for infants from low-income families in relationship to age, sex, ethnic group, and maternal antibody level. In *J Pediatr*, 708-15 edn.

Greenberg, A. S., Avila, D., Hughes, M., Hughes, A., McKinney, E. C. & Flajnik, M. F. (1995). A new antigen receptor gene family that undergoes rearrangement and extensive somatic diversification in sharks. *Nature* 374, 168-173.

Groothuis, J. R. & Simoes, E. A. (1993). Immunoprophylaxis and immunotherapy: role in the prevention and treatment of repiratory syncytial virus. In *Int J Antimicrob Agents*, pp. 97-103.

Hamers-Casterman, C., Atarhouch, T., Muyldermans, S., Robinson, G., Hamers, C., Songa, E. B., Bendahman, N. & Hamers, R. (1993). Naturally occurring antibodies devoid of light chains. *Nature* 363, 446-448.

Hmila, I., Saerens, D., Ben Abderrazek, R., Vincke, C., Abidi, N., Benlasfar, Z., Govaert, J., El Ayeb, M., Bouhaouala-Zahar, B. & Muyldermans, S. (2010). A bispecific nanobody to provide full protection against lethal scorpion envenoming. *Faseb J* 24, 3479-3489.

Huang, K., Incognito, L., Cheng, X., Ulbrandt, N. D. & Wu, H. (2010). Respiratory syncytial virus-neutralizing monoclonal antibodies motavizumab and palivizumab inhibit fusion. In *J Virol*, pp. 8132-8140.

Hultberg, A., Temperton, N. J., Rosseels, V., Koenders, M., Gonzalez-Pajuelo, M., Schepens, B., Ibañez, L. I., Vanlandschoot, P., Schillemans, J., Saunders, M., Weiss, R. A., Saelens, X., Melero, J. A., Verrips, C. T., Van Gucht, S. & de Haard, H. J. (2011). Llama-derived single domain antibodies to build multivalent, superpotent and broadened neutralizing anti-viral molecules. *PloS one* 6, e17665.

Ibañez, L. I., De Filette, M., Hultberg, A., Verrips, T., Temperton, N., Weiss, R. A., Vandevelde, W., Schepens, B., Vanlandschoot, P. & Saelens, X. (2011). Nanobodies with in vitro neutralizing activity protect mice against H5N1 influenza virus infection. *The Journal of infectious diseases* 203, 1063-1072.

Johnson, N., Cunningham, A. & Fooks, A. R. (2010). The immune response to the rabies infection and vaccination. In *Vaccine*, pp. 3896-3901.

Lafon, M., Edelman, L., Bouvet, J. P., Lafage, M. & Montchatre, E. (1990). Human monoclonal antibodies specific for the rabies virus glycoprotein and N protein. In *The Journal of general virology*, pp. 1689-1696.

Lauwereys, M., Arbadi Ghahroudi, M., Desmyter, A., Kinne, J., Holzer, W., De Genst, E., Wyns, L. & Muyldermans, S. (1998). Potent enzyme inhibitors derived from dromedary heavy-chain antibodies. In *EMBO J*, pp. 3512-3520.

Luke, C. J. & Subbarao, K. (2006). Vaccines for pandemic influenza. *Emerging infectious diseases* 12, 66-72.

McLellan, J. S., Yang, Y., Graham, B. S. & Kwong, P. D. (2011). Structure of respiratory syncytial virus fusion glycoprotein in the postfusion conformation reveals preservation of neutralizing epitopes. In *J Virol*, pp. 7788-7796., 17(9):1132-5.

Montano-Hirose, J. A., Lafage, M., Weber, P., Badrane, H., Tordo, N. & Lafon, M. (1993). Protective activity of a murine monoclonal antibody against European bat lyssavirus 1 (EBL1) infection in mice. In *Vaccine*, pp. 1259-1266.

Muyldermans, S., Atarhouch, T., Saldanha, J., Barbosa, J. A. & Hamers, R. (1994). Sequence and structure of VH domain from naturally occurring camel heavy chain immunoglobulins lacking light chains. In *Protein Eng*, pp. 1129-1135.

Nair, H., Nokes, D. J., Gessner, B. D., Dherani, M., Madhi, S. A., Singleton, R. J., O'Brien, K. L., Roca, A., Wright, P. F., Bruce, N., Chandran, A., Theodoratou, E., Sutanto, A., Sedyaningsih, E. R., Ngama, M., Munywoki, P. K., Kartasasmita, C., Simoes, E. A., Rudan, I., Weber, M. W. & Campbell, H. (2010). Global burden of acute lower respiratory infections due to respiratory syncytial virus in young children: a systematic review and meta-analysis. *Lancet* 375, 1545-1555.

Rasmussen, S. G., Choi, H. J., Fung, J. J., Pardon, E., Casarosa, P., Chae, P. S., Devree, B. T., Rosenbaum, D. M., Thian, F. S., Kobilka, T. S., Schnapp, A., Konetzki, I., Sunahara, R. K., Gellman, S. H., Pautsch, A., Steyaert, J., Weis, W. I. & Kobilka, B. K. (2011). Structure of a nanobody-stabilized active state of the beta(2) adrenoceptor. *Nature* 469, 175-180.

Rudge, J. S., Holash, J., Hylton, D., Russell, M., Jiang, S., Leidich, R., Papadopoulos, N., Pyles, E. A., Torri, A., Wiegand, S. J., Thurston, G., Stahl, N. & Yancopoulos, G. D. (2007). VEGF Trap complex formation measures production rates of VEGF, providing a biomarker for predicting efficacious angiogenic blockade. *Proceedings of the National Academy of Sciences of the United States of America* 104, 18363-18370.

Ruiz-Arguello, M. B., Martin, D., Wharton, S. A., Calder, L. J., Martin, S. R., Cano, O., Calero, M., Garcia-Barreno, B., Skehel, J. J. & Melero, J. A. (2004). Thermostability of the human respiratory syncytial virus fusion protein before and after activation: implications for the membrane-fusion mechanism. *The Journal of general virology* 85, 3677-3687.

Schepens, B., Ibañez, L. I., Hultberg, A., Bogaert, P., De Bleser, P., De Baets, S., Vervalle, F., Verrips, T., Melero, J., Vandevelde, W., Vanlandschoot, P. & Saelens, X. (2011). Nanobodies specific for Respiratory Syncytial Virus Fusion protein protect against infection by inhibition of fusion. *The Journal of infectious diseases*, 204, 1692-1701.

Seif, I., Coulon, P., Rollin, P. E. & Flamand, A. (1985). Rabies virulence: effect on pathogenicity and sequence characterization of rabies virus mutations affecting antigenic site III of the glycoprotein. In *J Virol*, pp. 926-934.

Stiehm, E. R., Keller, M. A. & Vyas, G. N. (2008). Preparation and use of therapeutic antibodies primarily of human origin. *Biologicals* 36, 363-374.

Swanson, K. A., Settembre, E. C., Shaw, C. A., Dey, A. K., Rappuoli, R., Mandl, C. W., Dormitzer, P. R. & Carfi, A. (2011). Structural basis for immunization with postfusion respiratory syncytial virus fusion F glycoprotein (RSV F) to elicit high neutralizing antibody titers. *Proceedings of the National Academy of Sciences of the United States of America* 108, 9619-9624.

Tayyari, F., Marchant, D., Moraes, T. J., Duan, W., Mastrangelo, P. & Hegele, R. G. (2011). Identification of nucleolin as a cellular receptor for human respiratory syncytial virus. *Nature medicine*.

Throsby, M., van den Brink, E., Jongeneelen, M., Poon, L. L., Alard, P., Cornelissen, L., Bakker, A., Cox, F., van Deventer, E., Guan, Y., Cinatl, J., ter Meulen, J., Lasters, I., Carsetti, R., Peiris, M., de Kruif, J. & Goudsmit, J. (2008). Heterosubtypic neutralizing monoclonal antibodies cross-protective against H5N1 and H1N1 recovered from human IgM+ memory B cells. *PloS one* 3, e3942.

Tomar, N. R., Singh, V., Marla, S. S., Chandra, R., Kumar, R. & Kumar, A. (2010). Molecular docking studies with rabies virus glycoprotein to design viral therapeutics. *Indian journal of pharmaceutical sciences* 72, 486-490.

Vene, S., Haglund, M., Vapalahti, O. & Lundkvist, A. (1998). A rapid fluorescent focus inhibition test for detection of neutralizing antibodies to tick-borne encephalitis virus. In *J Virol Methods*, pp. 71 - 75.

Verheesen, P., Roussis, A., de Haard, H. J., Groot, A. J., Stam, J. C., den Dunnen, J. T., Frants, R. R., Verkleij, A. J., Theo Verrips, C. & van der Maarel, S. M. (2006). Reliable and controllable antibody fragment selections from Camelid non-immune libraries for target validation. *Biochimica et biophysica acta* 1764, 1307-1319.

Vu, K. B., Ghahroudi, M. A., Wyns, L. & Muyldermans, S. (1997). Comparison of llama VH sequences from conventional and heavy chain antibodies. *Molecular immunology* 34, 1121-1131.

Wang, M. Z., Tai, C. Y. & Mendel, D. B. (2002). Mechanism by which mutations at his274 alter sensitivity of influenza a virus n1 neuraminidase to oseltamivir carboxylate and zanamivir. *Antimicrobial agents and chemotherapy* 46, 3809-3816.

Wang, P. & Yang, X. (2010). Neutralization efficiency is greatly enhanced by bivalent binding of an antibody to epitopes in the V4 region and the membrane-proximal external region within one trimer of human immunodeficiency virus type 1 glycoproteins. In *J Virol*, pp. 7114-7123.

Wiley, D. C., Wilson, I. A. & Skehel, J. J. (1981). Structural identification of the antibody-binding sites of Hong Kong influenza haemagglutinin and their involvement in antigenic variation. *Nature* 289, 373-378.

Wu, S. J., Schmidt, A., Beil, E. J., Day, N. D., Branigan, P. J., Liu, C., Gutshall, L. L., Palomo, C., Furze, J., Taylor, G., Melero, J. A., Tsui, P., Del Vecchio, A. M. & Kruszynski, M. (2007). Characterization of the epitope for anti-human respiratory syncytial virus F protein monoclonal antibody 101F using synthetic peptides and genetic approaches. *The Journal of general virology* 88, 2719-2723.

Wu, T. T., Johnson, G. & Kabat, E. A. (1993). Length distribution of CDRH3 in antibodies. In *Proteins*, pp. 1-7.

Yamada, S., Suzuki, Y., Suzuki, T., Le, M. Q., Nidom, C. A., Sakai-Tagawa, Y., Muramoto, Y., Ito, M., Kiso, M., Horimoto, T., Shinya, K., Sawada, T., Kiso, M., Usui, T., Murata, T., Lin, Y., Hay, A., Haire, L. F., Stevens, D. J., Russell, R. J., Gamblin, S. J., Skehel, J. J. & Kawaoka, Y. (2006). Haemagglutinin mutations responsible for the binding of H5N1 influenza A viruses to human-type receptors. *Nature* 444, 378-382.

Zhou, B., Zhong, N. & Guan, Y. (2007). Treatment with convalescent plasma for influenza A (H5N1) infection. *The New England journal of medicine* 357, 1450-1451.

9

Treatment of Herpes Simplex Virus with Lignin-Carbohydrate Complex Tablet, an Alternative Therapeutic Formula

Blanca Silvia González López[1], Masaji Yamamoto[2] and Hiroshi Sakagami[3]

[1]Laboratorio de Patología Bucal, Facultad de Odontología, Universidad Autónoma del Estado de México,
[2]Maruzen Pharmaceuticals Co., Ltd.,
[3]Meikai University School of Dentistry,
[1]México
[2,3]Japan

1. Introduction

Herpes simplex virus type 1 (HSV-1) commonly infects the mucosa and skin epithelial cells, and the virus remains latent in sensory neurons mainly in the trigeminal ganglia. Once a patient has been infected, the infection continues for life (Hunt, 2011a). Differences in HSV-1 prevalence have been reported around the world. According to Smith & Robinson (2002), the incidence in lower socioeconomic countries is higher. Primary infection, occur mainly in infants and young children, infections are usually mild or subclinical. Acute gingivoestomatitis is characterized by the appearance of multiple vesicular and ulcerative painful lesions in oral mucosa, with inflammation and bleeding of the gums, may also be associated with systemic symptoms (Arduino & Porter, 2008). Once the clinical infection concludes, the virus reaches peripheral nerves which supply sensation to the skin, migrating along the nerve axon to the dorsal root ganglia of the trigeminal or facial nerves and goes into latency stage (Esmann, 2001)

Recurrences of HSV-1 can be triggered by internal and external factors. The reactivation mechanism is unknown, the virus begins to replicate within the ganglion and grows down the nerves and out into the skin or mucous membranes (Koelle & Corey, 2008). After a prodromal of tingling, warmth or itching, the clinical lesion appear (Fatahzadeh & Schwartz 2007). The recurrence of oral HSV- 1 is developed almost always in the vermilion border of the lips but lesions can appear elsewhere around perioral skin (Siegel, 2002).

Prevention of infection can be achieved by avoiding the physical contact, kissing when the lesions are present, touching or using the articles that the patient has used (eating or drinking utensils, glasses, or straws). However, in order to prevent the recurrences, the control of external factors is recommended; avoiding the exposure to wind burn and ultraviolet radiation, using labial protectants and controlling the emotional stress (Paterson & Kwong, 2008).

On the other hand, internal factors that are related to the recurrence outbreaks such as, fever, illness, menstruation, gastrointestinal and respiratory infections, diseases as diabetes and hyperthyroidism, fatigue and factors that depress the immune system are difficult to control (Siegel, 2002; Paterson & Kwong, 2008).

Although different clinical assays have been developed in order to assess the efficacy of topical or oral antivirals, its effectiveness has not been demonstrated due to the immediate and complete termination of viral replication, the restoration of previously infected cells, and the inactivation of free virions (Hamuy & Berman 1998).

There is no treatment that can eradicate herpes virus, even though antiviral medications can reduce the frequency, duration, and severity of outbreaks (Emmert, 2006; Siegel, 2002; Sprurance, et al., 2003; Sprurance, et al., 2005)

1.1 Conventional treatment

According to Hunt (2011b), there are different phases of life cycle of virus; adsorption and penetration of the virus in the host cell, and early transcription, in which DNA polymerase, DNA binding proteins, thymidine kinase and ribonucleotide reductase are synthesized. These proteins are virally-coded, not host-coded enzymes, and therefore potentially weak in the virus life cycle, making them promising targets for anti-viral drugs.

The nucleoside analogues acyclovir, valacyclovir, are phosphorylated initially by viral thymidine kinase to eventually form a nucleoside triphosphate, and these molecules inhibit herpes simplex virus (HSV-1) polymerase, inhibiting replication of HSV-1 (Balzarini, 1994). The best anti-viral drugs are nucleoside analogs such as acyclovir (acycloguanosine). It gets into the cell across the plasma membrane as the nucleoside form and is then specifically phosphorylated inside the cell by herpes virus thymidine kinase to an active form. The advantages of nucleoside analogs are that they are only activated by the virus-infected cell and the activated form of the drug is rendered even more specific as a result of the viral DNA polymerase being more sensitive to the drug than the host enzyme (Hunt, 2001b)

In general, acyclovir compounds are safe and effective for treatment of HSV-1 reactivation and have good oral bioavailability (Chon & Elliott, 2007). However, topical administration of acyclovir at the acute stage of the lesion disease seems to be ineffective. On the other hand, its capability to avoid the recurrent episodes produces controversial efficacy (Elish, 2004; Spruance, et al., 2002). Emmert (2000) suggested that patients with mild and infrequent recurrences are not beneficiated with acyclovir treatment. There is general consensus that the therapy is most effective when started soon after symptoms occur.

Rare adverse effects include: coma, seizures, neutropenia, leukopenia, tremor, ataxia, encephalopathy, psychotic symptoms, crystalluria, anorexia, fatigue, hepatitis, Stevens-Johnson syndrome, toxic epidermal necrolysis and/or anaphylaxis (United States Food and Drug Administration, FDA, 2011). Also the appearance of virus strains resistant to frequently used anti-herpes virus drugs (Greco, et al., 2007 ; Stránská, et al., 2005; Ziyaeyan, et al, 2007)

1.2 Alternative treatment

It has been suggested that there are insufficient scientific evidences to support the use of alternative medicine in HSV-1 infection. Even though, anecdotal reports of alternative remedies claimed to be beneficial in the treatment of herpes infection, arguing that alternative medicine could be beneficial in the treatment of herpes infection through enhancing the immune system. The interest in alternative drugs having antiviral effect is increasingly, since HSV-1, might develop resistance to commonly used antiviral agents.

Besides, despite the fact that some patients manifested side effects, the majority of the natural remedies did not show a high prevalence of adverse or severe reactions.

There are a number of natural remedies used in the HSV-1 treatment; some of them have been the subject of scientific analysis, demonstrating *in vitro* and *in vivo* satisfactory results.

1.2.1 Some examples of traditional medicine

In an experimental-placebo study, the application of zinc oxide/glycine cream showed shorter duration of cold sore lesions and reduction in overall severity of signs and symptoms (Godfrey, et al., 2001). In a pilot study, Femiano, et al. (2005) reported similar results and a reduction of number of episodes of herpes labialis. Singh, et al. (2005) in a clinical trial, evaluated a combination of L-lysine with a mixture of botanicals and other nutrients, with satisfactory results. Since the early 90s, Kümel et al. (1990a, 1991b) explained that the zinc ions inactivate virus by inhibition of the virion glycoprotein's function after a nonspecific accumulation of zinc into many virion membrane components, thus inhibiting viral adsorption and penetration. Also, Arens & Travis (2000) demonstrated that zinc salts inactivated the clinical isolates of HSV *in vitro*.

Mårdberg et al., (2001), demonstrated that viruses with mutations at residues Arg129,130, Ile142, Arg143,145, Arg145,147, Arg151,155 and Arg155,160 had significantly impaired the heparan sulfate (HS) binding. Impairment of the HS-binding activity of glycoprotein C, by these mutations had profound consequences for virus attachment and infection of cells in which amounts of HS exposed on the cell surface had been reduced.

Recently Katsuyama et al., (2008) established that Butyroyl-arginine, an arginine derivative, strongly inactivates the enveloped virus, as HSV-1. The authors suggest that the ability of arginine to bind membranes may be responsible for the inactivation of viruses. Naito et al., (2009) also has demonstrated the inhibition of HSV-1 multiplication by ariginine.

Huleihel & Isanu (2002) reported that propolis could block the cell membrane receptors for HSV-1, blocking the penetration of viral particles into the cells and/or inducing the intracellular metabolic changes of host cells, which would in turn affect the viral replication cycle *in vitro*.

Ascorbic acid has been shown to inactivate HSV-1, prevent the virus reactivation, have anti-inflammatory properties and to enhance the immune function (Gaby, 2006; Hovi, et al., 1995; Yoon et al., 2000). Supplementation with flavonoids further increases the effectiveness of vitamin C (Terezhalmy, et al., 1978). According to Narayana, et al., (2001), flavonoids showed strong antiviral activity against HSV-1. Essential oils of ginger, thyme hyssop and sandalwood have been demonstrated to inactivate HSV-1 before it enters into the cells, even in acyclovir resistant HSV-1 (Schnitzler, et al., 2007). Melissa officinalis (*lemon balm)* contains rosmarinic acid, phenolic acids and tannins; rosmarinic acid has been reported to show anti-inflammatory and potent antioxidant action. Schnitzler, et al. (2008), demonstrated that balm oil affected the viruses *in vitro* before adsorption, although the mechanism of action is unclear. They suggest that the balm oil could bind the viral proteins involved in the host adsorption and penetration, or damage the virions envelop. Carson, et al. (2006) have reported that tea tree oil of *Melaleuca alternifolia* showed the greatest effect on free virus.

Surveys of alternative treatment for HSV-1 are difficult to perform, since numerous patients are needed the regular contact for long period until the completion of the study. Even so, we have applied the vitamin C-supplemented tablet of lignin-carbohydrate complex (LCC) prepared from the pine cone of *Pinus parviflora* Sieb et Zucc., to a sample of HSV-1 patients, and investigated its clinical effect for the first time, with satisfactory results (González et al., 2009). The inhibitory effect of pine cone lignin and ascorbic combination treatment depend on antioxidant and immunopotentiating activities of lignin and ascorbic acid (Sakagami, et al., 1992).

The goal of both conventional and alternative treatment is promoting faster healing, reduction of symptoms, as well as decreasing the frequency of recurrent episodes. There are different phases in the viral cycle, to which the medicaments could be applied, according to the properties and mechanism of action of each medication (Fig. 1)

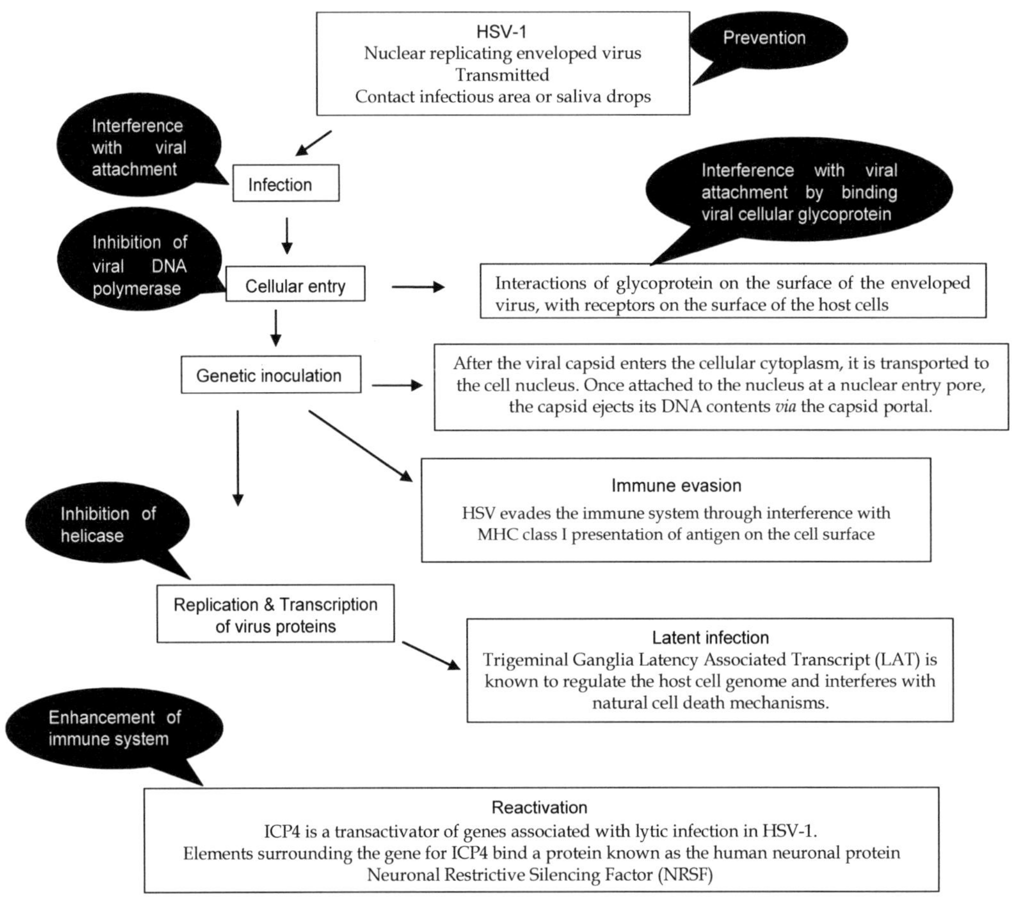

Fig. 1. A desirable effect of alternative treatment on HVS-1 virus cycle (Everett, 2006; Frick, 2003; Mettenleiter, et al., 2006; Newcomb, et al., 2007, Pinnoji, et al, 2007).

2. Functionality of LCC as alternative medicine

Lignin (polymers of phenylpropenoids), tannin and flavonoid are three major polyphenols in the natural kingdom (Table 1). So far, thousands of tannin and flavonoid-related compounds have been isolated from the methanol extracts of various plants and their complete structures have been elucidated. In contrast, lignins, extracted with alkaline solution, have been bound to polysaccharides (composed of glucose, arabinose, mannose, galactose, fucose, or uronic acids) to form lignin-carbohydrate complex (LCC) (Fig. 2).

		Component unit	MW (kDa)
Tannin	Hydrolysable Tannin	Esters of gallic acid and its oxidative derivatives with glucose or related sugars	0.5~4
	Condensed tannin	Flavan oligomers or polymers where their constituent monomeric flavans are connected mainly by C-4 - C-8 or C-4 - C-6 linkages	0.3~2
Flavonoid		Oxygen containing cyclic structure between two benzene rings	0.3~1
Lignin carbohydrate complex (LCC)		Complex of phenylpropenoid polymers and polysaccharide	10~200

Table 1. Representative polyphenols present in the natural kingdom.

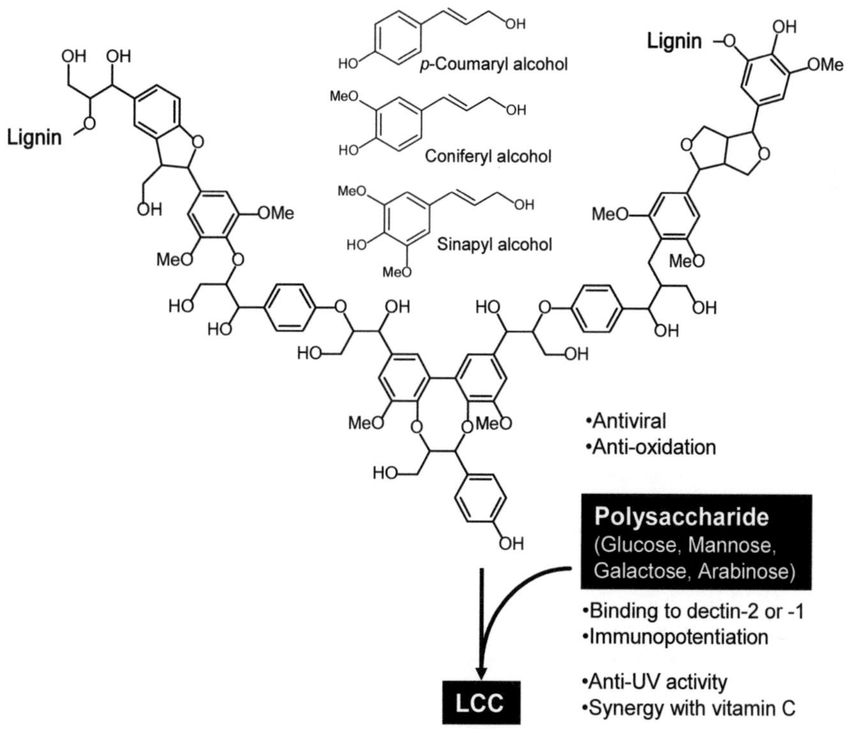

Fig. 2. Structure and function of lignin-carbohydrate complex (LCC)

This structural complexity of LCC has made it difficult to elucidate its complete structure. Varying the ratio of polysaccharide to phenylpropenoid polymer produces heterogeneity in the acidity, water-solubility, ethanol-insolubility, and molecular weight of LCC that might strongly affect its antiviral potency (Sakagami, et al., 2005, 2010b). However, this possibility has not been tested yet by any investigators. LCC was recoverable at much higher yield from the alkaline solution, in contrast to tannins and flavonoids (Fig. 3). The higher yield of LCC is very convenient for the mass-production in the factory.

2.1 Identification of LCC as an active antitumor principle of pine cone extract

We have paid attention to the folklore that intake of the hot water extract of pine cone of *Pinus parviflora* Sieb. et Zucc is effective for gastroenterological tumors. We isolated various polysaccharide fractions (Fig. 3), and investigated their antitumor activity against ascites sarcoma-180 cells (Sakagami, et al., 1987).

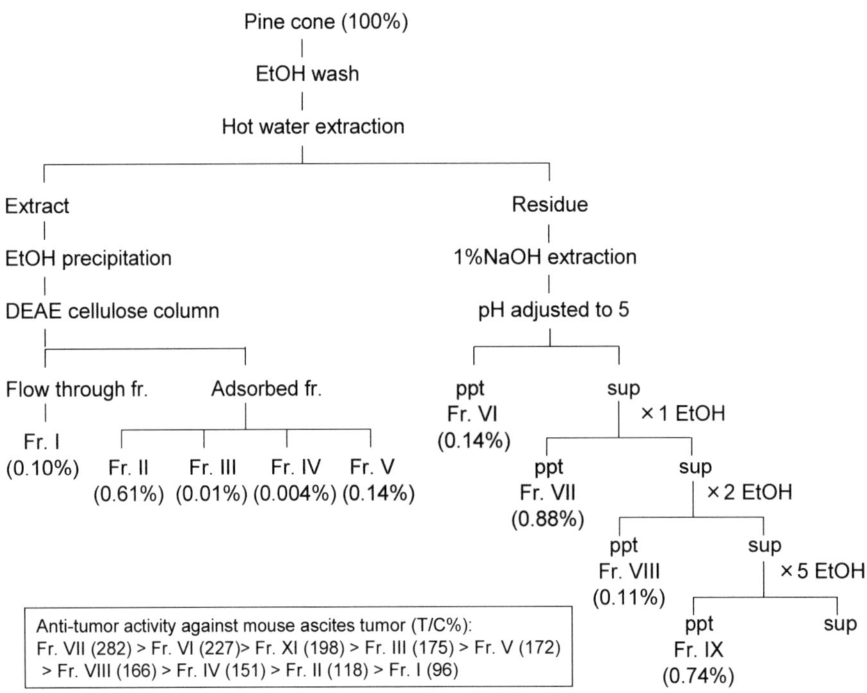

Fig. 3. Fractional preparation of LCC fractions from *Pinus parviflora* Sieb. et Zucc. Cited from Sakagami et al. (1987), with permission.

Pine cone was treated with ethanol to remove the sticky resin that contains cytotoxic substances, and then extracted with hot-water and then alkaline solution (1% NaOH). Polysaccharides in the hot water extract were precipitated by 86% ethanol, and then applied to DEAE-cellulose column chromatography. Neutral polysaccharide fraction (Fr. I) passed through the column, and then acidic polysaccharide fractions (Fr. II and III) rich in uronic acid were eluted from DEAE cellulose column chromatography with 0.5 and 2 M NaCl, respectively. The most acidic polysaccharides (Fr. VI and Fr. V) were eluted with 0.15M NaOH. The anti-tumor activity [evaluated by the survival ratio of treated group to control group (T/C%)] increased with the acidity: Fr. I (T/C=98%) < Fr. II (T/C=118%) < Fr. III (T/C=175%), Fr. IV (T/C=151 %) < Fr. V (T/C=172%) (Sakagami, et al., 1987). Higher anti-tumor activity was recovered by extraction with 1%NaOH, precipitated by acidification (pH 5) (Fr. VI) (T/C=227%), and also by ethanol precipitation (Fr. VII) (T/C=282%).

The most active acidic polysaccharide (IV) was subjected to spectral analysis, and identified as lignin-carbohydrate complex (LCC), based on the following evidences (Sakagami, et al., 1989). (i) UV absorption spectra：minimum absorption at 260 nm, maximum absorption at 280 nm, broad maximum absorption at 500 nm. (ii) IR spectra: hydroxyl group with hydrogen bonding (3400 cm^{-1}), aliphatic C-H (2700 cm^{-1}), carbonyl group conjugated to π-electron system (1700 ~ 1600 cm^{-1}), aromatic double bond (1600, 1500 cm^{-1}), C-O expansion and contraction (1400 ~ 1000 cm^{-1}), no ester bonding.(iii) ESR: one strong signal at g=2.003 under solid state at room temperature. Signal intensity was significantly reduced by oxidation and reduction.(iv) ^{1}H-NMR： When measured in 0.2%NaOD-D_2O, the presence of hydrogens in aromatic CH (δ6.5~7.5 ppm), >C=C< (δ4.5~5.5 ppm) and -O-CH-CH (δ3.0 ~ 4.0 ppm) was suggested. When the sample was acetylated by pyridine-acetic acid anhydride and dissolved in $CDCl_3$, the presence of acetyl group bound to phenolic OH (δ 2.3 ppm) or bound to alcoholic OH (δ 2.1 ppm) was confirmed. (v) Thin layer chromatography: Rf value of Fr. VI was the same with that of commercial alkali-lignin in various solvent systems (Table 2).

UV Absorption spectra	absorption peak at 260, 280, 500 nm (broad)
IR spectra	3400, 2700, 1700~1600, 1600, 1500, 1400~1000 cm^{-1}
ESR spectra	g=2.003 (strong signal)
^{1}H-NMR spectra	δ6.5~7.5, 4.5~5.5, 3.0~4.0 ppm
TLC	The same Rf value with alkali-lignin
Elementary analysis	C (43.21%), H (3.96%), N (2.61%), S (not detectable)
Neutral sugar/uronic acid	11.0%/1.7%
Composition of neutral sugar	Gal (44.7%), Glc (26.9%), Man (19.0%), Fuc (9.4%)
Molecular weight	10 kDa on gel filtration chromatography

Table 2. Identification of Fr. IV from pine cone of *Pinus parviflora* Sieb. et Zucc. as LCC, based on chemical analyses. Cited from Sakagami et al. (1987), with permission.

2.2 Distribution of LCC in the natural kingdom

Frs. VI and VII, prepared from the pine cones of *Pinus parviflora* Sieb. and Zucc. (T/C=227, 247%) showed higher antitumor activity in mice, than those prepared from *Pinus densiflora* Sieb. et Zucc (T/C=155, 245%), *Pinus thunbergii* Parl. (T/C=218, 191%), *Pinus elliottii* var. Elliotti (T/C=170, 217%), *Pinus taeda* L. (T/C=196, 179%), *Pinus caribaea* var. Hondurenses (T/C=114, 147%), *Pinus sylvestris* L. (T/C=180, 135%), or the pine seed shells of *Pinus parviflora* Sieb. et Zucc. (T/C=194. 220%), and *Pinus armandii* Franch (T/C=125%). Furthermore, the yields of Frs. VI and VII, prepared from *Pinus parviflora* Sieb. et Zucc. (0.51, 0.91%) were much higher than those from other pine cone sources [0.19±0.18 (0.001~0.48), 0.31±0.16 (0.06~0.48) %] (Harada, et al., 1988). These data suggest that acidic polysaccharides (Frs. VI and VII) are responsible for the legendary antitumor potential of the pine cone of *Pinus parviflora* Sieb. et Zucc.

LCCs from pine cone from *Pinus parviflora* Sieb et Zucc., and *Pinus elliottii* var. Elliotti [SI (selectivity index for measuring anti-HIV activity) =14, 28), bark of *Erythroxylum catuaba* Arr. Cam. (SI=43) (Manabe, et al., 1992), husk and mass of *Theobroma cacao* (SI= 311, 46) (Sakagami et al., 2008, 2011) and cultured extract of *Lentinus edodes* mycelia (LEM) (SI=>94) (Kawano et al. 2010) and mulberry juice (SI=7) (Sakagami et al., 2007, 2010b; Sakagami & Watanabe, 2011) showed higher anti-HIV activity than lower molecular weight polyphenols, such as tannins (SI=1-11) (Nakashima, et al., 1992b) and flavonoids (SI=1) (Fukai, et al., 2000), and natural and chemically modified glucans [*N,N*-dimethylaminoethyl paramylon, *N,N*-diethylaminoethyl paramylon, 2-hydroxy-3-trimethylammoniopropyl paramylon, sodium caroboxymethyl paramylon, carboxymethyl-TAK) (SI=1) except for sulfated polysaccharide (such as paramylon sulfate and dextran sulfate) (Koizumi, et al., 1993). Limited digestion of lignin structure by $NaClO_2$ resulted in significant loss of anti-HIV activity (from SI=14 to 3), whereas removal of the monosaccharide residues by acid-catalyzed hydrolysis did not significantly affect the anti-HIV activity (from SI= 14 to 13) (Lai et al., 1992) suggesting that that phenylpropenoid polymer, but not sugar moiety, is important for anti-HIV activity. This was confirmed by our finding that dehydrogenation polymers of phenylpropenoids without carbohydrate showed generally higher anti-HIV activity (SI=105) than LCCs (Nakashima, et al., 1992a). On the other hand, phenylpropenoid monomers (*p*-coumaric acid, ferulic acid, caffeic acid) were inactive, suggesting the importance of highly polymerized structure (Nakashima, et al., 1992a). The mechanism of anti-HIV activity induction has been suggested to be mediated by the inhibition of HIV adsorption to the cells (Nakashima, et al., 1992a). *In vitro*, LCCs have also been reported to inhibit the HIV-1 reverse transcriptase activity (Lai, et al., 1990, 1992) and HIV-1 protease activity (Ichimura, et al., 1999).

2.3 Anti-HSV activity *in vitro*

2.3.1 Inhibition of HSV-1 infection by Fr. VI

Inhibition of HSV infection was determined by plaque assay. Cells were inoculated with HSV-1 (200-400 plaques per well (3.5 cm diameter) 2 days after infection. Fr. VI showed potent anti-HSV-1 activity. Addition of Fr. VI during and after adsorption significantly reduced the number of plaques without affecting the morphology of the CV-1 cells. The plaque formation of HSV-1 was significantly inhibited by Fr. VI at a concentration of more than 0.1 μg/ml and completely inhibited by Fr. VI at more than 10 μg/ml (Fig. 4) (Fukuchi, et al., 1989a). Fr. VI inhibited the cytopathic effect of two different HSV-1 strains (HF and F) and HSV-2 strain G on two samples of cultured monkey kidney cells (CV-1 and Vero) and one sample of human adenocarcinoma cells (A-549). From the dose-response curves, the doses of Fr. VI that inhibited plaque formation by 50% (50% effective dose) in these cells were calculated to be 0.1-0.3 μg/ml (Fig. 4). When Fr. VI was adsorbed on and eluted from Sephadex LH-60, anti-HIV activity was slightly enhanced (Fr. VIb in Fig. 4).

Neither the growth rate nor the saturation density of CV-1 cells was significantly affected by up to 100 μg/ml of Fr. VI (Fig. 5). This indicates that the anti-HSV-1 effect of Fr. VI was not merely due to toxicity for the host cell.

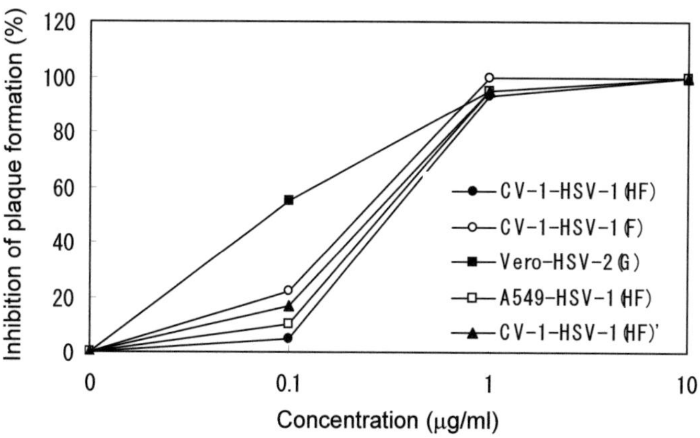

Fig. 4. Inhibition of HSV-1 plaque formation by Fr. VI and Fr. VIb in various cultured cells. The indicated doses of Fr. VI were added to the CV-1 cells at the time of infection with HSV-1 (HF) (•) or HSV-1 (F) (○), to the Vero cells at the time of infection with herpes virus simplex type 2 (G) (■), or to the A549 cells at the time of infection with HSV-1 (HF) (□). The CV-1 cells were also infected with HSV-1 (HF) in the presence of the indicated doses of Fr. VIb (▲). After washing with DME, these infected cells were overlaid with agarose, further incubated for 2 days in the presence of the same amounts of Fr. VI or Fr. VIb, and the number of plaques was then determined. Each value represents mean of triplicate determinations. Cited from Fukuchi, et al., (1989a), with permission.

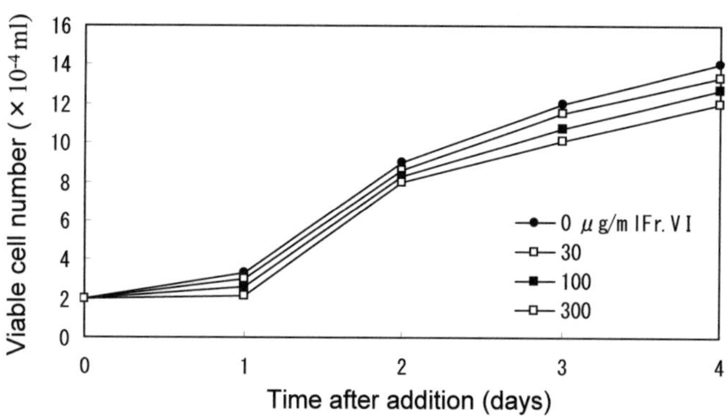

Fig. 5. Effect of Fr. VI on the growth of CV-1 cells. Each value represents mean of triplicate assays. Cited from Fukuchi, et al., (1989a), with permission.

2.3.2 Anti-HSV activity of LCCs from other plants, natural and chemically modified polysaccharides

Neutral polysaccharide (Fr. I) and uronic acid-rich polysaccharide (Fr. II) from pine cone extract of *Pinus parviflora* Sieb. et Zucc. had no anti-HSV activity at 10 μg/ml. Similarly, popular antitumor polysaccharides, such as paramylon, PSK, Schizophyllan, and chemically modified glucans (*N,N*-dimethylaminoethylparamylon, sodium carboxymethylparamylon, sodium paramylon sulfate, carboxymethyl TAK) were all inactive at 10 μg/ml. On the other hand, Fr. V tightly bound to DEAE-cellulose chromatography, and four LCC fractions (Frs.

VI-IX) almost completely inhibited the HSV-infection at 10 μg/ml (Table 3). LCC fractions (Frs. VI, VII) obtained from cones of other Japanese pine trees (*Pinus densiflora* Sieb. et Zucc., *Pinus thunbergii* Parl.), three Brazilian pine trees (*Pinus elliottii* var. Elliottii, *Pinus taeda* L., *Pinus caribaea* var. Hondurensus) and one Finnish pine tree (*Pinus sylvestris* L.), and from the seed shells of *Pinus parviflora* Sieb. et Zucc., and *Pinus armandii* Franch, also showed potent anti-HSV activity (Table 3).

Sample	Fr.	No. of plaques	% of inhibition
Neutral polysaccharide from cone of *Pinus parviflora* Sieb et Zucc.	I	310	0
Acidic polysaccharide from cone of *Pinus parviflora* Sieb et Zucc.	II	321	0
LCCs from pine cone of *Pinus parviflora* Sieb et Zucc.	V	0	100
	VI	0	100
	VII	33	89
	VIII	0	100
	IX	0	100
LCCs from cone of *Pinus densiflora* Sieb. et Zucc.	VI	0	100
	VII	9	97
LCCs from cone of *Pinus thunbergii* Parl.	VI	0	100
	VII	0	100
LCCs from cone of *Pinus elliottii* var. Elliottii	VI	2	99
	VII	0	100
LCCs from cone of *Pinus taeda* L.	VI	0	100
	VII	12	96
LCCs from cone of *Pinus caribaea* var. Hondurenses	VI	0	100
	VII	0	100
LCCs from cone of *Pinus sylvestris* L.	VI	0	100
	VII	0	100
LCCs from seed shell of *Pinus parviflora* Sieb et. Zucc.	VI	0	100
	VII	0	100
LCC from seed shell of *Pinus armandii* Franch	VI	0	100
Paramylon		310	0
PSK		320	0
Schizophyllan		325	0
N,N-dimethyaminoethylparamylon		306	0
Sodium carboxymethylparamylon		312	0
Sodium paramylon sulfate		299	2
Carboxymethyl-TAK		320	0
Alkali-lignin		0	100
Tannic acid		0	100
Saline (control)		305	–

Table 3. Anti-HSV activity of LCCs, natural and synthetic polysaccharides, added at 10 μg/ml. Each value represents mean of triplicate assays. Cited from Fukuchi, et al., (1989a), with permission.

2.3.3 Interference by Fr. VI of HSV-1 cellular adsorption

To determine the point of inhibition of HSV-1 infection, cells were treated with Fr. VI at various times before and after HSV-1 infection. Table 4 shows that: (i) no protective effect was observed when Fr. VI was not present in the adsorption medium, and (ii) pretreatment of the cells with Fr. VI for 6 days did not decrease the number of plaques.

Fr. VI (μg/ml)				
Before adsorption	During adsorption	After adsorption	No. of plaques	% of inhibition
0	0	0	229	–
10 (6 days)	0	0	204	11
0	10	0	0	100
0	0	10	230	0
10 (6 days)	0	10	188	18

Table 4. Dependence of anti-HSV activity induction by Fr. VI on treatment schedule. CV-1 cells were infected with HSV-1 strain HF. Fr. VI was added at the indicated stages. Each value represents mean of three separate assays. Cited from Fukuchi, et al., (1989a), with permission.

The results suggest that the protective effect of Fr. VI might be caused by its inhibition of virus adsorption. To test this possibility, the CV-1 cells were incubated with higher concentrations of radiolabeled virus particles (20,000 PFU) in the presence of Fr. VI, and the cell-bound radioactivity was measured. Table 5 shows Fr. VI at 10 μg/ml significantly inhibited the binding of the radiolabeled virus particles, even when the cells were incubated with higher concentrations of virus. Lignin similarly inhibited virus adsorption, but its effect was slightly lower than that of Fr. VI (Table 5).

		Cell-bound radioactivity	
Sample	Dose (μg/ml)	cpm	% of inhibition
Fr. VI	0	3007±168	–
	10	438±230	85
Lignin	0	5367±184	–
	10	2774±491	48
	100	193±53	96

Table 5. Inhibition of radiolabeled virus adsorption by Fr. VI and lignin. CV-1 cells were incubated for 1 hour at 37°C with the radioactive virus particle equivalent to 60,000 cpm (20,000 PFU/well) in the absence or presence of the indicated amounts of Fr. VI or lignin, and the cell-bound radioactivity was then determined. Each value represents mean ± S.D. of triplicate assays. Cited from Fukuchi, et al., (1989a), with permission.

We next investigated the effect of Fr. VI on virus penetration. Cells were first adsorbed for 1~2 hours with virus (200-400 PFU/well) at 4°C, a condition that allows virus adsorption but not virus penetration. The cells were treated with Fr. VI and the temperature was then raised to 37°C to initiate virus penetration. Fr. VI (1 μg/ml) did not inhibit plaque formation after completion of virus adsorption (data not shown). From the results, it was concluded that Fr. VI inhibits virus adsorption on target cells, but does not inhibit virus penetration.

We have previously reported that LCC also inhibited the adsorption of HIV to the cells (Nakashima, et al., 1992a, 1992b).

Recently, carboxylated lignins, synthesized using 4-hydroxy cinnamic acid scaffold by enzymatic oxidative coupling inhibited the entry of HSV-1 entry into the cells (Thakkar et al., 2010). Sulfated LCL (PPS-2b) (MW8500) also showed anti-HSV activity possibly by inhibiting the viral binding and penetration into host cells. Prunella cream formulated with a semi-purified fraction significantly reduced the skin lesion and mortality induced by HSV-1 infection in Guinea pigs (Zhang et al., 2007) The anti-HSV activity of sulfated lignins depended on their molecular weight, with the maximum at 39.4 kDa (Raghuraman et al. 2007).

2.4 Clinical effect of LCC-ascorbic acid tablet

The combination of alternative products can provide an effective therapy. To evaluate anti-HSV-1 activity of a pine cone LCC and ascorbic acid treatment, a clinical pilot study was carried out. We have modified the extraction method of LCC to achieve the mass production at the factory level (Fig. 6). Each LCC-ascorbic acid tablet contained a mixture of 50 mg pine cone extract powder JS, 50 mg ascorbic acid, 83 mg maltitol, 13 mg potato starch and 13 mg calcium stearate.

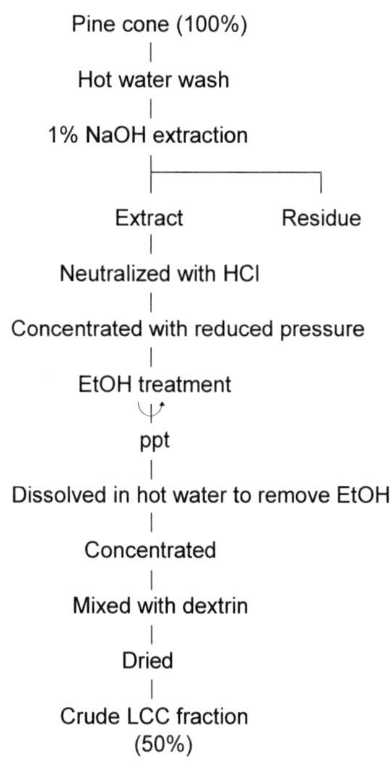

Fig. 6. Modified method for mass production of LCC at the factory level.

A pilot clinical study with pine cone lignin and ascorbic acid complex treatment against HSV-1-patients was carried out to evaluate the reduction of the duration with lesions, and the decrease of symptoms. A convenience sample of forty eight healthy patients of both genders between 4 and 61 years old (mean: 31±16.12 years), with active lesions of HSV-1, took part in the study. The patients were classified into the prodromic (16 patients), erytema (11 patients), papule edema (1 patient), vesicle/pustule (13 patients) and ulcer stages (7 patients). One mg of LCC-ascorbic acid tablet or solution was orally administered three times daily for a month. Clinical evaluations were made at least three times a week during the two first weeks after the onset and every six months during the subsequent year to identify recurrence episodes. The patients who began the LCC-ascorbic acid treatment within the first 48 hours did not develop HSV-1 characteristic lesions, whereas those patients who began the treatment later experienced a shorter duration of cold sore lesions and a decrease in the symptoms compared with previous episodes. The majority of the patients reported a reduction in the severity of symptoms and a reduction in the recurrence episodes after the LCC-ascorbic acid treatment compared with previous episodes, suggesting its possible applicability for the prevention and treatment of HSV-1 infection. Figs. 7, 8 and 9.

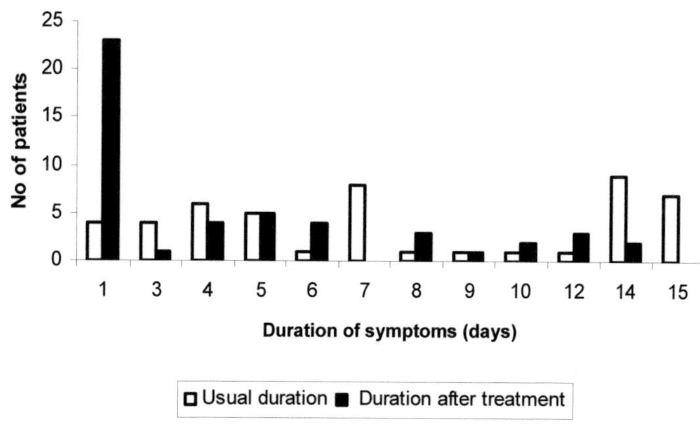

Fig. 7. Previous and new duration of lesions after pine cone ascorbic acid treatment. A significant difference in the duration of lesions was found between before and after treatment. Usual duration is based on patient report. Student's t 4.202 p =0.001. Cited from González et al. (2009) with permission.

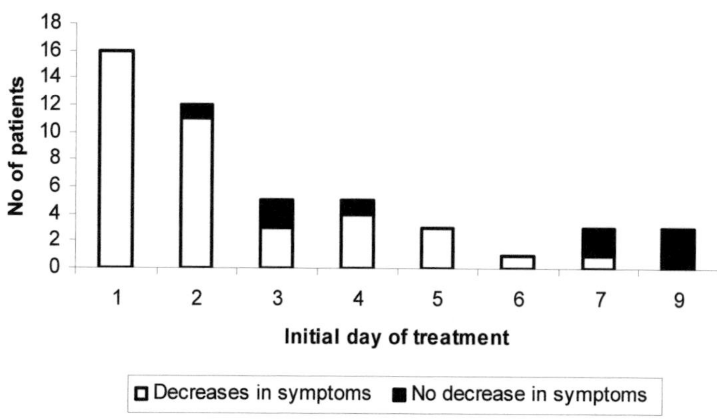

Fig. 8. Symptoms reduction according to the day of starting pine cone lignin and ascorbic acid complex treatment after onset. Symptoms were reduced notoriously when the treatment was taken in the first 48 h. after onset Kendall's Tau-b 0.456 p= 0.001. Cited from González, et al., (2009) with permission.

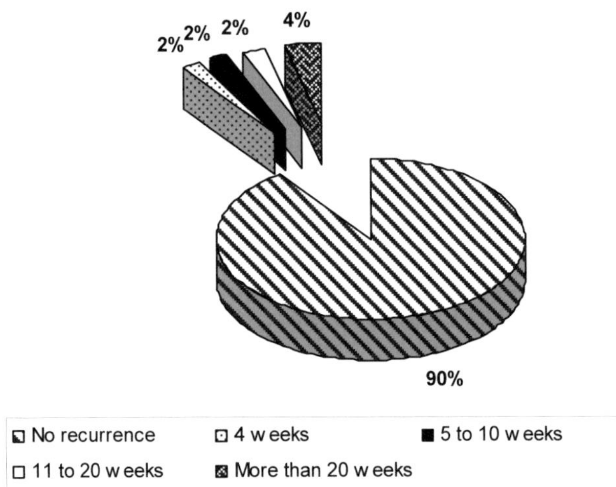

Fig. 9. Recurrence rate after pine cone lignin ascorbic acid complex treatment. Cited from González et al. (2009) with permission.

Majority of the patients reported the reduction in the severity of symptoms and in the recurrent episodes. This pilot study suggests possible applicability of LCC-vitamin C tablet for the prevention and treatment of HSV-1 infection (González, et al., 2009). However, it is not clear whether this clinical effect is due to the antiviral action of LCC itself or due to the combination effect of LCC + vitamin C.

We found significant differences between the usual and current duration after the pine cone lignin and ascorbic acid combination treatment and differences in the reduction of symptoms, taking into account the historical data provided by the patients. However, the small number of patients and the lack of a control group limited our ability to generalize the results to a larger population. To evaluate the effectiveness of pine cone lignin and ascorbic acid combination treatment, subsequent double-blind randomized controlled clinical trials must be done in a representative sample of patients who suffer from recurrent HSV-1.

2.5 Clinical effect of LCC tablet without vitamin C

In order to evaluate the effect of LCC obtained from pine " *Pinus parviflora* Sieb et Zucc." without ascorbic acid, on the treatment of infection by HSV type I, we already started a cross-sectional study on a sample of the patients, from the School of Dentistry of the Mexico State University. It has been planned to develop a double blind randomized clinical study in a larger, heterogeneous sample of captive population, incorporating students, professors and working personal of the Schools of Health Sciences of the University, the study will be carried out during three years.

Patients aged 18 or more who gave informed consent will enter into the study; they will be initially identified through an interview, and they will be asked to answer a questionnaire that includes signs and symptoms, the triggers and the treatments used. The patients will be randomized for treatment or placebo. No other antiviral drugs will be permitted during the study

The patients will be seen as soon as possible after the start of the outbreaks. The tablets will be delivered to patients with the instruction of taking a tablet 3 times a day for 30 days. The patients will be seen daily or at least three times during the episode until the complete healing had occurred. Any possible adverse effects will be recorded. When a recurrence occurs, the patients will repeat the treatment as previously described. The placebo group treatment protocol will be the same, but tablets without LCC will be administrated.

Until now we have identified 18 patients with a history of infection by HSV-1, who accepted to participate in the study, they signed the informed consent and answered the questionnaire. Among them only six patients have attended the clinic at the early stage of the disease, we carried out a clinical follow-up of patients to register the evolution of the disease (Table 6). In general the patients reported a reduction of the duration of the lesions and of the symptoms, according to their previous experience (Fig. 10-14).

One patient presented a light rash at the tenth day of LCC treatment. This disappeared without treatment, once the patient suspended the treatment. At present, it is not clear whether the reaction could be related with the LCC treatment. Alternatively, this may suggest that the combination of LCC and vitamin C is necessary to reduce such incidence.

Patient Gender/Age Female	Male	Date of initiation of treatment	Decrease of symptoms	Edema	Eritema	Vesicle	Erosion	Seudomebrane	Scab
49		Mar, 31	Apr, 03	Mar, 31	-	-	-	Apr, 06	Apr, 06
	23	Mar, 01	Mar, 02	-	Mar, 01	-	Mar, 08	Mar, 09	Mar, 09
	21	July, 10	July, 10	-	July, 11	July, 12	July , 12	July, 13	July, 13
53		Feb, 02	Feb, 02	Feb, 02	Feb, 03	Feb, 04	Feb, 04	Feb, 05	Feb, 05
57		Jan 10	Jan 10	-	-	Jan 12	Jan 12	Jan 13	Jan 14
	24*	Mar, 29	Mar, 30	Mar, 29	Mar, 31	Apr, 01	Apr, 01	Apr, 02	Apr, 02

*The patient presented a light skin rash.

Table 6. Evolution of the lesions of HSV-1 in five patients treated with LCC tablet without vitamin C.

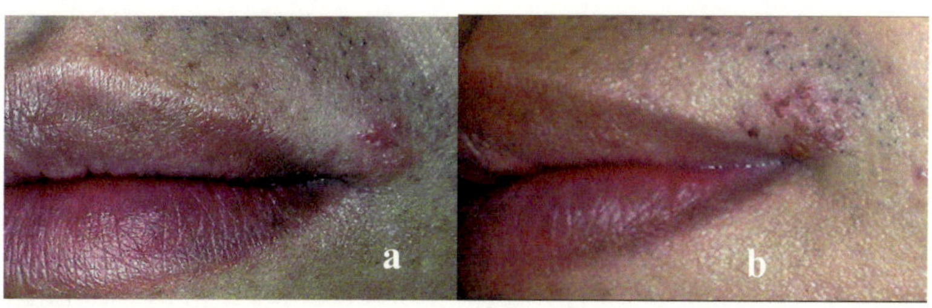

Fig. 10. Male 21 years old, a) Vesicles, b) Scab early stage

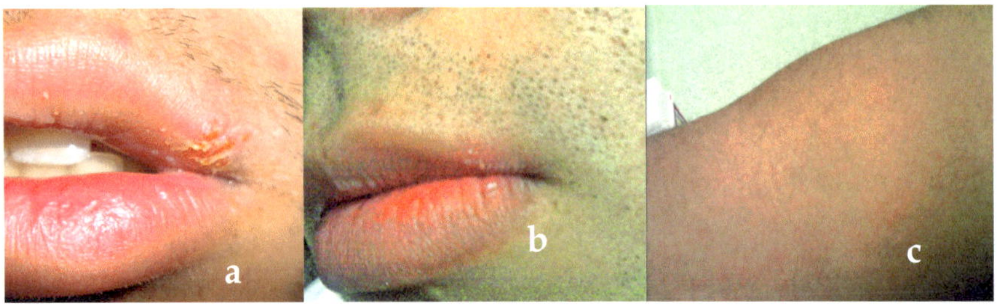

Fig. 11. Male 24 years old, a) Ulcerative stage, c) Seudomembrane stage, d) Skin rash

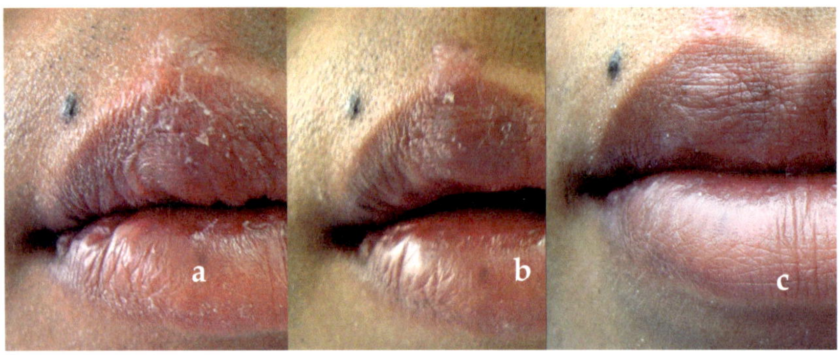

Fig. 12. Male, 25 years old. a) Erosion stage, b) Late scab stage, c) Complete healthy stage

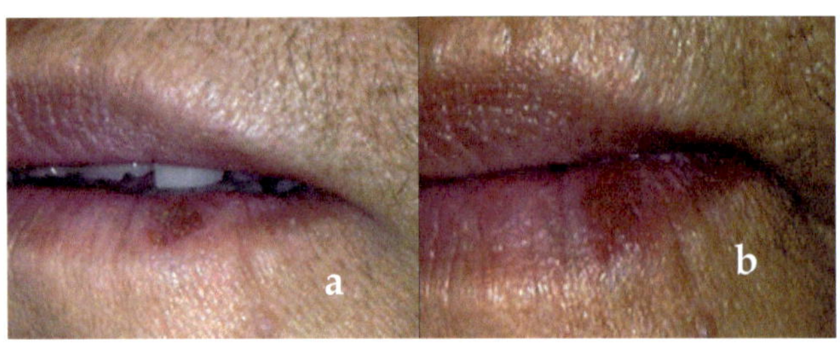

Fig. 13. Female 57 years old, a) Ulcerative stage, b) Scab early stage

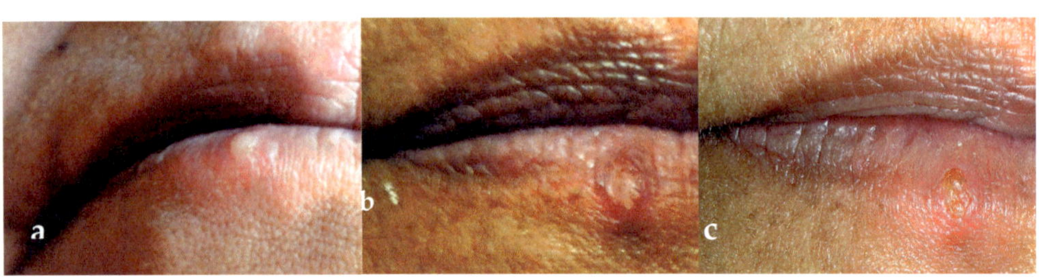

Fig. 14. Female 53 years old, a) Vesicle stage, b) Ulcerative stage, b) Seudomembrane stage

Fig. 10-14. Stages in the evolution of HSV-1 lesions in patients who received treatment with LCC. Only representative photographs were shown.

3. Conclusion

We have demonstrated that LCC from pine cone of *Pinus parviflora* Sieb. Zucc. showed anti-HSV activity *in vitro*, by inhibiting the viral adsorption to the cells. LCC shows broad antiviral spectrum. LCC exhibited high affinity with influenza virus, and in contact to LCC, influenza virus rapidly lose the virulence (Sakagami, et al., 1992). LCC showed much higher anti-HIV activity than tannins (Nakashima, et al., 1992a, 1992b), whereas both LCC and tannins showed potent anti-HSV activity (Fukuchi, et al., 1989a, 1989b). Since virus is one of major risk factor of oral cavity cancer (Sakagami, 2010a), anti-viral action of LCC may reduce the incidence of virus-triggered diseases such as cancer.

LCC shows also immunopotentiating activity. Administration with LCC induced antitumor, antimicrobial and anti-parasite activity, and enhanced the endogenous TNF production. At present, the receptors for LCC have not been identified. Recently, we have found LCC fraction isolated from *Lentinus edodes* mycelia extract (Fr4) enhanced the expression of dectin-2 (4.2-fold) and toll-like receptor (TLR)-2 (2.5-fold) prominently, but only slightly modified the expression of dectin-1 (0.8-fold), complement receptor 3 (0.9-fold), TLR1, 3, 4, 9 and 13 (0.8- to 1.7-fold), spleen tyrosine kinase (Syk)b, zeta-chain (TCR) associated protein kinase 70kDa (Zap70), Janus tyrosine kinase (Jak)2 (1.0- to 1.2-fold), nuclear factor (Nf)κb1, NFκb2, reticuloendotheliosis viral oncogene homolog (Rel)a, Relb (1.0- to 1.6-fold), Nfκbia, Nfκbib, Nfκbie, Nfκbi12 Nfκbiz (0.8- to 2.3-fold). On the other hand, LPS did not affect the expression of dectin-2 nor TLR-2. These data suggest the significant role of the activation of the dectin-2 signaling pathway in the action of LCC on macrophages (Kushida, et al., 2011). Identification of dectin-2 as LCC receptor awaits further confirmation with siRNA and gene over expression experiments.

The other intriguing property of LCC is the synergy with vitamin C. Ascorbate derivatives that produced the doublet signal of ascorbate radical (sodium-L-ascorbate, L-ascorbic acid, D-isoascorbic acid, 6-β-D-galactosyl-L-ascorbate, sodium 5,6-benzylidene-L-ascorbate) induced apoptosis in HL-60 cells, whereas ascorbate derivatives that did not produce radicals (L-ascorbic acid-2-phosphate magnesium salt, L-ascorbic acid 2-sulfate and dehydroascorbic acid) did not induce apoptosis (Sakagami, et al., 1996a, 1996b). High concentrations of LCC from the pine cone of *Pinus parviflola* Sieb et Zucc., pine cone of *Pinus elliottii* var. Elliotti, leaf of *Ceriops decandra* (Griff.) Ding Hou and, thorn apple of *Crataegu Cuneata* Sieb. et Zucc enhanced the radical intensity and cytotoxicity of sodium ascorbate. On the other hand, lower concentrations of LCC stimulated the superoxide anion (O_2^-), hydroxyl radical and 1,1-diphenyl-2-picrylhydrazyl (DPPH) radical scavenging activity of sodium ascorbate (Sakagami et al., 2000, 2005, 2008) . This suggests the possible application of LCC as stimulator of vitamin C action, especially in the field of UV protection and anti-aging research.

Solvent fractionation of alkaline extract of the leaves of *Sasa senanensis* Rehder (SE) demonstrated that (i) chlorophyllin in SE was recovered from the water layer, that contains majority of compounds (more than 81%) and inhibited the NO production by macrophages more potently than other *n*-hexane, diethyl ether and ethylacetate layers (Sakagami, et al., 2010c). Three-dimensional HPLC analysis demonstrated that the majority of SE components are recovered from one major peak. Furthermore, LCC isolated from SE showed the unique greenish color of chlorophyllin (absorption maximum = 452 nm) (Sakagami, et al., 2010c).

These data strongly suggest the possible association of chlorophyllin with LCC in the native state or during extraction with alkaline solutions. Biological significance of such association remains to be investigated.

4. Acknowledgment

This study was supported in part by Universidad Autónoma del Estado de México (González FE04/2009) and a Grant-in-Aid from the Ministry of Education, Science, Sports and Culture of Japan (Sakagami No.14370607, 2002-2004, Sakagami No. 19592156, 2007-2009).

5. References

Arduino, PG. & Porter, SR. (Feb, 2008). Herpes Simplex Virus Type 1 infection: overview on relevant clinic-pathological features. *Journal Oral Pathology Medicine*, Vol.37, No.2, pp. 107-21. ISSN: 1600-0714.

Arens, M. & Travis, S. (May, 2000). Zinc salts Inactivate Clinical isolates of herpes simplex virus in vitro. *Journal of clinical Microbiology,* Vol. 38, No.5, pp. 1758-1762. ISSN:0095-1137

Balzarini, J. (1994). Metabolism and mechanism of antiretroviral action of purine and pyrimidine derivatives. *Pharmacy World & Science*, Vol.15, No.16, pp. 113-26. ISSN: 0928-1231.

Bsoul, SA & Terezhalmy, GT. (May, 2004). Vitamin C in health and disease. Journal *Contemporary Dental Practice*, Vol.5, No.2, pp. 001-013 ISSN:1526-3711

Carson CF.; Hammer KA. & Riley, TV. (Jan 2006) Melaleuca alternifolia (Tea Tree) Oil: a review on antimicrobial and other medicinal properties. *Clinical Microbiology Reviews*, Vol.19, No.1, pp. 50-62. ISSN: 0893-8512.

Chon, T.; Nguyen, L. & Elliott, TC. (July, 2007). Clinical inquiries. What are the best treatments for herpes labialis?. *Journal of Family Practice,* Vol.56, No.2, pp. 576–8. ISSN: 0094-3509.

Elish, D.; Singh, F. & Weinberg, JM. (July, 2004). Therapeutic options for herpes labialis, II: Topical agents. *Cutis,* Vol.74, No.1, pp. 5-40. ISSN: 0011-4162.

Esmann, J. (Feb, 2001). The many challenges of facial herpes simplex virus infection. *Journal of Antimicrobial Chemotherapy*, VOL. 47 Topic T1, pp.17-27, ISSN 0305-7453.

Emmert, DH. (Mar, 2000). Treatment of Common Cutaneous Herpes Simplex Virus Infections. *American Academy of Family Physician*, Vol.61, No.6, pp. 1697-704, 1705-6. 1708. ISSN: 0002-838X. Retrieved from http://www.aafp.org/afp/20000315/1697.html

Everett, RD. (Aug, 2000). ICP0, a regulator of herpes simplex virus during lytic and latent infection. *Bioessays,* Vol.22, No.8, pp. 761–70. ISSN: 0265-9247.

Fatahzadeh, M. & Schwartz, RA. (Nov, 2007). Human herpes simplex labialis. *Journal Clinical and Experimental Dermatology*, Vol.32, No.6, pp. 625-630. ISSN: 1365-2230

Femiano, F.; Gombos, F, & Scully, C. (Aug, 2005). Recurrent herpes labialis: a pilot study of the efficacy of zinc therapy. *Journal of Oral Pathology & Medicine,* Vol. 34, No.7, pp. 423-425. ISSN: 0904-2512.

Frick DN. Helicases as antiviral drug target. (July-Aug, 2003) *Drug News and Perspectives,* Vol.16, No.6, pp. 352- 62 ISSN:0214-0934

Fukai, T., Sakagami, H.; Toguchi, M.; Takayama, F.; Iwakura, I.; Atsumi, T.; Ueha, T.; Nakashima, H. & Nomura, T. (July-Aug, 2000). Cytotoxic activity of low molecular weight polyphenols against human oral tumor cell lines. *Anticancer Research,* Vol.20, No.4, pp. 2525-2536. ISSN: 0250-7005.

Fukuchi, K; Sakagami, H.; Ikeda, M.; Kawazoe, Y.; Oh-hara, T.; Konno, K.; Ichikawa, S.; Hata, N.; Kondo, H.; & Nonoyama, M. (Mar-Apr, 1989a). Inhibition of herpes simplex virus infection by pine cone antitumor substances. *Anticancer Research,* Vol.9, No.2, pp. 313-317. ISSN: 0250-7005.

Fukuchi, K; Sakagami, H.; Okuda, T.; Hatano, T.; Tanuma, S.; Kitajima, K.; Inoue, Y.; Inoue ,S; Ichikawa, S.; Nonoyama, M. & Konno, K. (June-July, 1989b). Inhibition of herpes simplex virus infection by tannins and related compounds. *Antiviral Research,* Vol.11, No.(5-6), pp. 285-298. ISSN: 0166-3542.

Gaby, AR. Natural Remedies for Herpes Simplex. (June, 2006). *Alternative Medicine Review,* Vol.11,No.2,pp. 93-101. ISSN: 1089-5159. Retrieved from: http://www.encyclopedia.com/doc/1G1-148424510.html

González, BS.; Yamamoto, MA.; Utsumi, K.; Aratsu, C. & Sakagami, H. (Nov-Dec, 2009). Clinical Pilot study of lignin-ascorbic acid combination treatment of herpes simplex virus. *In Vivo,* Vol.23, No.6, pp. 1011-1016. ISSN: 0258-851X.

Godfrey, HR.; Godfrey, NJ.; Godfrey, JC. & Riley, D. (May-June, 2001). A randomized clinical trial on the treatment of oral herpes with topical zinc oxide/glycine. *Alternative Therapies in Health and Medicine,* Vol.7, No.3, pp. 49-56. ISSN: 1078-6791.

Greco, A.; Diaz, JJ.; Thouvenot, D. & Morfin, F. (Mar, 2007). Novel targets for the development of anti-herpes compounds. *Infectious Disorders - Drug Targets,* Vol.7, No.1, pp. 11-18. ISSN: 1871-5265

Hamuy, R. & Berman, B. (July-Aug, 1998). Treatment of herpes simplex virus infections with topical antiviral agents. *European Journal of Dermatology,* Vol.8, No.5, pp. 310–319. ISSN: 1167-1122.

Harada, H.; Sakagami, H.; Konno, K.; Sato T.; Osawa, N., Fujimaki, M. & Komatsu, N. (July-Aug, 1988). Induction of antimicrobial activity by antitumor substances from pine cone extract of *Pinus parviflora* Sieb. et Zucc. *Anticancer Research,* Vol.8, No.4, pp. 581-587. ISSN: 0250-7005.

Huleihel, M. & Isanu, V. Nov, 2002) Anti-herpes simplex virus effect of an aqueous extract of propolis. *Israel Medical Association Journal, 4 (suppl):* 923-927 ISSN: 1565-1088.

Hunt, R. (July, 2011a). *Microbiology and immunology On-Line.* Medical Microbiology Virology - Chapter Eleven Herpes viruses. (5th Edition), Murray PR, Rosenthal KS, Pfaller Michael AMD, ISBN: 978-0-323-05470-6, University of South Carolina. Retrieved from http://pathmicro.med.sc.edu/virol/herpes.htm

Hunt, R. (July,2011b). *Microbiology and immunology On-Line.* Medical Microbiology Virology - Chapter Nine Anti-viral Chemotherapy. (5th Edition), Murray PR, Rosenthal KS, Pfaller Michael AMD, ISBN: 978-0-323-05470-6, University of South Carolina. Retrieved from http://pathmicro.med.sc.edu/virol/herpes.htm

Hovi, T.; Hirvimies, A.; Stenvik, M.; Vuola, E. & Pippuri, R. (June,1995). Topical treatment of recurrent mucocutaneous herpes with ascorbic acid containing solution. *Antiviral Ressearch,* Vol, 27, No.3, pp.: 263-270, ISSN: 0166-3542

Ichimura, T.; Otake, T.; Mori, H. & Maruyama, S. (Dec, 1999). HIV-1 protease inhibition and anti-HIV effect of natural and synthetic water-soluble lignin-like substances.

Bioscience Biotechnology & Biochemistry, Vol.63, No.12, pp. 2202-2024. ISSN: 0916-8451.

Katsuyama, Y.; Yamasaki, H.; Tsujimoto, K.; Koyama HA., Ejima, D. & Arakawa, T. (Sept, 2008). Butyroyl-arginine as a potent virus inactivation agent. *International Journal of Pharmaceutics*, Vol. 362, No.1-2, pp. 92-98 ISSN: 0378-5173

Kawano, M.; Sakagami, H.; Satoh, K.; Shioda, S.; Kanamoto, T; Terakubo, S.; Nakashima, H. & Makino, T. (July-Aug,, 2010). Lignin-like activity of *Lentinus edodes mycelia* Extract (LEM). *In Vivo*, Vol.24, No.4, pp. 543-552. ISSN : 0258-851X.

Koelle, DM. & Corey, L. (Feb, 2008). Herpes simplex: insights on pathogenesis and possible vaccines. *Annual Review of Medicine*, Vol.59, pp. 381–395. ISSN: 0066-4219.

Koizumi, N.; Sakagami, H.; Utsumi, A.; Fujinaga, S.; Takeda, M.; Asano, K.; Sugawara, I.; Ichikawa, S.; Kondo, H.; Mori, S.; Miyatake, K.; Nakano, Y.; Nakashima, H.; Murakami, T.; Miyano, N. & Yamamoto,, N. (May, 1993). Anti-HIV (human immunodeficiency virus) activity of sulfated paramylon. *Antiviral Research*, Vol.21, No.1, pp. 1-14. ISSN: 0166-3542.

Kushida, T.; Makino, T.; Tomomura, M.; Tomomura, A.; & Sakagami, H. (Apr, 2011). Enhancement of dectin-2 gene expression by lignin-carbohydrate complex from *Lentinus edodes* extract (LEM) in mouse macrophage-like cell line. *Anticancer Research*, Vol.31, No.4, pp. 1241-1248. ISSN: 0250-7005.

Kümel, G.; Schrader, S.; Zentgraf, H. & Brendel, M. (July, 1991) Therapy of banal HSV lesions: molecular mechanisms of the antiviral activity of zinc sulfate. *Hautarzt*. Vol. 42, No. 7, pp.439-45. (Summary, Article in Germany) ISSN:0017-8470

Kümel, G.; Schrader, S.; Zentgraf, H.; Daus, H, & Brendel, M. (Dec 1990) The mechanism of the antiherpetic activity of zinc sulphate. *Journal of General Virology*, Vol. 71 No. 12, pp 2989-2997. ISSN: 0022-1317

Lai, PK.; Donovan, J.; Takayama, H.; Sakagami, H.; Tanaka, A.; Konno, K. & Nonoyama, M. (Feb, 1990). Modification of human immunodeficiency viral replication by pine cone extracts. *AIDS Research and Human Retroviruses*, Vol.6, No.2, pp. 205-217. ISSN: 1931-8405.

Lai, PK.; Oh-hara, T.; Tamura, Y.; Kawazoe, Y.; Konno, K.; Sakagami, H.; Tanaka, A. & Nonoyama, M. (1992). Polymeric phenylpropenoids are the active components in the pine cone extract that inhibit the replication of type-1 human immunodeficiency virus *in vitro*. *Journal of General and Applied Microbiology*, Vol.38, No.4, pp. 303-323. ISSN: 0022-1260.

Manabe, H.; Sakagami, H.; Ishizone, H.; Kusano, H.; Fujimaki, M.; Wada, C.; Komatsu, N.; Nakashima, H.; Murakami, T.; & Yamamoto N. (Mar-Apr, 1992). Effects of Catuaba extracts on microbial and HIV infection. *In Vivo*, Vol.6, No.2, pp. 161-166. ISSN: 0258-851X.

Mårdberg, K; Trybala, E.; Glorioso, JC. & Bergström, T.(Aug, 2001). Mutational analysis of the major heparin sulfate-binding domain of herpes simplex type 1 glycoprotein C. *Journal of General Virology*, Vol. 82, No.8, pp. 1941-1950 ISSN:14652099

Mettenleiter, TC.; Klupp, BG. & Granzow, H. (Aug , 2006). "Herpesvirus assembly: a tale of two membranes". *Current Opinion in Microbiology*, Vol.9, No.4, pp. 423–9. ISSN: 1369-5274

Naito, T.; Irie, H.;Tsujimoto, K.; Ikeda, K ; Arakawa, T. & Koyama, AH. (Apr., 2009). Antiviral effect of arginine against herpes simplex virus type 1. *International Journal of Molecular Medicine*, Vol.23, No 4, pp. 495-499. ISSN: 1107-3756

Nakashima, H.; Murakami, T.; Yamamoto, N.; Naoe, T.; Kawazoe, Y.; Konno, K. & Sakagami, H. (Aug, 1992a). Lignified materials as medicinal resources. V. Anti-HIV (human immunodeficiency virus) activity of some synthetic lignins. *Chemical and Pharmaceutical Bulletin*, Vol.40, No.8, pp. 2102-2105. ISSN: 1347-5223.

Nakashima, H.; Murakami, T.; Yamamoto, N.; Sakagami, H.; Tanuma, S.; Hatano, T.; Yoshida, T. & Okuda, T. (May, 1992b). Inhibition of human immunodeficiency viral replication by tannins and related compounds. *Antiviral Research*, Vol.18, No.1, pp. 91-103. ISSN: 0166-3542.

Narayana, KRAJ.; Sripal, M. & Chaluvadi, NR. (2001). Bioflavonoids classification, pharmacological, biochemical effects and therapeutic potential. *Indian Journal of Pharmacology*, Vol 33, pp. 2-16 ISSN:0253-7613

Newcomb, WW.; Booy, FP. & Brown, JC. (July, 2007). "Uncoating the herpes simplex virus genome". *Journal of Molecular Biology*. Vol.370,No.4: 633–42. ISSN: 1089-8638.

Paterson, J. & Kwong, M. (Apr, 2008). Recurrent Herpes Labialis, Assessment and Non-Prescription Treatment. *Glaxo Smithkline Consumer Healthcare*, ISSN: 1079-2082. Retrived from http://www.pharmacyresource.ca/recurrent_herpes_labialis.pdf

Pinnoji, RC.; Bedadala, GR.; George, B.; Holland, TC.; Hill, JM.; Hsia, SC. (June, 2007). "Repressor element-1 silencing transcription factor/neuronal restrictive silencer factor (REST/NRSF) can regulate HSV-1 immediate-early transcription via histone modification". *Journal of Virology* . Vol. 4, No.1, pp. 8149–56 56. ISSN: 0022-538X.

Raghuraman, A.; Tiwari, V.; Zhao, Q.; Shukla, D.; Debnath, AK. & Desai, UR. (May, 2007). Viral inhibition studies on sulfated lignin, a chemically modified biopolymer and a potential mimic of heparin sulfate. *Biomacromolecules*, Vol.8, No.5. pp. 1759-1763. ISSN: 1525-7797

Raj Narayana, NK.; Spiral, RM.; Chaluvadi, MR.; & Krishna DR. (June, 2000). Bioflavonoids classification, pharmacological, biochemical effects and therapeutic potential. *Indian Journal of Pharmacology*, Vol.33, pp. 2-16. ISSN: ISSN 0253-7613.

Sakagami, H.; Ikeda, M.; Unten, S.; Takeda, K.; Murayama, J.; Hamada, A.; Kimura, K.; Komatsu, N.; & Konno, K. (Nov-Dec, 1987). Antitumor activity of polysaccharide fractions from pine cone extract of *Pinus parviflora* Sieb. et Zucc. *Anticancer Research*, Vol.7, No.6, pp. 1153-1160. ISSN: 0250-7005.

Sakagami, H.; Oh-hara, T.; Kaiya T.; Kawazoe, Y.; Nonoyama, M.; & Konno, K. (Nov-Dec, 1989). Molecular species of the antitumor and antiviral fraction from pine cone extract. *Anticancer Research*, Vol.9, No.6, pp. 1593-1598. ISSN: 0250-7005.

Sakagami, H.; Konno, K.; Kawazoe, Y.; Lai, P.; & Nonoyama, M. (1992) Multiple immunological functions of extracts from the cone of Japanese white pine, Pinus parviflora Sieb. et Zucc. *Advances in Experimental Medicine and Biology*, Vol 319, No, pp.331-335. ISSN: 0065-2598

Sakagami, H.; Kuribayashi, N.; Iida, M.; Hagiwara, T.; Takahashi, H.; Yoshida, H.; Shiota, F.; Ohata, H.; Momose, K.; & Takeda M. (Mar, 1996a). The requirement for and mobilization of calcium during induction by sodium ascorbate and by hydrogen peroxide of cell death. *Life Sciences*, Vol.58, No.14, pp. 1131-1138. ISSN: 0024-3205.

Sakagami, H.; Satoh, K.; Ohata, H.; Takahashi, H.; Yoshida, H.; Iida, M.; Kuribayashi, N.; Sakagami, T.; Momose K. & Takeda, M. (Sep-Oct, 1996b). Relationship between ascorbyl radical intensity and apoptosis-inducing activity. *Anticancer Research*, Vol.16, No.5A, pp. 2635-2644. ISSN: 0250-7005.

Sakagami, H.; Satoh, K.; Hakeda, Y. & Kumegawa, M. (Feb, 2000). Apoptosis-inducing activity of vitamin C and vitamin K. *Cell Molecular Biology*, Vol.46, No.1, pp. 129-143. ISSN: 1939-4586.

Sakagami, H.; Hashimoto, K.; Suzuki, F.; Ogiwara, T.; Satoh, K.; Ito H.; Hatano, T.; Yoshida, T. & Fujisawa S. (Sep, 2005). Molecular requirements of lignin-carbohydrate complexes for expression of unique biological activities. *Phytochemistry*, Vol.66, No.17, pp. 2108-2120. ISSN: 0031-9422.

Sakagami, H.; Asano, K.; Satoh, K.; Takahashi, K.; Kobayashi, M.; Koga, N.; Takahashi, H.; Tachikawa, R.; Tashiro, T.; Hasegawa, A.; Kurihara, K.; Ikarashi, T.; Kanamoto, T.; Terakubo, S.; Nakashima, H.; Watanabe, S. & Nakamura, W. (May-June, 2007). Anti-stress, anti-HIV and vitamin C-synergized radical scavenging activity of mulberry juice fractions. *In Vivo*, Vol.21, No.3, pp. 499-506. ISSN: 0258-851X.

Sakagami, H.; Satoh, K.; Fukamachi, H.; Ikarashi, T.; Simizu, A.; Yano, K.; Kanamoto, T.; Terakubo, S.; Nakashima, H.; Hasegawa, H.; Nomura, A.; Utsumi, K.; Yamamoto, M.; Maeda, Y. & Osawa, K. (May-June, 2008). Anti-HIV and vitamin C-synergized radical scavenging activity of cacao husk lignin fractions. *In Vivo*, Vol.22, No.3, pp. 327-33. ISSN: 0258-851X.

Sakagami, H. (2010a). Chapter 5.1.8. Oral Cavity Cancer. *Cancer Report 2010*, Tuncer AM, Moore M, Qiao YL, Yoo K-Y, Tajima K, Ozgul N, Gultekin M, pp. 222-226, MN Medical & Nobel Publishing Company, Ankara, Turkey.ISBN:978-975-567-058-4.

Sakagami, H.; Kushida, T.; Oizumi, T.; Nakashima, H. & Makino, T. (Oct, 2010b). Distribution of lignin carbohydrate complex in plant kingdom and its functionality as alternative medicine. *Pharmacology & Therapeutics*, Vol.128, No.1, pp. 91-105. ISSN: 0163-7258.

Sakagami, H.; Zhou Li.; Kawano, M.; Thet, MM.; Takana, S.; Machino, M.; Amano, S.; Kuroshita, R.; Watanabe, S.; Chu, Q.; Wang, QT.; Kanamoto, T.; Terakubo, S.; Nakashima, H.; Sekine, K.; Shirataki, Y.; Hao, ZC.; Uesawa, Y.; Mohri, K.; Kitajima, M.; Oizumi, H. & Oizumi, T. (Sep-Oct, 2010c). Multiple Biological complex of alkaline extract of the leaves of *Sasa senanensis* Rehder. *In Vivo*, Vol.24, No.1, pp. 735-744. ISSN: 0258-851X.

Sakagami, H.; Kawano, M.; May Maw, T.; Hashimoto, K.; Satoh, K.; Kanamoto, T.; Terakubo, S.; Nakashima, H.; Haishima, Y.; Maeda, Y. & Sakurai, K. (Mar-Apr, 2011). Anti-HIV and immunomodulation activities of cacao mass lignin carbohydrate complex. *In Vivo*, Vol.25, No.2, pp. 229-236. ISSN: 0258-851X.

Sakagami, H. & Watanabe S. (2011). Beneficial effects of mulberry on human health. *Phytotherapeutics and Human Health: Pharmacological and Molecular Aspects*, Farooqui AA, pp. 257-273, Nova Science Publishers, Inc, Hauppauge, NY. ISBN: 978-1-61761-196-4.

Schnitzler, P.; Koch C. & Reichling, J. (2007) Susceptibility of drug-resistant clinical herpes simplex virus type 1 strains to essential oils of ginger, thyme, hyssop, and sandalwood. *Antimicrobial Agents and Chemotherapy*, Vol *51*, pp. 1859-1862. ISSN 0066-4804.

Schnitzler, P.; Schuhmacher, A.; Astani, A.; & Reichling, J. (Sep, 2008). Melissa officinalis oil affects infectivity of enveloped herpesviruses. *Phytomedicine,* Vol 15, No.9, pp 734-40. ISSN: 0944-7113.

Siegel, MA. (Sep, 002) Diagnosis and management of recurrent herpes simplex infections *Journal of the American Dental Association,* Vol 133, No 9, pp.,1245-1249 ISSN: 0002-8177.

Singh, BB.; Udani J.; Vinjamury S.; Der-Martirosian C.; Gandhi S.; Khorsan R.; Nanjegowda D. & Singh, V. (June, 2005) Safety and effectiveness of an L-lysine, zinc, and herbal-based product on the treatment of facial and circumoral herpes.(Original Research: Lysine / Herpes)." *Alternative Medicine Review. Thorne Research Inc.. HighBeam* retrieve from http://www.highbeam.com. ISSN: 1089-5159.

Smith, JS. & Robinson, NJ. (Oct, 2002). Age-specific prevalence of infection with herpes simplex virus types 2 and 1: a global review. *The Journal of Infectious Diseases,* Vol.15, No.186, Suppl 1:S3-28. ISSN: 1537-6613.

Spruance, SL.; Jones, T.; Blatter, MM.; Vargas, CM.; Barber, J.; Hill, J.; Goldstein, D. & Schultz, M. (Mar, 2003). High-Dose, Short Duration, Early Valaciclovir Therapy for Episodic Treatment of Cold Sores: Results of Two Randomized, Placebo-Controlled, Multicenter Studies. *Antimicrobial Agents and Chemotherapy,* Vol.47, No.3, pp. 1072-1080. ISSN: 1098-6596.

Spruance, SL.; Nett, R.; Mabury, T. Wolff, R. Johnson, J. & Spaulding, T. for the acyclovir cream study group. (July 2002) Acyclovir cream for treatment of herpes simplex labialis: Results of two randomized, double bind, vehicle-controlled, multicenter clinical trials. *Antimicrobial Agents and Chemotherapy,* Vol. 46, No.7, pp. 2238-2243, ISSN: 0066-4804

Spruance, SL. (Dec, 2005). Herpes Simplex Virus. Prophylactic chemotherapy with acyclovir for recurrent herpes simplex. *Journal of Medical Virology,* Vol.41, No.1, pp. 27-32. ISSN: 0146-6615.

Stránská, R.; Schuurman, R.; Nienhuis, E.; Goedegebuure, IW.; Polman, M.; Weel, JF.; Wertheim-Van Dillen, PM.; Berkhout, RJ. & van Loon, AM. (Jan, 2005). Survey of acyclovir-resistant herpes simplex virus in the Netherlands: prevalence and characterization. *Journal of Clinical Virology,* Vol.32, No.1, pp. 7-18. ISSN: 1386-6532.

Thakkar, JN.; Tiwari, V. & Dessai, UR. (Sep, 2010). Nonsulfated, cinnamic acid-based lignins are potent antagonists of HSV-1 entry into cells. *Biomacromolecules,* Vol.11, No. 5, pp. 1412-1416. ISSN: 1525-7797

Terezhalmy, G.T.; Bottomley, WK, & Pelleu, GB (1978). The use of water-soluble bioflavonoid ascorbic acid complex in the treatment of recurrent herpes labialis. *Oral Surgery, Oral Medicine, Oral Pathology, Oral Radiology, and Endodontic,* Vol.45, No.1, pp. 56-62, ISSN1528-395X.

United States Food and Drug Administration [FDA], (June, 2011), Retrieved from http://www.drugs.com/sfx/acyclovir-side-effects.html

Yoon, JC.; Cho, JJ.; Yoo, SM. & Ha, YM. (Feb, 2000). Antiviral activity of ascorbic acid against herpes simplex virus. *Journal Korean Society Microbiology,* Vol.35, No.1, pp. 1-8. ISSN: 0368-3494.

Zhang, Y., But, P.P., Ooi, V.E., Xu, H.X., Delaney, G.D., Lee, S.H. & Lee, S.F. (Sep. 2007). Chemical properties, mode of action, and in vivo anti-herpes activities of a lignin-carbohydrate complex from Prunella vulgaris. *Antiviral Research*, Vol. 75, No. 3, pp. 242-249. ISSN: 0166-3542

Ziyaeyan, M.; Alborzi, A.; Japoni, A.; Kadivar, M.; Davarpanah, MA.; Pourabbas, B. & Abassian, A. (Dec, 2007). Frequency of acyclovir-resistant herpes simplex viruses isolated from the general immunocompetent population and patients with acquired immunodeficiency syndrome. *International Journal of Dermatology*, Vol.46, No.12, pp. 1263-6. ISSN: 0011-9059.